Drug Design: Repurposing Techniques and Methodologies

Drug Design: Repurposing Techniques and Methodologies

Editor: Jesse Rodgers

AMERICAN
MEDICAL PUBLISHERS
www.americanmedicalpublishers.com

AMERICAN
MEDICAL PUBLISHERS
www.americanmedicalpublishers.com

Cataloging-in-publication Data

Drug design : repurposing techniques and methodologies / edited by Jesse Rodgers.
p. cm.
Includes bibliographical references and index.
ISBN 979-8-88740-076-1
1. Drugs--Design. 2. Drugs--Design--Data processing. 3. Drugs--Design--Methodology.
4. Drug development. 5. Pharmaceutical chemistry. I. Rodgers, Jesse.
RS420 .D78 2023
615.19--dc23

American Medical Publishers,
41 Flatbush Avenue,
1st Floor, New York,
NY 11217, USA

ISBN 979-8-88740-076-1 (Hardback)

Contents

Preface

This book has been an outcome of determined endeavour from a group of educationists in the field. The primary objective was to involve a broad spectrum of professionals from diverse cultural background involved in the field for developing new researches. The book not only targets students but also scholars pursuing higher research for further enhancement of the theoretical and practical applications of the subject.

Drug design refers to a type of inventive process of discovering novel medications based on the understanding of a biological target. Drug repurposing (DR) is the process of identifying new pharmacological indications from existing and old FDA approved drugs. It also uses newly produced drugs for treating conditions that are unrelated to its intended or original therapeutic use. It also entails discovering new therapeutic applications for previously known drugs, comprising abandoned, approved, withdrawn from use and experimental drugs. Traditional drug discovery is a costly, lengthy, risky and difficult procedure. The innovative technique of drug repositioning has the potential to be used instead of traditional drug discovery because it reduces the chance of failure, high financial cost and extended drug development time. There are two basic strategies of DR including on-target and off-target. This book explores all the important aspects of pharmacology and pharmaceutical sciences in the modern day. It covers repurposing techniques and methodologies for drug design. The readers would gain knowledge that would broaden their perspective in this area.

It was an honour to edit such a profound book and also a challenging task to compile and examine all the relevant data for accuracy and originality. I wish to acknowledge the efforts of the contributors for submitting such brilliant and diverse chapters in the field and for endlessly working for the completion of the book. Last, but not the least; I thank my family for being a constant source of support in all my research endeavours.

Editor

1

Drug Repurposing in Neurological Diseases: Opportunities and Challenges

Xiao-Yuan Mao

Abstract

Drug repurposing or repositioning refers to "studying of clinically approved drugs in one disease to see if they have therapeutic value and do not trigger side effects in other diseases." Nowadays, it is a vital drug discovery approach to explore new therapeutic benefits of existing drugs or drug candidates in various human diseases including neurological disorders. This approach overcomes the shortage faced during traditional drug development in grounds of financial support and timeline. It is especially hopeful in some refractory diseases including neurological diseases. The feature that structure complexity of the nervous system and influence of blood–brain barrier permeability often becomes more difficult to develop new drugs in neuropathological conditions than diseases in other organs; therefore, drug repurposing is particularly of utmost importance. In this chapter, we discuss the role of drug repurposing in neurological diseases and make a summarization of repurposing candidates currently in clinical trials for neurological diseases and potential mechanisms as well as preliminary results. Subsequently we also outline drug repurposing approaches and limitations and challenges in the future investigations.

Keywords: drug repurposing, brain injury, neurological diseases, therapeutics

1. Introduction

Neurological disorders are devastating diseases which usually occur in the brain, spinal cord, cranial nerves, peripheral nerves, and so on. It has reported that there are more than 600 kinds of neuropathological conditions including epilepsy, brain tumor, Parkinson's disease, Alzheimer's disease, and stroke. Nowadays, it is esti-mated that more than 1 billion people suffer from neurological disorders, seriously affecting people's life quality [1]. These kinds of diseases are especially prevalent in developing countries at any stage of age [2, 3]. There are several factors contribut-ing to etiology of neurological disorders such as aggravating tendency of aging population, irregular diet, and insufficient exercise [4].

Drug therapy is an important way for curing neurological diseases in the clinic. Nevertheless, serious neurological disorders such as Alzheimer's disease (AD) and Parkinson's disease (PD) are usually incurable in late stages of diseases with current therapeutic intervention [5, 6]. In the meantime, drug treatment often becomes less effective and causes serious side effects due to individual differences. Taking epilepsy as example, nearly 30% of epileptic patients are unable to obtain seizure control following treatment with marketed drugs [7, 8]. In addition, they have no significant effect on the improvement of cognitive dysfunction in patients with severe epilepsy [9]. Thus, it is essential for investigation of more effective and/or less toxic CNS targeted drugs.

Drug repurposing, also known as drug reprofiling or drug repositioning, includes the development of new uses and dosage forms for existing drugs or drug candidates. It is regarded as an economic and practical strategy [10]. Drug repurposing avoids the defects of new drug development. Compared to the drug repurposing, development of new drugs consumes much more time and huge investments. It is roughly reported that the cost from basic research for a new drug to clinical trials is 2.6 billion US dollars [11] and it often takes an average of 13–15 years [12]. Although more and more drug candidates are developed, many cases have failed in recent years [13]. Most of new drugs are withdrawn from the market due to unsatisfactory efficacy or intolerable side effects [14, 15]. Therefore, reusing existing drugs, namely, drug repurposing, has attracted great attention, as this approach has the capacity of saving cost and expediting drug development process.

The purpose of this chapter is to discuss the role of drug repurposing in human diseases especially neurological diseases and summarize repurposing candidates currently in clinical trials for neurological diseases and potential mechanisms as well as preliminary results. Subsequently we also list drug repurposing approaches and limitations and challenges in the future investigations.

2. Repurposed drugs in neurological diseases

Prior to development of repurposed drugs for neurological diseases therapeutics, it is emphasized how the drug reposition process is carried out. Generally, there are three stages in drug repurposing. First, diverse approaches including serendipitous clinical observation, cellular drug activity assays, in silico drug screens, and data mining of clinical drug interaction are employed to obtain drug candidates [16]. The detailed illustrations in grounds of methodologies are summarized as mentioned above [17]. Second, preclinical investigations including in vivo rodent models and in vitro cell lines for these drugs are conducted in neurological diseases [18]. Finally, large-scale and multicenter clinical trials are implemented for evaluat-ing efficacy and safety of repurposed drugs [19]. Up to date, there are plenty of drugs which are repurposed in neurological diseases through the above approaches. Then, in the following section, we also cite several repurposed drugs to elaborate how they function in neurological diseases. **Table 1** summarizes various repurposed drugs in the treatment of neurological disorders.

2.1 Verapamil

Verapamil, a classical calcium channel blocker, is mainly used in the treatment of hypertension, angina pectoris, arrhythmia, and other diseases, especially for paroxysmal supraventricular tachycardia [20]. It has been found that administration of verapamil greatly improves seizure control in drug-resistant epileptic patients via inhibiting P-glycoprotein (Pgp). Pgp is responsible for the transport of antiepileptic drug (AED) into the blood vessels through the blood–brain barrier (BBB). And there is evidence supporting that overexpression of Pgp in the brain represents a major mechanism underlying drug resistance in epileptic patients [21]. Verapamil is found to suppress Pgp expression and subsequently facilitates the entry of this

Name of drug	Original indication	Novel indication	Target	Summarization of evidence
Verapamil	Hypertension Angina pectoris Arrhythmia	Intractable epilepsy Subarachnoid hemorrhage Stroke Resistant depression	P-glycoprotein	I. Improving life quality in drug-resistant epileptic patients II. Preventing behavior phenotype in a mouse model of focal ischemia III. Showing no adverse effect in patients with stroke
Bumetanide	Liver disease Heart failure Stubborn edema Acute and chronic renal failure	Epilepsy Autism	NKCC1 protein	I. Improving anticonvulsant effect of phenobarbital in hypoxic rats II. Decreasing neuronal discharge in vitro and in vivo
Minocycline	Antibacterial	Epilepsy Spinal cord injury Brain inflammation Neurodegenerative diseases	Activated microglia IL-6, TNF-α TrkB/BDNF PPAR-γ/NF-κB LKB1/AMPK	I. Reducing seizure duration in rats II. Inhibiting inflammatory cytokines and cell death in kainic acid-induced epilepsy models
Fenfluramine	Simple obesity Diabetes Hypertension	Epilepsy Parkinson's disease	5-HT receptors	I. Alleviating epilepsy in patients with Dravet syndrome II. Anticonvulsant effects on photosensitive or induced convulsions
Propranolol	Hypertension Supraventricular tachycardia Prolonged Q-T interval Thyrotoxicosis	Migraine Traumatic brain injury Parkinson's disease	IL-6 β-adrenergic	I. Alleviating headache in patients with angina pectoris II. Reducing mortality within 24 h of admission in patients with TBI III. Preventing neuronal necrosis in a pig model of TBI
Sunitinib	Gastrointestinal stromal tumor Non-small-cell lung cancer Renal cell carcinoma	Glioma Pheochromocytoma Alzheimer's disease'	Acetylcholinesterase CGNs, SH-SY5Y	I. Penetrating the blood–brain barrier in clinical studies II. Alleviating glioma progression and glioma-induced neurodegeneration in vivo III. Preventing neuronal death induced by neurotoxins in vivo

Name of drug	Original indication	Novel indication	Target	Summarization of evidence
Angiotensin receptor blockers	Essential hypertension Renal disease Diabetes	Alzheimer's disease Episodic migraine	AT1 receptor Angiotensin II	I. Reducing Aβ accumulation and aggregation in vivo II. Alleviating AD in epidemiological studies and RCTs
Amantadine	Antiviral	Parkinson's disease Chronic traumatic brain injury	N-methyl-D-aspartate (NMDA) Anticholinergic	I. Improving motor symptoms in a female PD patient II. Activating the dopamine system in several preclinical data demonstrate

Table 1.
List of repurposed drugs in neurological disease.

drug into epileptogenic zones. As a marketed drug, verapamil treatment in patients with intractable epilepsy can doubtfully alleviate brain injury caused by repetitive seizures [22]. Actually, in clinical trials, verapamil has previously shown to exhibit great efficacy in intractable depression or mania via inhibiting the function of Pgp [23, 24]. Moreover, it is documented that verapamil has been approved to treat cerebral vasospasm secondary to subarachnoid hemorrhage due to its vasodilatory effects [25]. Intra-arterial (IA) treatment with verapamil, which was physiologically feasible, safe, and neuroprotective as a therapeutic adjunct in stroke, significantly reduces infarct volume and improved functional outcome [26], although there are still some mysteries about the mechanism.

2.2 Bumetanide

As a potent diuretic agent, bumetanide, which is mainly employed to cure liver disease, heart failure, and various kinds of stubborn edema in clinic [27], is a specific inhibitor of Na^+-K^+-$2Cl^-$ cotransporter isoform 1 (NKCC1) [28]. Mechanically, NKCC1 significantly modulates the content of intracellular Cl^-. Upregulation of NKCC1 leads to elevation of intracellular concentration of Cl^-, which is associated with pathogenesis of neurological diseases. It has been unequivocally proven that many of the available drugs have anti-seizure potential via activating GABAA-mediated hyperpolarization due to accumulation of neuronal Cl^- [29]. Indeed, current investigations have confirmed that bumetanide exerts antiepileptic effect via switching the GABA-mediated inhibitory postsynaptic potential in neurons from depolarization to hyperpolarization, resulting in decreased neuronal discharge [30, 31]. In addition, previous work reinforces that bumetanide can enhance the anticonvulsant effect of phenobarbital in hypoxic rats [32]. It suggests that the combination of phenobarbital and bumetanide may provide a promising therapeutic strategy for ceasing seizures in neonatal epilepsy and may increase the neuroprotective effect of hypothermia on asphyxiated newborns [33]. Persuasively, a current clinically pilot study further demonstrated that bumetanide, as a specific NKCC1 antagonist, considerably reduced seizure frequency in adult patients with temporal lobe epilepsy [34]. Additionally, as a consequence of a randomized controlled trial, bumetanide may also be effective for treatment of autism [35].

It should be considered that there are two obstacles for bumetanide treatment in neurological disorders [31, 36]. It has been shown that the highly potent diuretic effect of bumetanide can lead to hypokalemic alkalosis and the poor penetration into brain exists. This indicates that reuse of bumetanide in neurological diseases brings about opportunities and challenges in the future.

2.3 Minocycline

Minocycline is the second generation of semisynthetic broad-spectrum antibacterial tetracycline analogues. It has immunomodulatory, anti-inflammatory, and anti-apoptosis effects. Minocycline has neuroprotective effects in rodent models of ischemia, spinal cord injury, and infection [37]. It can efficiently penetrate the BBB and has a good effect on activated microglia, which indicates a possible role in the treatment of epilepsy. Minocycline may have synergistic effects with other compounds in manipulating epilepsy. Minocycline has been found to remarkably obviate epileptic conditions and reduce seizure-induced brain impairment at early stage [38]. In addition, minocycline also inhibits pro-inflammatory cytokines through caspase-dependent and caspase-independent pathways, thus inhibiting cell death in kainic acid-induced status epilepticus [39]. An obvious improvement of seizure phenotype is also observed in a rat model of amygdala kindling[40]. Additionally, increasing studies have reported the neuroprotective effects of minocycline in neurologic diseases, such as ischemic stroke, multiple sclerosis (MS), and traumatic brain injury (TBI) [41–43]. In in vivo animal model, minocycline promotes M2 microglia polarization via activation of tyrosine kinase receptor B (TrkB)/ brain-derived neurotrophic factors (BDNF) pathway and facilitates neurogenesis after intracerebral hemorrhage (ICH) [44]. In the process of acute cerebral infarct, minocycline also effectively inhibits oxidative stress via elevating the activity of superoxide dismutase (SOD) and activating the liver kinase B1 (LKB1)/adenosine 5′-monophosphate (AMP)-activated protein kinase (AMPK) signaling pathway [45]. However, repurposing of minocycline in treating neurological diseases requires to be re-evaluated as there is a clinical study showing serious neurodegeneration TBI [46].

2.4 Fenfluramine

Fenfluramine, which has been successfully applied in obesity, diabetes, and hypertension [47], is a potent 5-hydroxytryptamine (5-HT) releaser activating multiple 5-HT receptor subtypes. Of note, elevation of extracellular 5-HT levels inhibits focal and generalized seizures, while depletion of 5-HT lowers the threshold of epileptic seizures [48]. Therefore, 5-HT agonist fenfluramine is assessed for treat-ment of epilepsy. In a small-scale retrospective study, it has reported that adjuvant treatment with fenfluramine has evidently obtained seizure control in patients with Dravet syndrome. As the side effects is not serious, it does not lead to the termina-tion of treatment [49]. This drug may have anticonvulsant effects on other severe epilepsy syndromes, especially those characterized by photosensitive or induced convulsions [50, 51]. Encouragingly, a recent investigation has unveiled that fenflu-ramine significantly reduces convulsive seizure frequency compared with placebo and exhibits good tolerance [52]. It indicates that fenfluramine could be functioned as a potent novel therapeutic regime for patients with Dravet syndrome. It is note-worthy that fenfluramine also alleviates L-DOPA-induced dyskinesia via stimulation of 5-HT1A receptor in PD [53].

2.5 Propranolol

Propranolol as a β-adrenoceptor antagonist (b-blocker) has been commonly used in hypertension, supraventricular tachycardia, prolonged Q-T interval, and thyrotoxicosis in clinic [54]. Since 1996, in patients who were being treated for angina pectoris, Rabkin et al. has disclosed the therapeutic effect of propranolol on migraine headache [55]. Meanwhile, further clinical studies have noted that admin-istration of propranolol within 24 h of admission after TBI triggers lower mortality [56]. The evidence also arises from a recent study that propranolol blocks the upreg-ulation of IL-6 and prevents neuronal cell necrosis in CA1 and CA3 hippocampus in a pig model of TBI [57]. Given that propranolol has neuroprotective potential in neuropathological conditions, it is likely to serve as a neuroprotective drug in epi-lepsy. Additionally, both clinical and experimental studies have demonstrated the potential of propranolol to resist dyskinesia in PD, as modulation of β-adrenergic receptors (βAR), which is abundantly, expressed in striatum, is involved L-DOPA-induced dyskinesia (LID) [58, 59].

2.6 Sunitinib

Sunitinib, which is an oral, small molecule receptor tyrosine kinase inhibitor approved by the US Food and Drug Administration, has been currently implemented in the treatment of various cancers such as gastrointestinal stromal tumor

(GIST), non-small-cell lung cancer, and renal cell carcinoma [60]. Clinical evidence has revealed that oral administration of sunitinib penetrates the BBB and subsequently facilitates the entry into central nervous system [61]. Furthermore, on the basis of its potent antiangiogenic and antitumoral characteristics, it has discovered that sunitinib can alleviate glioma-induced neurodegeneration and glioma progression in vivo models [60]. Meanwhile, sunitinib has been found to exert therapeutic effects on learning and memory deficits in a mouse model of AD through inhibition of acetylcholinesterase (AChE) [62]. Additionally, sunitinib has also demonstrated to prevent neuronal death induced by neurotoxins via inhibiting NO overproduction in cerebellar granule neurons (CGNs) and SH-SY5Y cells following exposure with low potassium or 1-methyl-4-phenylpyridiniumion (MPP^+)-induced neuronal apoptosis [63]. It indicates that sunitinib may improve brain dysfunction via inhibition of oxidative stress.

2.7 Angiotensin receptor blockers

In in vitro studies, angiotensin receptor blockers (ARBs) are generally known to treat essential hypertension by influencing the level of angiotensin II (Ang II) via two distinct pathways, namely, through interrupting the AT_1 receptor and augmentation of Ang II processing which plays a critical role in cognition regula-tion [64]. For example, valsartan, which has previously been found to penetrate BBB and elicit antihypertensive responses in the brain, has been demonstrated to reduce Aβ accumulation and aggregation in vivo and in vitro [65]. Actually, similar situation exists in losartan and telmisartan, which are also classical ARBs [66, 67]. Overall, it indicates ARBs are potential candidates for treating AD. Significantly, several clinically epidemiological studies and RCTs certify the efficacy of ARBs in AD. A large-scale retrospective cohort study has revealed an obvious reduction of dementia in patients treated with ARBs compared with other cardiovascular agents [68]. Likewise, the further UK-based study also reports a similar trend, with a 50% reduction in AD after ARBs treatment [69]. In brief, ARBs, the conventional cardiovascular medicine, have been confirmed to exert a vital effect in AD, and it is further deserved to identify the most suitable dosage in clinic.

2.8 Amantadine

Amantadine is a classic antiviral compound which has been found to moderately ameliorate impaired motor behavior in Parkinson's disease [70]. Intriguingly, in 1969, it was coincident that Schwab et al. found an improvement of motor symptoms in a female PD patient, who took 200 mg amantadine daily for antiviral prophylaxis [71]. Subsequently, three potential mechanisms have been proposed to explain the efficacy of amantadine in PD. Several preclinical data demonstrate an activation of the dopamine system's both presynaptic and postsynaptic actions [72], and amantadine also inhibits the N-methyl-D-aspartate (NMDA) subtype of glutamate receptors [72, 73]. The mild anticholinergic effect is also involved [74]. Surprisingly, PD is well known to be frequently associated with depression, and antagonism of NMDA receptors is also a promising target for new antidepressants, although there is no definite evidence to certify its efficacy in depressive disorder.

3. Approaches to drug repurposing

There are three important stages in the field of drug repurposing: generation of candidate compounds, preclinical investigation, and clinical trial. Determination of appropriate drugs for potential indications is crucial for production of candidate compounds. At present, two approaches are widely used for drug repurposing including experimental screening approaches and molecular docking by computer. In the following items, we make a detailed description of these two methods in drug repurposing process.

3.1 Experimental approaches

Experimental screening approaches are usually regarded as the first stage in the process of drug discovery and drug repurposing. Proteomic techniques such as affinity chromatography and mass spectrometry have been widely employed to identify drug candidates [75]. Nowadays, drug target analysis and drug repurposing are inseparable. Drug repurposing is distinct from drug discovery in terms of altera-tion of drug target. Cellular thermo stability assay technique can predict the affinity of drug ligands by mapping the contact patterns of intracellular targets [76]. The molecular on and off targets have been disclosed for many clinically approved drugs via this method. Especially in the field of kinases, new targets of well-known drugs are obtained through affinity matrices [77, 78]. For example, imatinib, a tyrosine kinase inhibitor, has been successfully reused in the treatment of gastrointestinal stromal tumors [79].

In addition, chemical compounds with disease-related effects can be defined in the model through phenotype screening [80]. Phenotype screening has always been more successful than target screening in the facet of drug development [81, 82]. In the case of drug repurposing, if the compounds selected through phenotypical assays are approved clinical drugs or ongoing clinical trials, they are probable to reuse. Several drugs approved for tobacco dependence have been evaluated, and it has been found that topiramate changes nicotine- or ethanol-induced behavior in zebrafish models [83]. However, there are some challenges that the efficacy of drug candidates in in vitro experiments require to be validated in human diseases [84].

3.2 Computational approaches

Molecular docking by a computer is also an important method for evaluating drug target binding kinetics and drug residence times of existing drugs or drug candidates [85]. Large amounts of computational drug repositioning methods choose transcriptomic data to identify potential new indications for drugs. Furthermore, these methods have applied techniques such as comparison of gene expression profiles between a disease model and drug-treated condition [86], network integration [87], prediction of drug-protein interactions [88], and utilization of genotype–phenotype associations. Recently, a proteotranscriptomic-based computational drug repositioning method named Drug Repositioning Perturbation Score/Class (DRPS/C) for Alzheimer's disease occurs on the basis of inverse associations between disease-induced or drug-induced gene and protein perturbation patterns [89]. Briefly, these approaches can be applicable to discovery of drug targets or biomarkers.

It should be considered that for many neurological disorders, drugs require good penetration into BBB. Then, the therapeutic approaches of targeting brain have been classified as invasive and noninvasive categories [90, 91]. The invasive approaches contain the temporary increase of BBB permeability, and noninvasive approaches involve modification of drug molecule via physiological, chemical, or colloidal carrier system approach. Meanwhile, these methods are also related to computational approaches. Influx clearance into the brain (K_{in}), which is the unidirectional influx constant from the blood to brain, can be used to calculate the transport of drugs in the brain. Similar computational approaches conclude the permeability surface area (PS), brain/plasma ratio (K_p), brain uptake index (BUI), and apparent permeability (P_{app}) [92–95]. Consequently, drug repurposing in neurological diseases covers various manners to participate in integrating the role of transporters and pathophysiological complexity of BBB to establish a suitable model for high-throughput screening.

4. Concluding remarks and perspectives

Drug repurposing is a vital strategy for developing new therapeutic values of existing drugs or drug candidates due to its ability to save time and reduce cost [96]. This type of innovative concept will undoubtedly expedite the drug development process. Meanwhile, some limitations need to be considered during drug repurposing process in neurological diseases. Owing to complex molecular and cellular signaling mechanisms in neuropathological states, drug repurposing may be difficult. Additionally, drugs not only respond to a single target but also affect multiple targets [97], causing a variety of adverse reactions. A comprehensive assessment of the advantages and disadvantages of these side effects can help us understand drug repositioning from a more all-round perspective [98, 99].

In order to overcome limitations faced during drug repurposing, we make proposals in the following descriptions. Firstly, it is foremost to establish a comprehensive data analysis platform to maximize data sharing. Information science services and artificial intelligence can help unlock and reanalyze the large amount of data accumulated by approved drugs or drug candidates to clinical trials. These data may be stored in a diversified way. Storage locations, formats, and types may vary, including different storage locations, formats, and types. The data obtained from clinical trials and biological databases are too large and complex that the traditional data processing methods cannot deal with it, which leads to the bottleneck in the research process [99]. Big data can significantly improve our understanding of the disease and make more accurate disease-related strategies. However, there is a big gap between generating biomedical data and data analysis [99, 100]. To ensure the efficiency of research, it takes time, energy, and expertise to find technical solutions to integrate them. Secondly, it is encouraged to provide more financial support for clinical trials of drug repurposing, including technical support. The preclinical research of drug repurposing requires financial support to obtain the data in clinical trials. In this case, drugs that can be developed to treat rare diseases are more likely to apply in clinical neurological diseases therapeutics [101]. Finally, in order to facilitate drug repurposing process, we advocate it is indispensable to solve patent restrictions and take reasonable supervision. All applications of drug repurposing should be accompanied by a risk management plan. Drug's safety can be supported by clinical trial data or post marketing data.

In conclusion, drug repurposing is a novel approach for expediting drug development process in neurological diseases. Repurposed drugs may provide an efficient avenue for improving a plethora of pathological conditions including neurological disorders. In the future, it is essential to exploit molecular mechanisms during drug repurposing processes due to the possibility that targets of repurposed drugs in neurological diseases are distinct from original targets in treating other diseases, in order to make these drugs more effective and safe.

Acknowledgements

The authors apologize to all the investigators whose work cannot be cited in this paper due to space constraint. This work was partly supported by the National Natural Science Foundation of China (No. 81974502 and 81671293).

Abbreviations

CNS	central nervous system
AD	Alzheimer's disease
PD	Parkinson's disease
AED	antiepileptic drug
BBB	blood–brain barrier
Pgp	P-glycoprotein
NKCC1	Na^+-K^+-2Cl-cotransporter isoform 1
GABAA	gamma-aminobutyric acid
MS	multiple sclerosis
TBI	traumatic brain injury
TrkB	tyrosine kinase receptor B
BDNF	brain-derived neurotrophic factors
ICH	intracerebral hemorrhage
SOD	superoxide dismutase
LKB1	liver kinase B1
AMPK	adenosine 5′-monophosphate (AMP)-activated protein kinase
5-HT	5-hydroxytryptamine
LID	L-DOPA-induced dyskinesia
βAR	β-adrenergic receptors
AChE	acetylcholinesterase
CGNs	cerebellar granule neurons
ARBs	angiotensin receptor blockers
Ang II	angiotensin II
NMDA	N-methyl-D-aspartate

Author details

Xiao-Yuan Mao[1,2,3,4]

1 Department of Clinical Pharmacology, Xiangya Hospital, Central South University, Changsha, P.R. China

2 Hunan Key Laboratory of Pharmacogenetics, Institute of Clinical Pharmacology, Central South University, Changsha, P.R. China

3 Engineering Research Center of Applied Technology of Pharmacogenomics, Ministry of Education, Changsha, P.R. China

4 National Clinical Research Center for Geriatric Disorders, Changsha, Hunan, P.R. China

*Address all correspondence to: xiaoyuanm@csu.edu.cn; maoxiaoyuan2011@163.com

References

[1] Cottler LB, Zunt J, Weiss B, Kamal AK, Vaddiparti K. Building global capacity for brain and nervous system disorders research. Nature. 2015;**527**:S207-S213. DOI: 10.1038/nature16037

[2] Chin JH, Vora N. The global burden of neurologic diseases. Neurology. 2014;**83**:349-351. DOI: 10.1212/wnl.0000000000000610

[3] Whiteford HA et al. Global burden of disease attributable to mental and substance use disorders: Findings from the global burden of disease study 2010. Lancet. 2013;**382**:1575-1586. DOI: 10.1016/s0140-6736(13)61611-6

[4] Nugent RA, Yach D, Feigl AB. Non-communicable diseases and the Paris declaration. Lancet. 2009;**374**:784-785. DOI: 10.1016/s0140-6736(09)61589-0

[5] Lane CA, Hardy J, Schott JM. Alzheimer's disease. European Journal of Neurology. 2018;**25**:59-70. DOI: 10.1111/ene.13439

[6] Radder DLM et al. Physical therapy and occupational therapy in Parkinson's disease. The International Journal of Neuroscience. 2017;**127**:930-943. DOI: 10.1080/00207454.2016.1275617

[7] Shorvon SD. The epidemiology and treatment of chronic and refractory epilepsy. Epilepsia. 1996;**37**(Suppl 2): S1-S3. DOI: 10.1111/j.1528-1157.1996.tb06027.x

[8] Löscher W, Brandt C. Prevention or modification of epileptogenesis after brain insults: Experimental approaches and translational research. Pharmacological Reviews. 2010;**62**: 668-700. DOI: 10.1124/pr.110.003046

[9] Holmes GL, Noebels JL. Th e epilepsy s pectrum: Targeting future research challenges. Cold Spring Harbor Perspectives in Medicine. 2016;**6**:1-12. DOI: 10.1101/cshperspect.a028043

[10] Hemphill CS, Sampat BN. Evergreening, patent challenges, and effective market life in pharmaceuticals. Journal of Health Economics. 2012;**31**:327-339. DOI: 10.1016/j.jhealeco.2012.01.004

[11] DiMasi JA, Grabowski HG, Hansen RW. Innovation in the pharmaceutical industry: New estimates of R&D costs. Journal of Health Economics. 2016;**47**:20-33. DOI: 10.1016/j.jhealeco.2016.01.012

[12] Strittmatter SM. Overcoming drug development bottlenecks with repurposing: Old drugs learn new tricks. Nature Medicine. 2014;**20**:590-591. DOI: 10.1038/nm.3595

[13] Scannell JW, Blanckley A, Boldon H, Warrington B. Diagnosing the decline in pharmaceutical R&D efficiency. Nature Reviews. Drug Discovery. 2012;**11**:191- 200. DOI: 10.1038/nrd3681

[14] DiMasi JA, Feldman L, Seckler A, Wilson A. Trends in risks associated with new drug development: Success rates for investigational drugs. Clinical Pharmacology and Therapeutics. 2010;**87**:272-277. DOI: 10.1038/clpt.2009.295

[15] Arrowsmith J, Miller P. Trial watch: Phase II and phase III attrition rates 2011-2012. Nature Reviews. Drug Discovery;**12**:569, 2013. DOI: 10.1038/nrd4090

[16] O'Connor KA, Roth BL. Finding new tricks for old drugs: An efficient route for public-sector drug discovery. Nature Reviews. Drug Discovery. 2005;**4**:1005-1014. DOI: 10.1038/nrd1900

[17] Kumar R et al. Exploring the new horizons of drug repurposing: A vital tool for turning hard work into smart work. European Journal of Medicinal Chemistry. 2019;**182**:111602. DOI: 10.1016/j.ejmech.2019.111602

[18] Turanli B et al. Drug repositioning for effective prostate cancer treatment. Frontiers in Physiology. 2018;**9**:500. DOI: 10.3389/fphys.2018.00500

[19] Lago SG, Bahn S. Clinical trials and therapeutic rationale for drug repurposing in schizophrenia. ACS Chemical Neuroscience. 2019;**10**:58-78. DOI: 10.1021/acschemneuro.8b00205

[20] Delaney B, Loy J, Kelly AM. The relative efficacy of adenosine versus verapamil for the treatment of stable paroxysmal supraventricular tachycardia in adults: A meta-analysis. European Journal of Emergency Medicine: Official Journal of the European Society for Emergency Medicine. 2011;**18**:148-152. DOI: 10.1097/MEJ.0b013e3283400ba2

[21] Robey RW, Lazarowski A, Bates SE. P-glycoprotein—A clinical target in drug-refractory epilepsy? Molecular Pharmacology. 2008;**73**:1343- 1346. DOI: 10.1124/mol.108.046680

[22] Summers MA, Moore JL, McAuley JW. Use of verapamil as a potential P-glycoprotein inhibitor in a patient with refractory epilepsy. The Annals of Pharmacotherapy. 2004;**38**:1631-1634. DOI: 10.1345/aph.1E068

[23] de Klerk OL et al. Locally increased P-glycoprotein function in major depression: A PET study with [11C]verapamil as a probe for P-glycoprotein function in the blood-brain barrier. The International Journal of Neuropsychopharmacology. 2009;**12**:895-904. DOI: 10.1017/s1461145709009894

[24] Barton BM, Gitlin MJ. Verapamil in treatment-resistant mania: An open trial. Journal of Clinical Psychopharmacology. 1987;**7**:101-103

[25] KeuskampJ,MuraliR,ChaoKH. High-dose intraarterial verapamil in the treatment of cerebral vasospasm after aneurysmal subarachnoid hemorrhage. Journal of Neurosurgery. 2008;**108**:458-463. DOI: 10.3171/jns/2008/108/3/0458

[26] Fraser JF et al. Intra-arterial verapamil post-thrombectomy is feasible, safe, and neuroprotective in stroke. Journal of Cerebral Blood Flow and Metabolism: Official Journal of the International Society of Cerebral Blood Flow and Metabolism. 2017;**37**:3531-3543. DOI: 10.1177/0271678x17705259

[27] Xiong L et al. Evaluation of severe myalgia induced by continuous-infusion bumetanide in patients with acute heart failure. Pharmacotherapy. 2019;**39**:854- 860. DOI: 10.1002/phar.2297

[28] Kaila K, Price TJ, Payne JA, Puskarjov M, Voipio J. Cation-chloride cotransporters in neuronal development, plasticity and disease. Nature Reviews. Neuroscience. 2014;**15**:637-654. DOI: 10.1038/nrn3819

[29] Hochman DW. The extracellular space and epileptic activity in the adult brain: Explaining the antiepileptic effects of furosemide and bumetanide. Epilepsia. 2012;**53**(Suppl 1):18-25. DOI: 10.1111/j.1528-1167.2012.03471.x

[30] Rheims S et al. Excitatory GABA in rodent developing neocortex in vitro. Journal of Neurophysiology. 2008;**100**:609-619. DOI: 10.1152/jn.90402.2008

[31] Löscher W, Puskarjov M, Kaila K. Cation-chloride cotransporters NKCC1 and KCC2 as potential targets for novel antiepileptic and antiepileptogenic treatments.

Neuropharmacology. 2013;**69**:62-74. DOI: 10.1016/j.neuropharm.2012.05.045

[32] Dzhala VI, Brumback AC, Staley KJ. Bumetanide enhances phenobarbital efficacy in a neonatal seizure model. Annals of Neurology. 2008;**63**:222-235. DOI: 10.1002/ana.21229

[33] Liu Y, Shangguan Y, Barks JD, Silverstein FS. Bumetanide augments the neuroprotective efficacy of phenobarbital plus hypothermia in a neonatal hypoxia-ischemia model. Pediatric Research. 2012;**71**:559-565. DOI: 10.1038/pr.2012.7

[34] Eftekhari S et al. Bumetanide reduces seizure frequency in patients with temporal lobe epilepsy. Epilepsia. 2013;**54**:e9-e12. DOI: 10.1111/j.1528-1167.2012.03654.x

[35] Lemonnier E et al. A randomised controlled trial of bumetanide in the treatment of autism in children. Translational Psychiatry. 2012;**2**:e202. DOI: 10.1038/tp.2012.124

[36] Töllner K et al. A novel prodrug-based strategy to increase effects of bumetanide in epilepsy. Annals of Neurology. 2014;**75**:550-562. DOI: 10.1002/ana.24124

[37] Rosenblat JD, McIntyre RS. Efficacy and tolerability of minocycline for depression: A systematic review and meta-analysis of clinical trials. Journal of Affective Disorders. 2018;**227**:219- 225. DOI: 10.1016/j.jad.2017.10.042

[38] Abraham J, Fox PD, Condello C, Bartolini A, Koh S. Minocycline attenuates microglia activation and blocks the long-term epileptogenic effects of early-life seizures. Neurobiology of Disease. 2012;**46**:425-430. DOI: 10.1016/j. nbd.2012.02.006

[39] Heo K et al. Minocycline inhibits caspase-dependent and -independent cell death pathways and is neuroprotective against hippocampal damage after treatment with kainic acid in mice. Neuroscience Letters. 2006;**398**:195-200. DOI: 10.1016/j.neulet.2006.01.027

[40] Beheshti Nasr SM, Moghimi A, Mohammad-Zadeh M, Shamsizadeh A, Noorbakhsh SM. The effect of minocycline on seizures induced by amygdala kindling in rats. Seizure. 2013;**22**:670-674. DOI: 10.1016/j.seizure.2013.05.005

[41] Kumar A et al. NOX2 drives M1-like microglial/macrophage activation and neurodegeneration following experimental traumatic brain injury. Brain, Behavior, and Immunity. 2016;**58**:291-309. DOI: 10.1016/j.bbi.2016.07.158

[42] Perego C et al. Macrophages are essential for maintaining a M2 protective response early after ischemic brain injury. Neurobiology of Disease. 2016;**96**:284-293. DOI: 10.1016/j.nbd.2016.09.017

[43] Wan S et al. Microglia activation and polarization after intracerebral hemorrhage in mice: The role of protease-activated receptor-1. Translational Stroke Research. 2016;**7**:478-487. DOI: 10.1007/s12975-016-0472-8

[44] Miao H, Li R, Han C, Lu X, Zhang H. Minocycline promotes posthemorrhagic neurogenesis via M2 microglia polarization via upregulation of the TrkB/BDNF pathway in rats. Journal of Neurophysiology. 2018;**120**:1307-1317. DOI: 10.1152/jn.00234.2018

[45] Cai Z, Wang C, Chen Y, He W. An antioxidant role by minocycline via enhancing the activation of LKB1/AMPK signaling in the process of cerebral ischemia injury. Current Molecular Medicine. 2018;**18**:142-151.

DOI: 10.2174/1566524018666180907161504

[46] Scott G et al. Minocycline reduces chronic microglial activation after brain trauma but increases neurodegeneration. Brain: A Journal of Neurology. 2018;**141**:459-471. DOI: 10.1093/brain/awx339

[47] Aman MG, Kern RA. Review of fenfluramine in the treatment of the developmental disabilities. Journal of the American Academy of Child and Adolescent Psychiatry. 1989;**28**:549-565. DOI: 10.1097/00004583-198907000-00014

[48] Bagdy G, Kecskemeti V, Riba P, Jakus R. Serotonin and epilepsy. Journal of Neurochemistry. 2007;**100**:857-873. DOI: 10.1111/j.1471-4159.2006.04277.x

[49] Ceulemans B et al. Successful use of fenfluramine as an add-on treatment for Dravet syndrome. Epilepsia. 2012;**53**:1131-1139. DOI: 10.1111/j.1528-1167.2012.03495.x

[50] Boel M, Casaer P. Add-on therapy of fenfluramine in intractable self-induced epilepsy. Neuropediatrics. 1996;**27**:171- 173. DOI: 10.1055/s-2007-973781

[51] Pierce JG, Mithal DS. Fenfluramine: New treatment for seizures in Dravet syndrome. Pediatric Neurology Briefs. 2020;**34**:8. DOI: 10.15844/pedneurbriefs-34-8

[52] Lagae L et al. Fenfluramine hydrochloride for the treatment of seizures in Dravet syndrome: A randomised, double-blind, placebo-controlled trial. Lancet. 2020;**394**:2243-2254. DOI: 10.1016/s0140-6736(19)32500-0

[53] Bishop C et al. MDMA and fenfluramine reduce L-DOPA-induced dyskinesia via indirect 5-HT1A receptor stimulation. The European Journal of Neuroscience. 2006;**23**:2669-2676. DOI: 10.1111/j.1460-9568.2006.04790.x

[54] Bidabadi E, Mashouf M. A randomized trial of propranolol versus sodium valproate for the prophylaxis of migraine in pediatric patients. Paediatric Drugs. 2010;**12**:269-275. DOI: 10.2165/11316270-000000000-00000

[55] Rabkin R, Stables DP, Levin NW, Suzman MM. The prophylactic value of propranolol in angina pectoris. The American Journal of Cardiology. 1966;**18**:370-383. DOI: 10.1016/0002-9149(66)90056-7

[56] Ko A et al. Early propranolol after traumatic brain injury is associated with lower mortality. The Journal of Trauma and Acute Care Surgery. 2016;**80**:637-642. DOI: 10.1097/ta.0000000000000959

[57] Armstead WM, Vavilala MS. Propranolol protects cerebral autoregulation and reduces hippocampal neuronal cell death through inhibition of interleukin-6 upregulation after traumatic brain injury in pigs. British Journal of Anaesthesia. 2019;**123**:610-617. DOI: 10.1016/j.bja.2019.07.017

[58] Barnum CJ et al. Effects of noradrenergic denervation on L-DOPA-induced dyskinesia and its treatment by α- and β-adrenergic receptor antagonists in hemiparkinsonian rats. Pharmacology, Biochemistry, and Behavior. 2012;**100**:607-615. DOI: 10.1016/j.pbb.2011.09.009

[59] Waeber C, Rigo M, Chinaglia G, Probst A, Palacios JM. Beta-adrenergic receptor subtypes in the basal ganglia of patients with Huntington's chorea and Parkinson's disease. Synapse. 1991;**8**:270-280. DOI: 10.1002/syn.890080405

[60] Hatipoglu G et al. Sunitinib impedes brain tumor progression and reduces

tumor-induced neurodegeneration in the microenvironment. Cancer Science. 2015;**106**:160-170. DOI: 10.1111/cas.12580

[61] Addeo R, Caraglia M. The oral tyrosine kinase inhibitors lapatinib and sunitinib: New opportunities for the treatment of brain metastases from breast cancer? Expert Review of Anticancer Therapy. 2011;**11**:139-142. DOI: 10.1586/era.10.190

[62] Huang L et al. Sunitinib, a clinically used anticancer drug. Is a potent AChE inhibitor and attenuates cognitive impairments in mice. ACS Chemical Neuroscience. 2016;**7**:1047-1056. DOI: 10.1021/acschemneuro.5b00329

[63] Cui W et al. Sunitinib produces neuroprotective effect via inhibiting nitric oxide overproduction. CNS Neuroscience & Therapeutics. 2014;**20**:244-252. DOI: 10.1111/cns.12203

[64] Wright JW, Harding JW. Brain renin-angiotensin—a new look at an old system. Progress in Neurobiology. 2011;**95**:49-67. DOI: 10.1016/j.pneurobio.2011.07.001

[65] Wang J et al. Valsartan lowers brain beta-amyloid protein levels and improves spatial learning in a mouse model of Alzheimer disease. The Journal of Clinical Investigation. 2007;**117**:3393- 3402. DOI: 10.1172/jci31547

[66] Mogi M et al. Telmisartan prevented cognitive decline partly due to PPAR-gamma activation. Biochemical and Biophysical Research Communications. 2008;**375**:446-449. DOI: 10.1016/j. bbrc.2008.08.032

[67] Danielyan L et al. Protective effects of intranasal losartan in the APP/PS1 transgenic mouse model of Alzheimer disease. Rejuvenation Research. 2010;**13**:195-201. DOI: 10.1089/ rej.2009.0944

[68] Li NC et al. Use of angiotensin receptor blockers and risk of dementia in a predominantly male population: Prospective cohort analysis. British Medical Journal (Clinical Research Edition). 2010;**340**:b5465. DOI: 10.1136/bmj.b5465

[69] Davies NM, Kehoe PG, Ben-Shlomo Y, Martin RM. Associations of anti-hypertensive treatments with Alzheimer's disease, vascular dementia, and other dementias. Journal of Alzheimer's Disease. 2011;**26**:699-708. DOI: 10.3233/jad-2011-110347

[70] Müller T, Kuhn W, Möhr JD. Evaluating ADS5102 (amantadine) for the treatment of Parkinson's disease patients with dyskinesia. Expert Opinion on Pharmacotherapy. 2019;**20**:1181-1187. DOI: 10.1080/14656566.2019.1612365

[71] Schwab RS, England AC Jr, Poskanzer DC, Young RR. Amantadine in the treatment of Parkinson's disease. JAMA. 1969;**208**:1168-1170

[72] Bailey EV, Stone TW. The mechanism of action of amantadine in parkinsonism: A review. Archives Internationales de Pharmacodynamie et de Thérapie. 1975;**216**:246-262

[73] Chase TN, Bibbiani F, Oh JD. Striatal glutamatergic mechanisms and extrapyramidal movement disorders. Neurotoxicity Research. 2003;**5**:139-146. DOI: 10.1007/bf03033378

[74] Nastuk WL, Su P, Doubilet P. Anticholinergic and membrane activities of amantadine in neuromuscular transmission. Nature. 1976;**264**:76-79. DOI: 10.1038/264076a0

[75] Brehmer D et al. Cellular targets of gefitinib. Cancer Research. 2005;**65**:379-382

[76] Martinez Molina D et al. Monitoring drug target engagement in cells and

tissues using the cellular thermal shift assay. Science (New York, N.Y.). 2013;**341**:84-87. DOI: 10.1126/science.1233606

[77] Klaeger S et al. Chemical proteomics reveals ferrochelatase as a common off-target of kinase inhibitors. ACS Chemical Biology. 2016;**11**:1245-1254. DOI: 10.1021/acschembio.5b01063

[78] Troutman S et al. Crizotinib inhibits NF2-associated schwannoma through inhibition of focal adhesion kinase 1. Oncotarget. 2016;7:54515-54525. DOI: 10.18632/oncotarget.10248

[79] Blanke CD et al. Long-term results from a randomized phase II trial of standard- versus higher-dose imatinib mesylate for patients with unresectable or metastatic gastrointestinal stromal tumors expressing KIT. Journal of Clinical Oncology : Official Journal of the American Society of Clinical Oncology. 2008;**26**:620-625. DOI: 10.1200/jco.2007.13.4403

[80] Moffat JG, Vincent F, Lee JA, Eder J, Prunotto M. Opportunities and challenges in phenotypic drug discovery: An industry perspective. Nature Reviews. Drug Discovery. 2017;**16**:531-543. DOI: 10.1038/nrd.2017.111

[81] Swinney DC, Anthony J. How were new medicines discovered? Nature Reviews. Drug Discovery. 2011;**10**:507-519. DOI: 10.1038/nrd3480

[82] Eder J, Sedrani R, Wiesmann C. The discovery of first-in-class drugs: Origins and evolution. Nature Reviews. Drug Discovery. 2014;**13**:577-587. DOI: 10.1038/nrd4336

[83] Cousin MA et al. Larval zebrafish model for FDA-approved drug repositioning for tobacco dependence treatment. PLoS One. 2014;**9**:e90467. DOI: 10.1371/journal.pone.0090467

[84] Horvath P et al. Screening out irrelevant cell-based models of disease. Nature Reviews. Drug Discovery. 2016;**15**:751-769. DOI: 10.1038/nrd.2016.175

[85] De Benedetti PG, Fanelli F. Computational modeling approaches to quantitative structure-binding kinetics relationships in drug discovery. Drug Discovery Today. 2018;**23**:1396-1406. DOI: 10.1016/j.drudis.2018.03.010

[86] Chen B et al. Reversal of cancer gene expression correlates with drug efficacy and reveals therapeutic targets. Nature Communications. 2017;**8**:16022. DOI: 10.1038/ncomms16022

[87] Luo Y et al. A network integration approach for drug-target interaction prediction and computational drug repositioning from heterogeneous information. Nature Communications. 2017;**8**:573. DOI: 10.1038/s41467-017-00680-8

[88] Yang L, Agarwal P. Systematic drug repositioning based on clinical side-effects. PLoS One. 2011;**6**:e28025. DOI: 10.1371/journal.pone.0028025

[89] Lee SY et al. A proteotranscriptomic-based computational drug-repositioning method for Alzheimer's disease. Frontiers in Pharmacology. 2019;**10**:1653. DOI: 10.3389/fphar.2019.01653

[90] Gabathuler R. Approaches to transport therapeutic drugs across the blood-brain barrier to treat brain diseases. Neurobiology of Disease. 2010;**37**:48-57. DOI: 10.1016/j.nbd.2009.07.028

[91] Alam MI et al. Strategy for effective brain drug delivery. European Journal of Pharmaceutical Sciences: Official Journal of the European Federation for Pharmaceutical Sciences. 2010;**40**:385-403. DOI: 10.1016/j.ejps.2010.05.003

[92] van Rooy I et al. In vivo methods to study uptake of nanoparticles into the brain. Pharmaceutical Research. 2011;**28**:456-471. DOI: 10.1007/s11095-010-0291-7

[93] Reichel A. Addressing central nervous system (CNS) penetration in drug discovery: Basics and implications of the evolving new concept. Chemistry & Biodiversity. 2009;**6**:2030-2049. DOI: 10.1002/cbdv.200900103

[94] Bonate PL. Animal models for studying transport across the blood-brain barrier. Journal of Neuroscience Methods. 1995;**56**:1-15. DOI: 10.1016/0165-0270(94)00081-q

[95] Artursson P. Epithelial transport of drugs in cell culture. I: A model for studying the passive diffusion of drugs over intestinal absorptive (Caco-2) cells. Journal of Pharmaceutical Sciences. 1990;**79**:476-482. DOI: 10.1002/jps.2600790604

[96] Raju TN et al. Lancet. 2000;**355**:1022. DOI: 10.1016/s0140-6736(05)74775-9

[97] Vogt I, Mestres J. Drug-target networks. Molecular Informatics. 2010;**29**:10-14. DOI: 10.1002/minf.200900069

[98] Reddy AS, Zhang S. Polypharmacology: Drug discovery for the future. Expert Review of Clinical Pharmacology. 2013;**6**:41-47. DOI: 10.1586/ecp.12.74

[99] Yildirim MA, Goh KI, Cusick ME, Barabási AL, Vidal M. Drug-target network. Nature Biotechnology. 2007;**25**:1119-1126. DOI: 10.1038/nbt1338

[100] Chen Y, Elenee Argentinis JD, Weber G. IBM Watson: How cognitive computing can be applied to big data challenges in life sciences research. Clinical Therapeutics. 2016;**38**:688-701. DOI: 10.1016/j.clinthera.2015.12.001

[101] Eisenstein M. Big data: The power of petabytes. Nature. 2015;**527**:S2-S4. DOI: 10.1038/527S2a

2

Drug Repurposing in Dermatology: Molecular Biology and Omics Approach

Farid A. Badria and Abdullah A. Elgazar

Abstract

The withdrawal of several blockbuster drugs due to severe adverse effects and the failure of several developed drugs in clinical trials raised questions about the efficacy of current approaches of drug discovery. Moreover, the limitation of resources and the long and costive process of drug discovery made a lot of pharmaceutical companies to employ drug repurposing strategies to get new insights about activities that were not considered during their initial discovery. The development of therapeutics for treatment of dermatological condition is not considered as priority although it affects the lifestyle of thousands of people around the world. Serendipity and observations have contributed significantly in this field but immerse efforts have been exerted to find systematic methods to identify new indications for drugs, especially with the unprecedented progress in molecular biol-ogy and omics. So, in this chapter, we will emphasize on different approaches used for drug repositioning and how it was applied to find new therapeutics for different dermatoses.

Keywords: drug repositioning, alopecia, psoriasis, acne, hirsutism, hyperpigmentation

1. Introduction

In the early years of this century, it was expected that revolutionary development in industry and technology will allow an unprecedented opportunities for drug discovery and development; however, the disappointing rate of drug approval in the last 20 years shed the light on the urgent need to reassess the efficiency of current strategies of drug discovery.

Despite the large amount of investment that has been put in drug development, several drug candidates fail to pass due to pharmacokinetic issues or severe side effects that mainly are not demonstrated until clinical phases, which lead to extreme economic loss to pharmaceutical companies that might spend more than billion dollars in the process.

These facts were not overlooked by pharmaceutical industries or academia; so, they started to apply a new strategy that embraces new application of approved drugs rather than starting from scratch, which is known as drug repositioning. While the term was first coined in 2004, the approach has already led to the discov-ery of several therapeutic agents in the last century; however, serendipity, trials, and errors were the main players in most of these cases.

This means that harnessing our highly advanced tools of molecular biology and computational techniques would guarantee the rediscovery of new indications for already approved drugs, which will not only increase our arsenal of therapeutic agents but also will drastically decrease the time and costs of the whole process.

Moreover, this approach could help for finding therapeutic solutions for orphan diseases or clinical conditions that affects low number of population which are usually neglected by pharmaceutical corps as in the case of dermatologic therapeutics due to the low prevalence of many dermatoses and the inappropriate estimation of the burden of psychological and physical impact of skin disorders on the quality of lifeIndeed, the field of dermatology covers wide range of disorders, but this means that drug repurposing strategy may be uniquely successful, hence the broad variety of pathophysiological process affecting the skin. In that aspect, the liver research laboratory (FAB-Lab, Faculty of Pharmacy, Mansoura University, Mansoura, Egypt) has utilized several approaches for not only optimization and enhancing the therapeutic effect of commonly available natural products but also recognizing novel application for them so that one therapeutic agent could be used for treatment of several or complex conditions (**Table 1**). In this chapter, we will review different strategies for drug repositioning and their application in dermatological and cosmeceutical field.

No.	Studies for discovery of new indications for natural products		Ref
	Compounds	**Indication**	
1.	Compounds from frankincense	Anti-herpes	[1]
2.	Frankincense oil	Immunomodulatory activity	[2]
3.	Myrrh standardized extract	Schistosomicidal	[3]
4.	Free-B-ring flavonoids	Colon cancer	[4]
5.	Anti-neoplaston A-10	Immune-modulatory in breast cancer patients	[5]
6.	Ricinine alkaloids analogs	Oral squamous cell carcinoma	[6]
7.	Stemmadenine alkaloid derivative	Antiproliferative activity against different cancers	[7]
8.	Curcumin	Iron accumulation in liver	[8]
9.	Cucurbitacin B	Chemo-sensitization of cisplatin-resistant ovarian cancer	[9]
10.	Bi-aryl methyl eugenol analogs	Breast cancer invasion inhibitors	[10]
	Studies for discovery of new target for natural products		
	Compounds/extract	**Targets**	
1.	Flavonoids containing an alpha-keto group	Tyrosinase inhibitors	[11]
2.	Cycloartane glycoside	Lactate dehydrogenase inhibitor	[12]
3.	Betulinic acid analogs	Topoisomerase inhibitors	[13]
4.	Gingerol derivatives	LTA_4H inhibitory activity	[14]
5.	Curcumin derivative	Alpha-amylase inhibitory	[15]
6.	Glycyrrhizin derivative	Acetylcholinesterase inhibitory activity	[16]

Table 1.
Studies of natural product repositioning in FAB-Lab.

2. Drug repositioning strategies

Drug repositioning is achieved by understanding of molecular mechanisms of drug action and by identification of the interacting proteins of the drug. In many cases, molecular mechanism of drug action is poorly understood or completely unknown. The drug action can be observed by identification of drug targets and their specific interactions, drug-induced change in expression of a specific gene and the associated pathways, and change in disease phenotypes.

Current approaches for drug repositioning come from the so-called "drug action spectrum" concept as shown in **Figure 1**, which is based on three paradigms, namely, target-centric, drug-centric, and disease-centric repositioning. The first and second modules are closely related and usually applied interchangeably; the target-centric module focuses on finding new indication for the already established target; for example, the discovery of the role of androgenic receptor in hair loss allowed the repurposing of finasteride for treatment of androgenic alopecia.

Drug-centric module aims in finding a new target for therapeutic agent, experimental or abandoned drugs; for example, the notorious thalidomide, which was firstly indicated for treatment of nausea and caused the phocomelia crisis, has been repurposed for treatment of myeloma and several dermatological conditions related to immune diseases.

These types of repositioning use computational ligand- and structure-based techniques [12, 13], chemical proteomics [16, 17], and off-target screening to identify potential therapeutic applications; so, we will explain the theory behind its approach and its application in drug repositioning.

In the third module, the repurposing depends on the similarity of pathophysiological nature of diseases; for example, different types of cancers or different autoimmune diseases which allow the expansion of drug to a closely related indication so that extensive analysis of the associated molecular targets may not be required. Nevertheless, this type of repositioning strategy is the most observed type

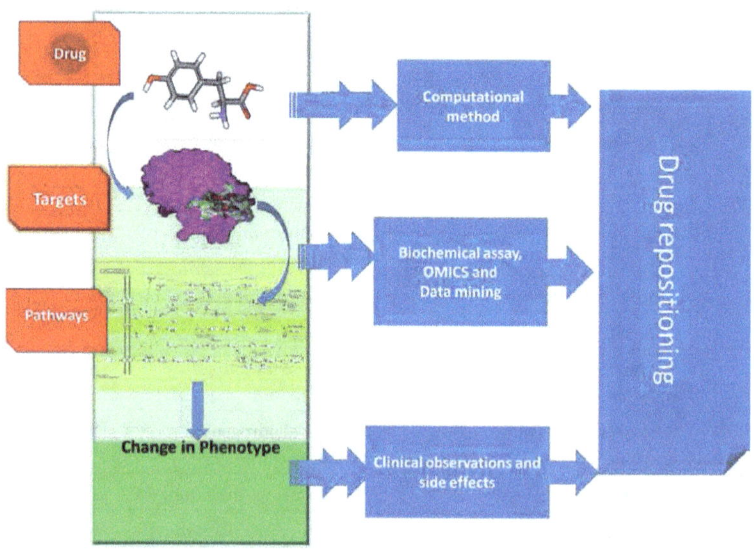

Figure 1.
The concept of drug action spectrum in drug repositioning is based on three paradigms, namely, drug-centric, target-centric, and disease-centric repositioning. In the first and second approaches, computational approaches are used extensively to identify novel targets for compounds that were used for different applications. Omics, data mining, and meta-analysis of clinical trials could also be used to analyze the relationship between diseases and novel molecular targets that was previously investigated in different diseases.

in drug repurposing field; it is worthy to note that retrospective analysis of several repurposing cases could be explained exclusively by drug-target interaction [18].

The main tools used for applying disease-centric repositioning are gene or protein expression profiling [14, 15], phenotypic screening [11], clinical observations [19], side effect analysis [20], and data mining and neural networks [21, 22]. In the following section, we will shed the light on the application of these tools in drug repositioning, especially in dermatology.

2.1 Application of drug-target interaction in drug repositioning

2.1.1 Ligand- and structure-based approaches

Ligand-based approaches are usually employed when no structural information about the target under investigation is available. They are not only used for virtual screening but also for lead optimization [17]. The key concept in ligand-based approaches is to determine common structural features or descriptors that could be found in compounds with the same pharmacological activity; therefore, pharmacophoric function groups which are necessary to maintain the activity could be elucidated (**Figure 2**) [19].

In structure-based approach, the 3D structure of biological target is used to recognize how an active compound bind to its active site; hence, molecular docking could be used for identifying other drugs that can bind to the active site in similar fashion [20]. It is worthy to note that such approach could be used also for identifying the ability of drugs to bind to diverse types of targets, which is known as target fishing or inverse docking; this could be achieved by docking drug of interest against database of targets of clinical significance (**Figure 3**) [21].

Indeed, drug repositioning cases derived from this approach are still limited, but it has been extensively used to give insights on the mode of action of natural products and the rationale behind their use in traditional medicine. For example, ricinoleic acid **(1)**, acteoside **(2)**, amentoflavone **(3)**, quercetin-3-O-rutinoside **(4)**, and hinokiflavone **(5)** were expected to be prostaglandin D2 synthase inhibitors by inverse docking, which could explain their use in herbal preparation for hair loss treatment [22]; another study revealed that the anti-inflammatory effect of *Bryophyllum pin-natum* is due to the ability of quercetin 3-O-α-L-arabinopyranosyl-(1 → 2)-O-α-L-rhamnopyranoside **(6)** to inhibit PDE4B, a prominent target in the pathogenesis of psoriatic arthritis, and atopic dermatitis [23, 24]; also, the antiaging effect of allicin was linked to its ability to act as leukocyte elastase inhibitor [25].

Bagherzadeh et al. applied pharmacophore and structure-based virtual screening to identify tyrosinase inhibitor from zinc database; among them, five compounds showed the potential to be used as potent inhibitor according to molecular

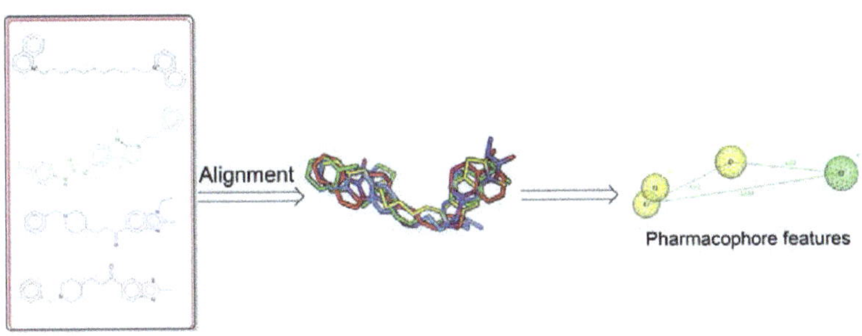

Figure 2.
Ligand-based approaches depend on the elucidation of structural features that could be found in set of active drugs (fingerprint) so that compounds possessing the same pharmacophores could be identified.

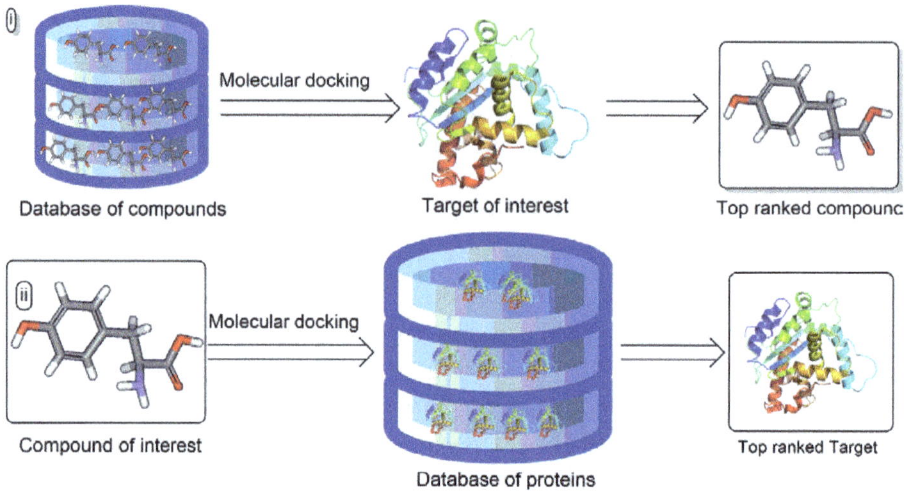

Figure 3.
Structure-based virtual screening employ two main approaches: (i) molecular docking where databases of thousands of compounds could be docked to the active site of target of interest to identify the top ranked compounds and (ii) inverse docking, as the name suggests, where compound of interest is docked against a panel of different targets to identify new potential targets.

dynamic simulation [26]. Interestingly, Choi et al. used structure-based virtual screening for repurposing thiopurine drugs such as mercaptopurine **(7)** as tyrosinase inhibitors for treatment of hyperpigmentation [27]. The chemical structure of compounds **(1–7)** is shown in **Figure 4**.

2.1.2 Off-target-based repositioning

The ability of most of drugs to induce side effects is originated from their binding with other targets that might share certain homology with the original targets,

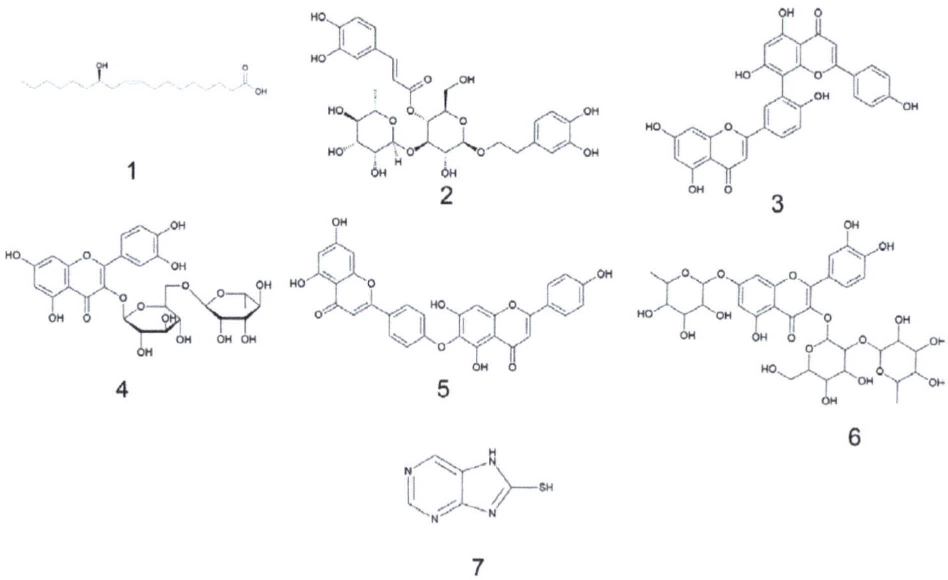

Figure 4.
Chemical structure of ricinoleic acid **(1)**, *acteoside* **(2)**, *amentoflavone* **(3)**, *quercetin-3-O-rutinoside* **(4)**, *hinokiflavone* **(5)**, *quercetin 3-O-α-L-arabinopyranosyl-(1 → 2)-O-α-L-rhamnopyranoside* **(6)**, *and mercaptopurine* **(7)**.

so it could be quite handful to use this drugs in treatment of diseases where these targets are dysregulated.

Spironolactone **(8)** is an antagonist to aldosterone; so, it is used for treatment of hypertension due to its diuretic effect; however, its steroidal nature allows it to act as a competitive antagonist at androgenic receptor; so, it was suggested to be used in treatment of androgenic alopecia; however, its effects on hair growth patterns in males might be not clinically preferable. On the other hand, it proved to be significantly effective in treatment of polycystic ovary syndrome and hirsutism in females, due to its ability to inhibit hair regrowth in androgen-dependent regions of the body, which was proven by several clinical trials.

Another intriguing example for off-targets drug repositioning is doxepin **(9)** which is a tricyclic antidepressant; it prevents reuptake of serotonin and norepinephrine, leading to an increase in the synaptic concentrations of those neurotransmitters. Nevertheless, there are several off-target effects that are associated with the use of this class of drugs, which are mainly mediated by muscarinic and histamine receptors. This could be explained by its high affinity to H_1 receptor which is much higher than hydroxyzine by 56 times and diphenhydramine 800 times; such observation opened the gate to the FDA approval for treatment of dermatological conditions such as pruritus, psychodermatosis, and chronic urticaria as topical and systemic agents.

Off-target effects are also influenced by the route of administration; sodium valproate **(10)**, an anti-epileptic drug, inhibits the cellular sodium influx by blocking voltage-dependent sodium channels and induces chloride influx by gamma hydroxyl butyric acid (GABA)-mimetic effect. It also reduces the release of GABA, thereby attenuating neuronal excitation induced by glutamate receptors. It was reported by several clinical trials that oral administration of valproate could induce hair loss in dose-dependent manner by decreasing biotinidase activity leading to alopecia induced by biotin deficiency.

However, sodium valproate topical treatment induced hair growth in male C3H mice model, which could be explained by its ability to inhibit glycogen synthase kinase 3β and activation of Wnt/β-catenin pathway, which in turn, is associated with hair regeneration and anagen induction. This result was supported by randomized interventional study, where 7.2% spray of sodium valproate applied twice daily on scalp up to 24 weeks showed the efficacy of valproate spray on androgenic alopecia.

Dapsone **(11)**, which is known to be one of the few agents used to fight leprosy, was developed as an antistreptococcal agent by targeting dihydropteroate synthetase in bacteria; it was only matter of time until its anti-inflammatory effect was noticed due to its effect on numerous neutrophil-mediated and autoimmune processes; so, it is now used for recurring neutrophilic dermatosis, cicatricial pemphigoid, linear IgA dermatosis, IgA pemphigus, erythema elevatum diutinum, acropustulosis infantilis, and prurigo pigmentosa [28].

Finally, thalidomide **(12)** is a distinguishable case in drug repositioning; it was used for treatment of morning sickness in pregnant women after its withdrawal due its teratogenic effect; such side effect was studied thoroughly and explained by the ability of the drug to inhibit vascular endothelial growth factor (VEGF) which has a significant role in angiogenesis and embryo development; so, this drug was repositioned for treatment of multiple myeloma; also, it was found that thalidomide is a strong inhibitor for tumor necrosis factor alpha (TNF-α) and was approved by FDA for management of erythema nodosum leprosum [29, 30]. The chemical structure of compounds **(8–13)** is presented in **Figure 5**.

2.1.3 New target indication-based repositioning

In this approach, data analysis based on omics is used to identify new function instead of finding new targets for certain chemical entity; hence, it might be the

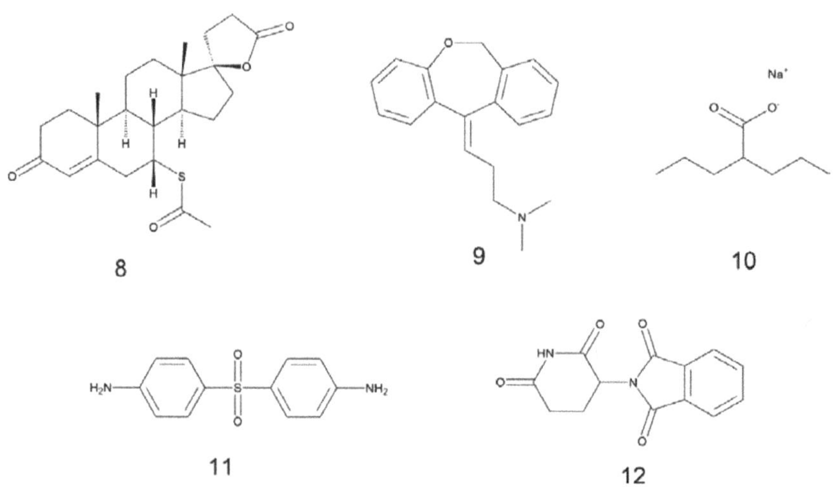

8 9 10

11 12

Figure 5.
Chemical structure of spironolactone (**8**), *doxepin* (**9**), *sodium valproate* (**10**), *dapsone* (**11**), *and thalidomide* (**12**).

most challenging approach as it depends on the advances of molecular biology tools which can reveal the role of already known target in completely different diseases.

Finasteride **(13)** is a drug that was developed for treatment of benign prostatic hyperplasia, by acting as 5α-reductase enzyme inhibitor; this enzyme was found later to be contributing in the development of androgenic alopecia; hence, finasteride at low doses was repositioned to treatment of baldness in men.

Another example is the repositioning of eflornithine **(14)**, which was used for treatment of African trypanosomiasis by inhibiting ornithine decarboxylase; several years later, the homolog enzyme in humans was found to be responsible for hair growth and eflornithine was suggested as potential treatment of hirsutism in woman due to its ability to reduce hair growth. This observation was supported by several clinical trials and is currently marketed as topical preparation.

Zileuton **(15)** is a 5-lipoxygenase inhibitor which is used for treatment of asthma, by blocking the biosynthesis of leukotriene B4, which contributes significantly in tissue inflammation in acne; so, several studies on the experimental and clinical levels have been performed to understand its mode of action, as well as safety of this compound in the management of acne vulgaris. Zileuton demonstrated a significant efficiency in patients with moderate acne, whereas a decrease in inflammatory lesions was noticed in comparison to the placebo group. Also, the tolerability and safety of zileuton were satisfactory in all conducted clinical studies [31]. The chemical structure of compounds **(13–15)** is shown in **Figure 6**.

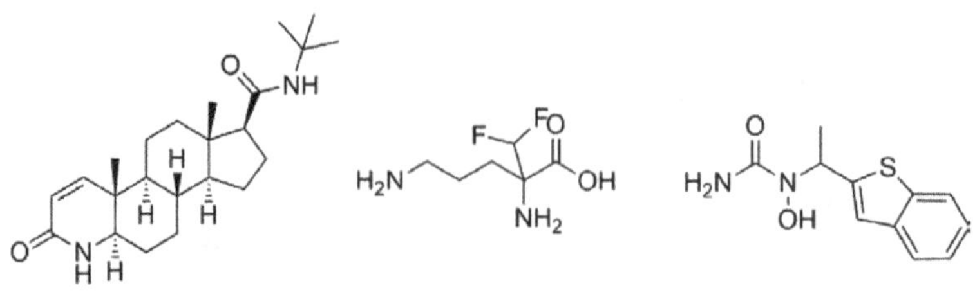

13 14 15

Figure 6.
Chemical structure of finasteride (**13**), *eflornithine* (**14**), *and zileuton* (**15**).

2.2 Disease-centered drug repositioning

2.2.1 Application of data mining and omics in drug repositioning

In disease-centered paradigm, the observation and analysis of data from phenotypic assays, clinical trials, and literature could be an important resource for drug repositioning, as previously mentioned, this type of repositioning is oriented toward the clinical outcomes rather than the exact molecular mechanism behind the drug switch; from other angle, the researcher aims to find certain fingerprint on the genetic or proteomic level to support the repositioning hypothesis; for example, the transcriptomic analysis of different types of autoimmune diseases could reveal similar pattern of gene expression, which means that the same drug could be used for different types of immunity-related condition.

Qu et al. applied integrative clinical transcriptomic analyses for finding new drugs for treatment of psoriasis. First, gene expression analysis of samples collected from psoriasis patient and normal volunteers were used to identify molecular targets associated with the disease, and then, connectivity map analysis revealed potential drugs for the identified targets, which were resveratrol **(16)**, tiabendazole **(17)**, monobenzone **(18)**, parthenolide **(18)**, doxycycline **(19)**, and methotrexate **(20)** [32].

Also, Patrick et al. gathered drug-related information from more than 20 million articles using machine learning based on word embedding to build a model that highlights drug-disease relationship in order to repurpose drugs for treatment of immune-mediated dermatological conditions, where prednisone **(21)**, triamcinolone **(22)**, budesonide **(23)**, hydroxychloroquine **(24)**, and leflunomide **(25)** were among the top five predicted drugs for treatment of psoriasis [33]. The chemical structure of compounds **(15–25)** is demonstrated in **Figure 7**.

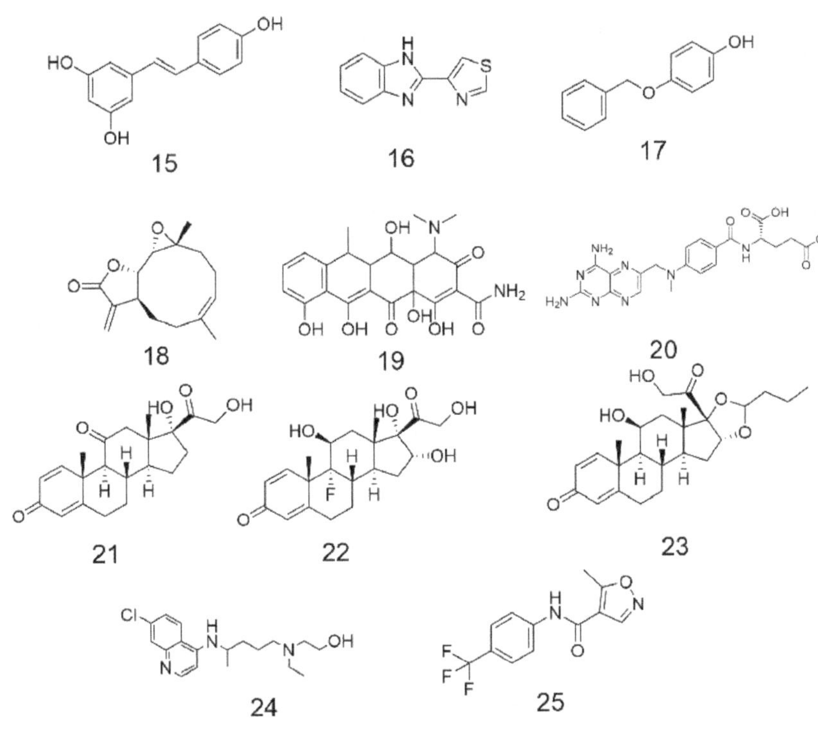

Figure 7.
Chemical structure of resveratrol (16), *tiabendazole* (17), *monobenzone* (18), *parthenolide* (18), *doxycycline* (19), *methotrexate* (20) *prednisone* (21), *triamcinolone* (22), *budesonide* (23), *hydroxychloroquine* (24), *and leflunomide* (25).

2.2.2 Clinical observation-based drug repurposing

Bimatoprost **(26)**, a prostaglandin analog, was used for treatment of glaucoma patient, but several clinical observations reported the occurrence of eyelash hypertrichosis; so, it was used for induction of eyelash regrowth in alopecia areata and for cosmeceutical purposes [34, 35].

Phenytoin **(27)** is one of the first discovered antiepileptic drugs; after its introduction to the market, gingival hyperplasia was reported as a side effect for the treatment, which triggered dermatologist to evaluate its ability to heal wounds; so, phenytoin has been evaluated by several clinical studies, where it proved to be useful in treatment of wounds in topical and oral forms; however, the exact mechanism of action is still ambiguous [36].

Bevacizumab, a monoclonal antibody that is used for treatment of several types of cancer, was observed to achieve complete remission of psoriasis in metastatic colon cancer without any other treatment for psoriasis [37]; a case which was reported again in another study that described the same effect in metastatic renal cell cancer, psoriasis, and psoriatic arthritis patient, which means the bevacizumab could be repurposed for treatment of these dermatoses; also, it sheds the light on the importance of (VEGF) as a target for treatment of inflammatory skin conditions [38].

The Janus kinase (JAK) inhibitor, tofacitinib **(28)**, was developed originally for management of rheumatoid arthritis, ulcerative colitis and other autoimmune diseases, but it was repurposed for psoriasis and atopic dermatitis since JAK was found to be contributing in the pathogenesis of these diseases, and currently, several clinical trials were performed to assess its clinical significance and concluded that response rates in tofacitinib-treated group were significantly higher compared to that in placebo [39–41].

Metformin **(29)**, a type-2 diabetes medication, reduces insulin resistance; however, its mechanism is not completely understood; so, it was suggested as a treatment of several dermatological conditions associated with insulin resistance such as acanthosis nigricans and acne; this was supported by several clinical trials where the patients showed complete resolution. It also was employed in treatment of hyperpigmentation due to its inhibitory effect on tyrosinases, the key enzymes in melanin biosynthesis. The anti-melanogenic effect of metformin was demonstrated experimentally on human skin biopsies and reconstituted human epidermis; also, clinical trials showed that metformin efficacy is comparable to TCC in treating melasma [42–44].

Finally, minoxidil **(30)**, which is a well-known case in drug repositioning, was initially used for treatment of hypertension since its strong vasodilator effect but during clinical trials, hair regrowth was noticed in patients with androgenic alopecia such effect is contributed by stimulating the vascular bed nearby the hair follicles which lead to better environment for hair growth. It was suggested that the ability of minoxidil to activate cytoprotective prostaglandin synthase-1 and stimulate adipose-derived stem cells (ASCs) [45, 46].

2.2.3 Phenotypic screening for drug repositioning

Niclosamide (NCL) **(31)** is an anti-helminthic drug that has been utilized for long time with considerable safety profile; several studies reported its anti-inflammatory and anticancer activities, highlighting the potential of repurposing for different indications; Thatikonda et al. used imiquimod (IMQ)-induced BALB/c mouse model to evaluate the efficacy of NCL for treatment of psoriasis, where it alleviated epidermal hyperplasia and inflammation induced by IMQ via down-regulating p65, STAT3, NFATc-1, and NF-κB transcription factors along with Ki-67, ICAM-1, and Akt protein expression [47].

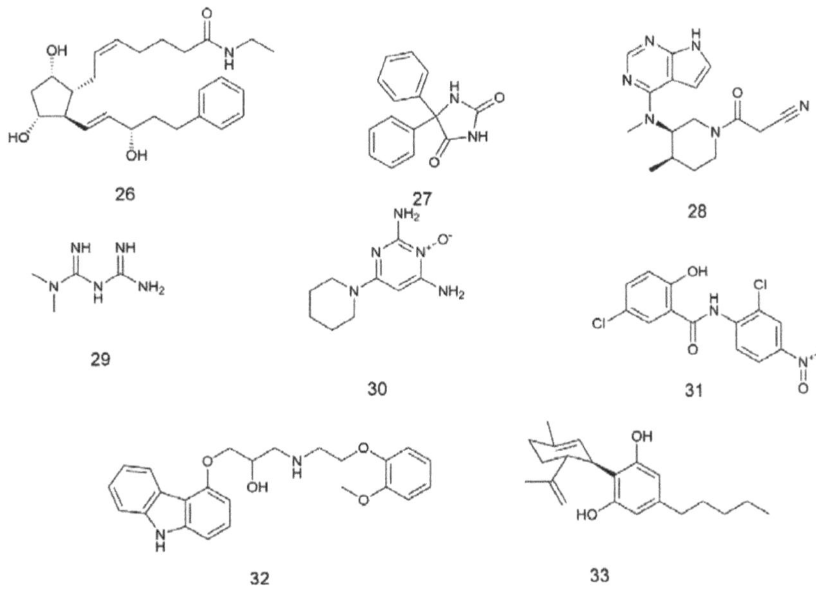

Figure 8.
Chemical structure of bimatoprost (26), *phenytoin* (27), *tofacitinib* (28), *metformin* (29), *minoxidil* (30), *niclosamide* (31), *carvedilol* (32), *and cannabidiol (CBD)* (33).

Hall et al. used zebrafish neutrophil migration assay, for evaluation of the suppressive effect of 1280 approved drugs on recruitment of neutrophils; where drugs showing prominent anti-inflammatory activity were further tested in atopic dermatitis animal model, among them 11 drugs which was not reported previously as anti-inflammatory agent [48].

Chang et al. used in vivo model of chemically induced murine skin tumorigenesis to confirm the hypothesis of repositioning of beta blocker for treatment of skin cancer, since several studies showed that stress-related catecholamine hormone expression can affect tumor progression [49].

Carvedilol **(32)**, when administrated orally and topically, prevented DMBA-induced epidermal hyperplasia, suggesting that it may serve as a new agent for protecting against skin cancer [50], which was supported by another study that demonstrated the preventive effect of carvedilol applied topically after UV exposure; so, it can be repositioned as prophylactic agent against skin inflammation and cancer [51]Cannabidiol (CBD) **(33)** is a nonpsychoactive phytocannabinoid found in *Cannabis sativa*. It is approved recently for the treatment of seizures associated with two uncommon and serious forms of epilepsy, Dravet syndrome, and Lennox-Gastaut syndrome. Oláh et al. reported that CBD-treated human sebocytes and human skin organ in vitro showed strong antiproliferative, lipostatic, and anti-inflammatory effects mediated by a plethora of receptors, ion channels, and other components of the endocannabinoid system [52]. These findings were confirmed later by clinical trial showing that CBD administrated as an ointment is an effective and noninvasive option for enhancing the quality of life in patients with some skin disorders, especially those with inflammatory background [53]. The chemical structure of compounds **(26–33)** is depicted in **Figure 8**.

3. Concluding remarks and future perspective

Drug repositioning is an important strategy to maximize the benefits from already approved drugs; it will not only contribute to reduction of time and cost for drug discovery but also could help to develop new therapeutics for orphan and ignored diseases. While historic cases of drug repositioning were inspired by serendipity and observations, more systematic approaches became well established by time. In silico and data mining tools could help to analyze the large amount of data available from omics, phenotypic assay, and clinical investigations by revealing novel relationship between drugs, targets, and different pathways of diseases as described in this chapter; the integration of different tools of drug repurposing will allow the identification of safe and effective therapeutics for treatment of dermatological condition and enhance the quality of life of patients.

Author details

Farid A. Badria[1*] and Abdullah A. Elgazar[2]

1 Department of Pharmacognosy, Faculty of Pharmacy, Mansoura University, Mansoura, Egypt

2 Department of Pharmacognosy, Faculty of Pharmacy, Kafrelsheikh University, Kafrelsheikh, Egypt

*Address all correspondence to: faridbadria@gmail.com

References

[1] Badria FA, Abu-Karam M, Mikhaeil BR, Maatooq GT, Amer M. Antiherpes activity of isolated compounds from frankincense. Biosciences, Biotechnology Research Asia. 2016;**1**(1): 1-10

[2] Badria FA, Mikhaeil BR, Maatooq GT, Amer MM. Immunomodulatory triterpenoids from the oleogum resin of *Boswellia carterii* Birdwood. Zeitschrift für Naturforschung C, A Journal of Biosciences. 2003;**58**(7-8):505-516

[3] Badria F, Abou-Mohamed G, El-Mowafy A, Masoud A, Salama O. Mirazid: A new schistosomicidal drug. Pharmaceutical Biology. 2001;**39**(2):127-131

[4] Ibrahim A, Sobeh M, Ismail A, Alaa A, Sheashaa H, Sobh M, et al. Free-B-ring flavonoids as potential lead compounds for colon cancer therapy. Molecular and Clinical Oncology. 2014;**2**(4):581-585

[5] Badria F, Mabed M, Khafagy W, Abou-Zeid L. Potential utility of antineoplaston A-10 levels in breast cancer. Cancer Letters. 2000;**155**(1):67-70

[6] El-Naggar MH, Abdel Bar FM, Choudhary H, Javadi M, Shimizu K, Kunnumakkara AB, et al. Synthesis of new selective cytotoxic ricinine analogues against oral squamous cell carcinoma. Natural Product Research. 2019:1-12. DOI: 10.1080/14786419.2019.1663513

[7] Abdul-Hameed ZH, Alarif WM, Omer A, El Omri A, Ayyad S-EN, Badria FA, et al. Selective anti-proliferative activity of indole alkaloids from *Rhazya stricta* Decne leaves. 2019;**16**(12):941-947

[8] Badria FA, Ibrahim AS, Badria AF, Elmarakby AA. Curcumin attenuates iron accumulation and oxidative stress in the liver and spleen of chronic iron-overloaded rats. PLoS One. 2015;**10**(7):e0134156

[9] El-Senduny FF, Badria FA, El-Waseef AM, Chauhan SC, Halaweish F. Approach for chemosensitization of cisplatin-resistant ovarian cancer by cucurbitacin B. Tumour biology: The Journal of the International Society for Oncodevelopmental Biology and Medicine. 2016;**37**(1):685-698

[10] Abdel Bar FM, Khanfar MA, Elnagar AY, Badria FA, Zaghloul AM, Ahmad KF, et al. Design and pharmacophore modeling of biaryl methyl eugenol analogs as breast cancer invasion inhibitors. Bioorganic & Medicinal Chemistry. 2010;**18**(2):496-507

[11] Badria FA, El Gayyar MA. A new type of tyrosinase inhibitors from natural products as potential treatments for hyperpigmentation. Bollettino Chimico Farmaceutico. 2001;**140**(4):267-271

[12] El-attar E, Galala A, Gohar A, Badria F. Cycloartane glycoside: A new lactate dehydrogenase inhibitor, from the aerial part of agriculture waste of watermelon. World Journal of Pharmaceutical Sciences. 2015;**3**(4): 689-695

[13] Bar FMA, Khanfar MA, Elnagar AY, Liu H, Zaghloul AM, Badria FA, et al. Rational design and semisynthesis of betulinic acid analogues as potent topoisomerase inhibitors. Journal of Natural Products. 2009;**72**(9):1643-1650

[14] El-Naggar MH, Mira A, Abdel Bar FM, Shimizu K, Amer MM, Badria FA. Synthesis, docking, cytotoxicity, and LTA(4) H inhibitory activity of new gingerol derivatives as potential colorectal

cancer therapy. Bioorganic & Medicinal Chemistry. 2017;**25**(3):1277-1285

[15] Eman Elattar AAG, Saad H-EA, Badria FA. Alpha-amylase inhibitory effect and docking studies of some new curcumin-triazole derivatives. Acta Scientific Nutritional Health. 2019;**3**(11):124-129

[16] Abdel Bar FM, Elimam DM, Mira AS, El-Senduny FF, Badria FA. Derivatization, molecular docking and in vitro acetylcholinesterase inhibitory activity of glycyrrhizin as a selective anti-Alzheimer agent. Natural Product Research. 2019;**33**(18):2591-2599

[17] Franke L, Schwarz O, Müller-Kuhrt L, Hoernig C, Fischer L, George S, et al. Identification of natural-product-derived inhibitors of 5-lipoxygenase activity by ligand-based virtual screening. Journal of Medicinal Chemistry. 2007;**50**(11):2640-2646

[18] Parisi D, Adasme MF, Sveshnikova A, Moreau Y, Schroeder M. Drug repositioning or target repositioning: A structural perspective of drug-target-indication relationship for available repurposed drugs. Computational and Structural Biotechnology Journal. 2019:715094

[19] Koes DR, Camacho CJ. ZINCPharmer: Pharmacophore search of the ZINC database. Nucleic Acids Research. 2012;**40**(W1):W409-W414

[20] Schulz-Gasch T, Stahl M. Binding site characteristics in structure-based virtual screening: Evaluation of current docking tools. Journal of Molecular Modeling. 2003;**9**(1):47-57

[21] AbdulHameed MDM, Chaudhury S, Singh N, Sun H, Wallqvist A, Tawa GJ. Exploring polypharmacology using a ROCS-based target fishing approach. Journal of Chemical Information and Modeling. 2012;**52**(2):492-505

[22] Fong P, Tong HH, Ng KH, Lao CK, Chong CI, Chao CM. In silico prediction of prostaglandin D2 synthase inhibitors from herbal constituents for the treatment of hair loss. Journal of Ethnopharmacology. 2015;**175**:470-480

[23] Li H, Zuo J, Tang W. Phosphodiesterase-4 inhibitors for the treatment of inflammatory diseases. Frontiers in Pharmacology. 2018;**9**:1048

[24] Lourenço EMG, Fernandes JM, Carvalho VF, Grougnet R, Martins MA, Jordão AK, et al. Identification of a selective PDE4B inhibitor from *Bryophyllum pinnatum* by target fishing study and in vitro evaluation of quercetin 3-O-α-L-arabinopyranosyl-(1→2)-O-α-L-rhamnopyranoside. Frontiers in Pharmacology. 2019;**10**:1582

[25] Pangastuti A, Indriwati SE, Amin M. Investigation of the anti-aging properties of allicin from *Allium sativum* L bulb extracts by a reverse docking approach. Tropical Journal of Pharmaceutical Research. 2018;**17**(4):635-639

[26] Bagherzadeh K, Shirgahi Talari F, Sharifi A, Ganjali MR, Saboury AA, Amanlou M. A new insight into mushroom tyrosinase inhibitors: Docking, pharmacophore-based virtual screening, and molecular modeling studies. Journal of Biomolecular Structure & Dynamics. 2015;**33**(3):487-501

[27] Choi J, Lee YM, Jee JG. Thiopurine drugs repositioned as tyrosinase inhibitors. International Journal of Molecular Sciences. 2017;**19**(1):77

[28] Wozel G, Blasum C. Dapsone in dermatology and beyond. Archives of Dermatological Research. 2014;**306**(2):103-124

[29] Wu JJ, Huang DB, Pang KR, Hsu S, Tyring SK. Thalidomide: Dermatological

indications, mechanisms of action and side-effects. The British Journal of Dermatology. 2005;**153**(2):254-273

[30] Perri AJ III, Hsu S. A review of thalidomide's history and current dermatological applications. Dermatology Online Journal. 2003;**9**(3):5

[31] Zouboulis CC. Zileuton, a new efficient and safe systemic anti-acne drug. Dermato-Endocrinology. 2009;**1**(3):188-192

[32] Qu XA, Freudenberg JM, Sanseau P, Rajpal DK. Integrative clinical transcriptomics analyses for new therapeutic intervention strategies: A psoriasis case study. Drug Discovery Today. 2014;**19**(9):1364-1371

[33] Patrick MT, Raja K, Miller K, Sotzen J, Gudjonsson JE, Elder JT, et al. Drug repurposing prediction for immune-mediated cutaneous diseases using a word-embedding-based machine learning approach. The Journal of Investigative Dermatology. 2019;**139**(3):683-691

[34] Law SK. Bimatoprost in the treatment of eyelash hypotrichosis. Clinical Ophthalmology. 2010;**4**:349-358

[35] Tosti A, Pazzaglia M, Voudouris S, Tosti G. Hypertrichosis of the eyelashes caused by bimatoprost. Journal of the American Academy of Dermatology. 2004;**51**(5 Suppl):S149-S150

[36] Keppel Hesselink JM. Phenytoin repositioned in wound healing: Clinical experience spanning 60 years. Drug Discovery Today. 2018;**23**(2):402-408

[37] Akman A, Yilmaz E, Mutlu H, Ozdogan M. Complete remission of psoriasis following bevacizumab therapy for colon cancer. Clinical and Experimental Dermatology. 2009;**34**(5):e202-e204

[38] Datta-Mitra A, Riar NK, Raychaudhuri SP. Remission of psoriasis and psoriatic arthritis during bevacizumab therapy for renal cell cancer. Indian Journal of Dermatology. 2014;**59**(6):632

[39] Purohit VS, Ports WC, Wang C, Riley S. Systemic tofacitinib concentrations in adult patients with atopic dermatitis treated with 2% tofacitinib ointment and application to pediatric study planning. Journal of Clinical Pharmacology. 2019;**59**(6):811-820

[40] Howell MD, Kuo FI, Smith PA. Targeting the Janus kinase family in autoimmune skin diseases. Frontiers in Immunology. 2019;**10**:2342

[41] Kvist-Hansen A, Hansen PR, Skov L. Systemic treatment of psoriasis with JAK inhibitors: A review. Dermatology and Therapy. 2020;**10**(1):29-42

[42] Bubna AK. Metformin - For the dermatologist. Indian Journal of Pharmacology. 2016;**48**(1):4-10

[43] Banavase Channakeshavaiah R, Andanooru Chandrappa NK. Topical metformin in the treatment of melasma: A preliminary clinical trial. Journal of Cosmetic Dermatology. 2019

[44] Lehraiki A, Abbe P, Cerezo M, Rouaud F, Regazzetti C, Chignon-Sicard B, et al. Inhibition of melanogenesis by the antidiabetic metformin. The Journal of Investigative Dermatology. 2014;**134**(10):2589-2597

[45] Michelet JF, Commo S, Billoni N, Mahé YF, Bernard BA. Activation of cytoprotective prostaglandin synthase-1 by minoxidil as a possible explanation for its hair growth-stimulating effect. The Journal of Investigative Dermatology. 1997;**108**(2):205-209

[46] Choi N, Shin S, Song SU, Sung JH. Minoxidil promotes hair growth through stimulation of growth factor release from adipose-derived

stem cells. International Journal of Molecular Sciences. 2018;**19**(3):691

[47] Thatikonda S, Pooladanda V, Godugu C. Repurposing an old drug for new use: Niclosamide in psoriasis-like skin inflammation. Journal of Cellular Physiology. 2020;**235**(6):5270-5283

[48] Hall CJ, Wicker SM, Chien AT, Tromp A, Lawrence LM, Sun X, et al. Repositioning drugs for inflammatory disease - Fishing for new anti-inflammatory agents. Disease Models & Mechanisms. 2014;**7**(9):1069-1081

[49] Yang EV, Eubank TD. The impact of adrenergic signaling in skin cancer progression: Possible repurposing of β-blockers for treatment of skin cancer. Cancer Biomarkers: Section A of Disease Markers. 2013;**13**(3):155-160

[50] Chang A, Yeung S, Thakkar A, Huang KM, Liu MM, Kanassatega RS, et al. Prevention of skin carcinogenesis by the β-blocker carvedilol. Cancer Prevention Research (Philadelphia, Pa.). 2015;**8**(1):27-36

[51] Huang KM, Liang S, Yeung S, Oiyemhonlan E, Cleveland KH, Parsa C, et al. Topically applied carvedilol attenuates solar ultraviolet radiation induced skin carcinogenesis. Cancer Prevention Research (Philadelphia, Pa.). 2017;**10**(10):598-606

[52] Oláh A, Tóth BI, Borbíró I, Sugawara K, Szöllõsi AG, Czifra G, et al. Cannabidiol exerts sebostatic and antiinflammatory effects on human sebocytes. The Journal of Clinical Investigation. 2014;**124**(9):3713-3724

[53] Palmieri B, Laurino C, Vadalà M. A therapeutic effect of cbd-enriched ointment in inflammatory skin diseases and cutaneous scars. La Clinica Terapeutica. 2019;**170**(2):e93-e99

3

Drug Repurposing (DR): An Emerging Approach in Drug Discovery

Mithun Rudrapal, Shubham J. Khairnar and Anil G. Jadhav

Abstract

Drug repurposing (DR) (also known as drug repositioning) is a process of identifying new therapeutic use(s) for old/existing/available drugs. It is an effective strategy in discovering or developing drug molecules with new pharmacological/therapeutic indications. In recent years, many pharmaceutical companies are developing new drugs with the discovery of novel biological targets by applying the drug repositioning strategy in drug discovery and development program. This strategy is highly efficient, time saving, low-cost and minimum risk of failure. It maximizes the therapeutic value of a drug and consequently increases the success rate. Thus, drug repositioning is an effective alternative approach to traditional drug discovery process. Finding new molecular entities (NME) by traditional or *de novo* approach of drug discovery is a lengthy, time consuming and expensive venture. Drug repositioning utilizes the combined efforts of activity-based or experimental and *in silico*-based or computational approaches to develop/identify the new uses of drug molecules on a rational basis. It is, therefore, believed to be an emerging strategy where existing medicines, having already been tested safe in humans, are redirected based on a valid target molecule to combat particularly, rare, difficult-to-treat diseases and neglected diseases.

Keywords: drug repurposing, drug discovery, *in silico* repositioning, activity-based repositioning, target-based screening, therapeutic indication

1. Introduction

Drug repurposing (DR) is also known as drug repositioning, drug re-tasking, drug reprofiling, drug rescuing, drug recycling, drug redirection, and therapeutic switching. It can be defined as a process of identification of new pharmacological indications from old/existing/failed/investigational/already marketed/FDA approved drugs/pro-drugs, and the application of the newly developed drugs to the treatment of diseases other than the drug's original/intended therapeutic use. It involves establishing new therapeutic uses for already known drugs, including approved, discontinued, abandoned and experimental drugs [1–3]. Traditional drug discovery is a time-consuming, laborious, highly expensive and high risk process. The novel approach of drug repositioning has the potential to be employed over traditional drug discovery program by mitigating the high monetary cost, longer duration of development and increased risk of failure. It confers reduced risk of failure where a failure rate of ~45% is associated due to safety or toxicity issues in traditional drug discovery program with additional benefit of saving up to 5–7 years in average drug development time [4, 5]. In recent years, the drug repositioning strategy has gained considerable momentum with about one-third of the new drug approvals correspond to repurposed drugs which currently generate around 25% of the annual revenue for the pharmaceutical industry [6]. It has been accounted that approximately 30% of the US Food and Drug Administration (FDA) approved drugs and biologics (vaccines) are repositioned drugs. According to recent estimates, pharmaceutical industries have significantly placed the market for repurposed drugs at $24.4 billion in 2015 with projected growth up to $31.3 billion in 2020. The first example of drug repositioning was an accidental discovery/ serendipitous observations in the 1920s. After about a century of development, more approaches were developed for accelerating the process of drug repositioning. Some most successful and best-known drugs that have been emerged out of the DR approach are sildenafil, minoxidil, aspirin, valproic acid, methotrexate etc. [7]. For example, sildenafil originally developed for the treatment of hypertension and angina pectoris has currently been used to treat erectile dysfunction.

2. Traditional drug discovery vs. drug repurposing

The traditional approach to drug discovery involves *de novo* identification and of new molecular entities (NME), which include five stages: discovery and preclinical, safety review, clinical research, FDA review, and FDA post-market safety monitoring. It is a time-consuming and costly process with high risk of failure [8]. On the other hand, there are only four stages in drug repositioning, which include compound identification, compound acquisition, development, and FDA post-market safety monitoring [9] (**Figure 1**). With the advancement of bioinformatics/cheminformatics tools and availability of huge biological and structural database, drug repositioning has significantly decreased the time and cost of the drug development with reduction in risk of failure. In recent years, the use of *in silico* techniques along with the application of structure-based drug design (SBDD) and artificial intelligence (AI) technology has further accelerated the drug purposing process [10, 11].

However, the repositioning strategy of using approved therapeutics for new therapeutic indications has demonstrated success particularly through prior serendipitous observations. The discovery of drugs by this approach is certainly advantageous as depicted above over traditional drug discovery program as described below. For example, sildenafil (Viagra), a phosphodiesterase-5 (PDE5) inhibitor initially developed for coronary artery disease (angina) by Pfizer (1985) has been repurposed for the treatment of erectile dysfunction. It potentially reduced the development cost at shorter development time. Metformin (Glucophage), an oral anti-diabetic medication used widely in type 2 diabetes mellitus has been developed as a cancer therapeutic which is currently under phase II/phase III clinical trials [1, 12]Drug repositioning has several advantages in comparison with traditional approaches to drug discovery. When comparing with traditional drug discovery program, a significant reduction of the time spent in R&D can be observed. In traditional approach, it is estimated that 10–16 years are spent for the develop-ment of a new drug, while in DR the estimated time is between 3 and 12 years. It only costs $1.6 billion to develop a new drug using a drug repositioning strategy, while the drug development through traditional strategy costs around $12 billion. Moreover, researchers only need 1–2 years to identify new drug targets and about an average of 8 years to develop a repositioned drug [6, 7]. A repositioned drug does not require the initial 6–9 years typically required for the development of new drugs

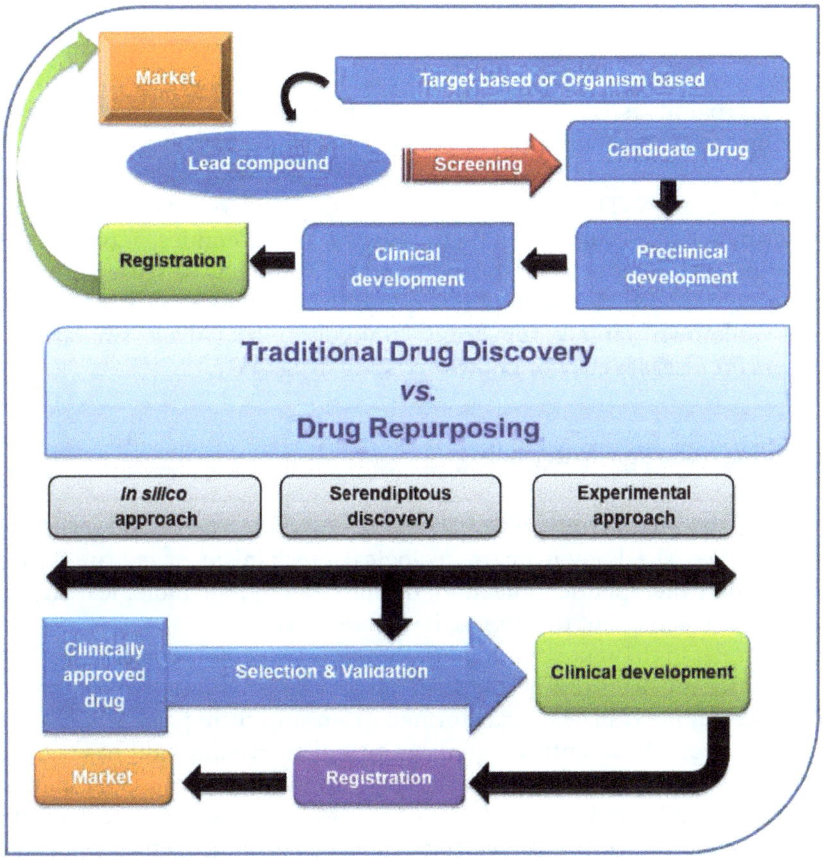

Figure 1.
Traditional drug discovery vs. drug repurposing.

by traditional process, but instead enters directly to preclinical testing and clinical trials, thus reducing the overall risk, time and cost of development. Reports suggest that repurposed drugs require approximately 3–12 years for gaining approval from FDA and/or European Medicines Agency (EMA) and at reduced 50–60% cost. At the beginning of a repositioning project, a range of pre-clinical (pharmacological, toxicological, etc.), and clinical efficacy and safety information is already available, as the candidate drug has already undergone through the early stages of drug development such as structural optimization, preclinical and/or clinical trials, in addition to the possibility of the candidate drug being an approved drug, having its clinical efficacy and safety profile. In this way, there is a reduction of the risks associated with failures in the early stages of development, which are high in traditional approaches, as well as a significant reduction of cost with the possible increase in clinical safety and therefore, high success rate [13, 14].

Due to the availability of previously collected pharmacokinetic, toxicological, clinical and safety data at the start of a repurposing development project, the advantages that are encountered with drug repurposing over traditional drug discovery approach are reduced time of development, lower cost of development and reduced risks of failure in the clinical development.

It has been estimated that the time required for development of a repositioned drug varies from 3 to 12 years (which is about 10–17 years in traditional discovery program) with substantially lower costs, which ensures the repositioning company's significant savings in terms of time and capital. The average cost required to bring a new drug to market is USD 1.24 billion by traditional drug development process, whereas in drug repurposing it costs around ≤60% expenditure of traditional drug discovery. Some other advantages are as follow. The primary focus of traditional dis-covery program is to discover drugs to treat chronic and complex diseases, whereas by drug repositioning approach, development of drugs for rapidly emerging and re-emerging infectious diseases, difficult to treat diseases and neglected diseases (NTDs) are focused. Due to the availability of bioinformatics or cheminformatics approaches, huge omics (proteomics, transcriptomics, metabolomics, genomics etc.) data and database resources, disease targeted-based repositioning methods can be used to explore the unknown mechanisms of action (such as unknown targets for drugs, unknown drug–drug similarities, new biomarkers for diseases etc.) of known/existing drugs [13].

3. Strategies of drug repurposing

There are two main strategies of DR, viz., on-target and off-target (**Figure 2**). In on-target DR, the known pharmacological mechanism of a drug molecule is applied to a new therapeutic indication. In this strategy, the biological target of the drug molecule is same, but the disease is different [12].

For example, in the repositioning of minoxidil (*Rogaine*), an on-target profile is observed, since the drug acts on the same target and produces two different therapeutic effects. Minoxidil was transformed from an antihypertensive vasodilator anti hair loss drug. As an antihypertensive vasodilator, minoxidil has the property of widening blood vessels and opening potassium channels, which allows more oxygen, blood, and nutrients to the hair follicles and this pharmacological action helps its use in the treatment of male pattern baldness (androgenic alopecia).

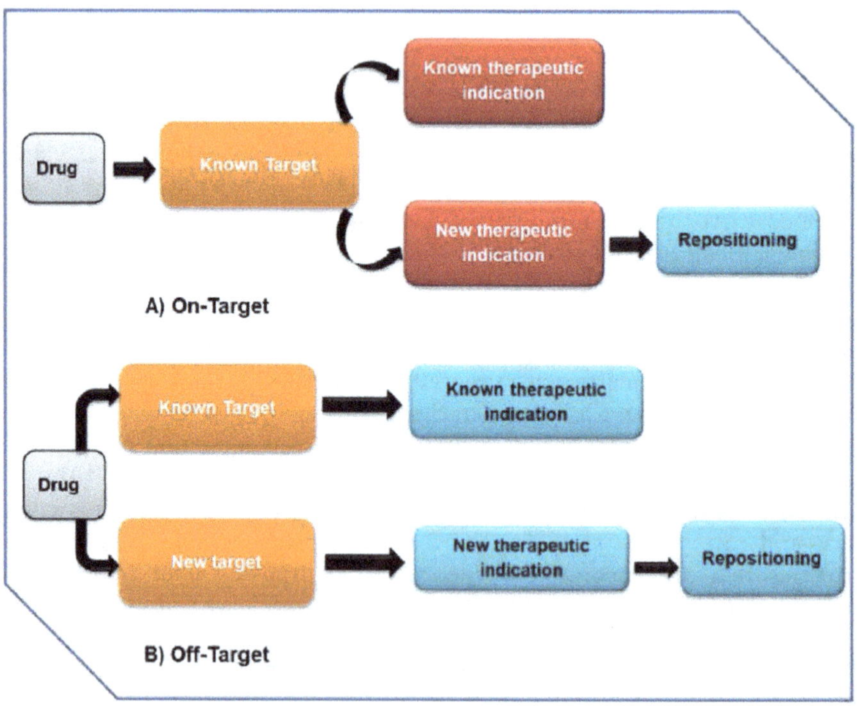

Figure 2.
On-target and off-target strategies of drug repositioning.

On the other hand, in the off-target profile, the pharmacological mechanism is unknown. Drugs and drugs candidates act on new targets, out of the original scope, for new therapeutic indications. Therefore, both the targets and the indications are new [1]. Aspirin (*Colsprin*) is good example of the off-target profile. Aspirin has been traditionally used as NSAID in the treatment of various pain and inflammatory disorders. It also suppresses blood coagulation (clot formation) by inhibiting the normal functioning of platelets (antiplatelet drug). It is, therefore, used in the treatment of heart attacks and strokes. Another new use of aspirin in the treatment of prostate cancer has also been reported.

4. Approaches of drug repurposing

Drug repositioning has two alternative and complementary approaches, one is experiment-based approach and the other is *in silico*-based approach.

The experiment-based approach is also known as activity-based repositioning which refers to the screening of original drugs for new pharmacological indications based on experimental assays. It involves protein target-based and cell/organism-based screens in *in vitro* and/or *in vivo* disease models without requiring any structural information of target proteins. Several approaches of experimental repositioning are target screening approach, cell assay approach, animal model approach and clinical approach [15, 16].

In contrast, *in silico* repositioning carries out virtual screening of public databases of huge drug/chemical libraries using computational biology and bioinformatics/cheminformatics tools. In this approach, the identification of potential bioactive molecules is achieved based upon the molecular interaction between drug molecule and protein target [17].

The differences between activity- and *in silico*-based approaches of drug repositioning are summarized in **Table 1**.

Over the past few decades, the *in silico* approach has gained wide popularity with significant success in drug discovery program. Many pharmaceutical companies and drug discovery research laboratories have already successfully incorporated the *in silico* tools and techniques for the drug discovery from structurally diverse chemical spaces since a large amount of information on the chemical structure bioactive compounds, structure of proteins and pharmacophore models are available in the public domain. Moreover, *in silico* repositioning has some advantages over the experimental-based approach, which includes reduced time and cost of development and low risk of failure. The limitation of this method is that it requires

Activity-based approach	*In silico*-based approach
Experimental (*in vitro* and *in vivo*) screening	Computational (virtual) screening
Target-based and cell/organism-based screening assay	Protein target-based screening
Requires no structural information of target proteins and drug-induced cell/disease phenotypic information	Requires structural information of target proteins and drug-induced cell/disease phenotypic information
Time and labor consuming	Time and labor efficient
Lower rate of false positive hits during the screening	Higher rate of false positive hits during the screening

Table 1.
Differences between activity- and in silico*- based approaches of drug repositioning [17, 18].*

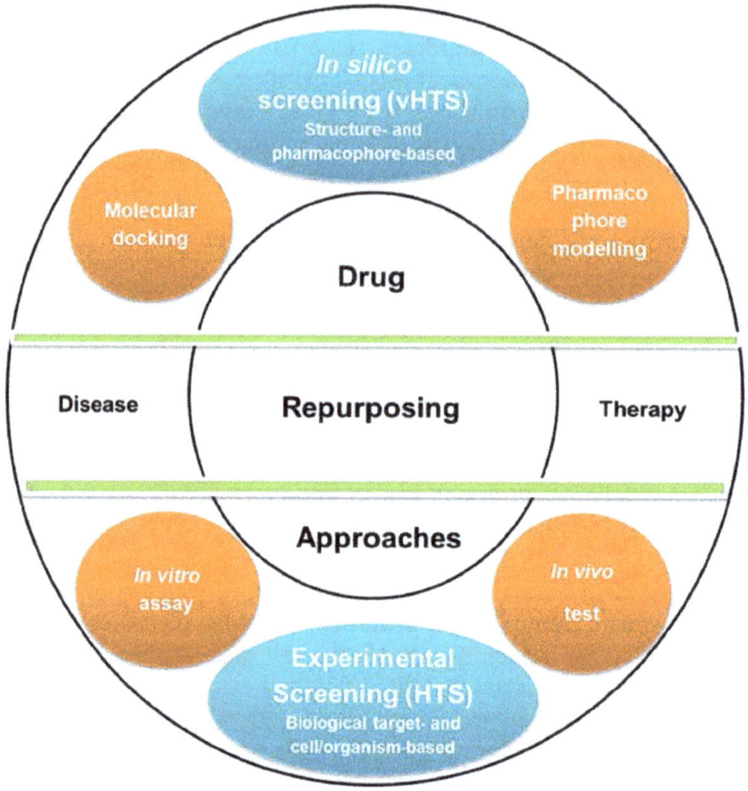

Figure 3.
Approaches of drug repositioning.

precise structural information about drug targets and in case, the protein target is not available, disease specific phenotypic or genotypic profiles of drugs are required [19]. **Figure 3** represents the approaches of drug repositioning.

In recent years, discovery scientists and researchers have combined *in silico* and experimental approaches to identify new therapeutic indications for existing drugs, called mixed approach. In the mixed approach, the result of computational methods is validated by pre-clinical biological experiments (*in vitro* and *in vivo* tests) and clinical studies. The simultaneous application of computational and experimental methodologies in a systematic manner offer a robust and logical approach to the discovery of new indications, demonstrating a greater efficiency than the discovery based on serendipity. Further, mixed approach offers opportunities for developing repositioned drugs more effectively and rapidly. This approach is credible and yet, reliable [20].

5. Methodologies of drug repurposing

The methodologies adopted in DR can be divided into three broad groups depending on the quantity and quality of the pharmacological, toxicological and biological activity information available. These are mainly (i) drug-oriented, (ii) target-oriented, and (iii) disease/therapy-oriented.

In the drug-oriented methodology, the structural characteristics of drug molecules, biological activities, adverse effects and toxicities are evaluated. This strategy is meant for identifying molecules with biological effects based on cell/

animal assays. This type of repositioning methodology is based on traditional pharmacology and drug discovery principles, where studies are usually conducted to determine the biological efficacy of drug molecules without really knowing about the biological targets. Significant successes in DR have been achieved with this orientation profile, through serendipity or clinical observation, such as discoveries with sildenafil [21].

Target-based methodology comprise *in silico* screening or virtual high-throughput screening (vHTS) of drugs or compounds from drug libraries/compound databases such as ligand-based screening or molecular docking followed by *in vitro* and *in vivo* high-throughput and/or high-content screening (HTS/HCS) of drugs against a selective protein molecule or a biomarker of interest. In this method, there is a significant success rate in drug discovery as compared to drug-oriented method, because most biological targets directly represent the disease pathways/mechanisms [22].

The application of disease/therapy-oriented methodology in DR is relevant when there is more information on the disease model is available. In this case, DR can be guided by the disease and/or treatment based upon availability of information given by proteomics (disease specific target proteins), genomics (disease specific genetic data), metabolomics (disease specific metabolic pathways/profile) and phenotypic data (off-target mechanism, pharmacological targets, disease pathways, pathological conditions, adverse and side effects etc.) concerning the disease process. It, therefore, requires construction of specific disease networks, recognizing genetic expression, considering key targets, identifying disease causing protein molecules related to cell and metabolic pathways of interest in the disease model [23].

Figure 4 delineates the methodologies and steps involved in drug repositioning.

Drug-based phenotypic screening and target-based methods account for more than 50% of the FDA approved small drug molecules and biologics. Phenotypic drug screening methods identify drug candidates from small molecule libraries

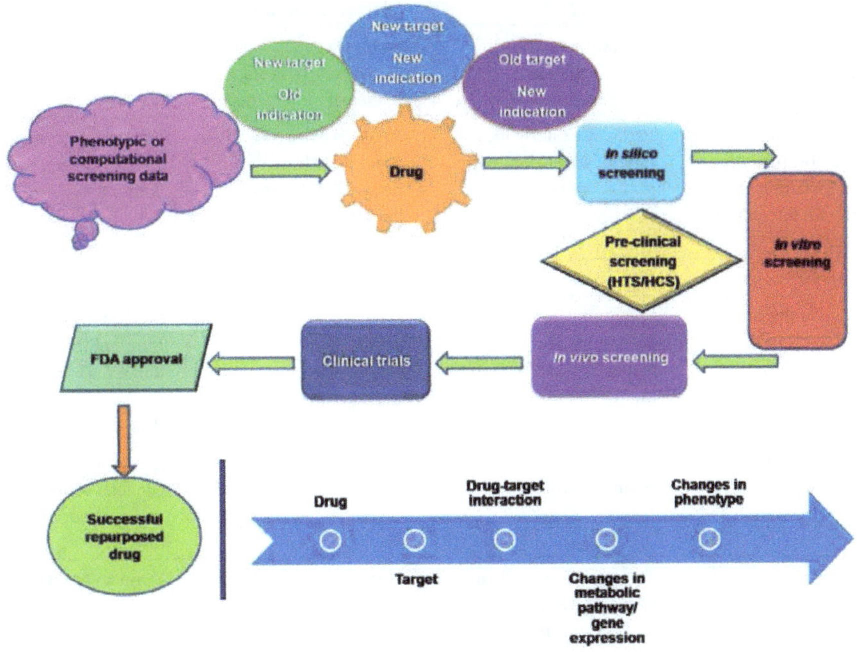

Figure 4.
Methodologies and steps involved in drug repositioning.

by serendipitous observations. Target-based methods discover drugs based upon known target molecules. The treatment/therapy-based repositioning methodology is similar to disease-based methodology [23].

A detailed enumeration of various methodologies employed in drug repositioning along with suitable examples is given in **Table 2**.

Methodology	Type of method, category	Method/specific approach	Example(s)
Drug-oriented			
Phenotypic screening	Blinded/ Target-based, Screening	*In vitro* and *in vivo* HTS/HCS screening	Sildenafil (erectile dysfunction), rituximab (breast cancer)
Target 3D structure, chemical structure, information of drugs and ligands	Target-based, Cheminformatics	*In silico* screening, ligand-based screening and molecular docking, fragment-based screening	Fluorouracil (lung cancer), etoposide (bladder cancer)
Drug-target information, chemical structure, information of targets and drugs	Knowledge-based, Bioinformatics/ Chem-informatics	Drug–target prediction	Simvastatin, ketoconazole (breast cancer)
Clinical trial information and adverse effects	Knowledge-based, Bioinformatics	Drug similarity studies	—
FDA approval labels	Knowledge-based, Bioinformatics	Drug similarity studies	—
Disease-oriented			
Available Pathway information	Knowledge-based, Bioinformatics	Discovery of disease mechanism and address of key targets	Vismodegib (skin cancer)
Disease omics/ genetics data	Signature-based Bioinformatics	Studying gene signatures/ genomics to identify key targets	—
Disease omics data, available pathway information, and protein interaction network	Pathway or network-based, Network biology	Analysis of disease-specific pathways and networks to identify key targets	Sunitinib, dasatinib (breast cancer, brain tumor)
Therapy-oriented			
Drug omics data	Signature- based or Signature- and network-based, Bioinformatics and/or Network biology	Studying gene signatures	Sirolimus (acute lymphoblastic leukemia), Fasudil (neurodegenerative disorders)
Disease omics and drug omics data	Signature based, Bioinformatics	Similarities between drugs and diseases	Cimetidine (lung cancer), topiramate (inflammatory bowel disease)
Drug omics data, disease pathway and protein interaction network	Targeted- mechanism based, Network biology and Systems biology	Elucidating targeted pathways	Daunorubicin, clomifene (breast cancer)

Table 2.
Some available methods of drug repositioning [23, 24].

Several available repositioning methods depicted above in **Table 2** are described briefly as follows:

Blinded search or screening methods involve serendipitous identification from biological tests/experimental screens aimed at specific disease models and drugs. The advantage of these methods is that they possess higher flexibility for screening a large number of drugs or diseases.

Target-based methods carry out *in vitro* and *in vivo* high-throughput and/or high-content screening (HTS/HCS) of drug molecules for a protein target or a biomarker of interest and *in silico* screening of compounds or drugs from large compound libraries, such as ligand-based screening or molecular docking. In these methods, there is a higher possibility of finding useful drugs/drug leads as compared to blinded search methods. It also requires less time for the entire screening process to complete.

Knowledge-based methods utilize bioinformatics or cheminformatics approaches to gather the available information of drug profile, chemical structures of targets and drugs, drug-target networks, clinical trial information including adverse effects, signaling or metabolic pathways. This information content of knowledge-based methods is rich enough as compared to blinded or target-based methods. The known information can be used to predict therefore, be used to predict the unknown new mechanisms, such as unknown targets for drugs, unknown drug–drug similarities, new biomarkers for diseases etc.

Signature-based methods use gene signatures derived from disease omics data (genomics data) with or without treatments to discover unknown off-targets or unknown disease mechanisms. Genomics data are publicly available as databases. The advantage of these methods is that they are useful to explore unknown mechanisms of action of drugs. In comparison to knowledge-based methods, signature-based methods investigate drug mechanisms at more molecular-level, such as changes in expression of genes by using computational approaches.

Pathway- or network-based methods make use of disease omics data, available signaling or metabolic pathways, and protein interaction networks to reconstruct disease-specific path- ways that provide the key targets for repositioned drugs. The advantage of these methods is that they can narrow down general signaling networks from a large number of proteins to a specific network with a few proteins (or target molecules).

Targeted mechanism-based methods integrate treatment omics data, available signaling pathway information and protein interaction networks to describe the unknown mechanisms of action of drugs. The advantage of these methods is that they are not only used to discover the mechanisms related to diseases or drugs, but also to identify those directly related to treatments of drugs to specific diseases [23–25].

6. Repositioned drugs

Drug repositioning is an alternative approach to traditional drug discovery. With increasing market demand many pharmaceutical companies are developing new drugs or new therapeutic uses from existing/old/available drugs by drug repositioning approaches in less time, yet at low cost. In drug discovery program, the repositioning is usually essentially carried out in two stages as described follows. In the first stage, the *in silico* screening of approved drugs against a particular disease target is carried out, which is followed by the second step, in which the selected identified molecules are further experimentally investigated both *in vitro* and *in vivo* in specific disease models of interest. After successful preclinical studies in the second stage of repositioning, identified drug candidates enter the clinical trials in human subjects [24, 25]. **Figure 5** delineates several potential strategies (with suitable examples) of drug repositioning.

Table 3 depicts examples of some repositioned drugs already developed or currently under development from various approved (FDA) or marketed drugs and investigational new drugs (IND). Some repositioned drugs currently under clinical trials in COVID-19 are also included in the list.

Colchicine, a well-known anti-inflammatory drug used in the treatment of gout and pericarditis, is currently under clinical trial for treating COVID-19 patients. This drug has been proved to be effective in preventing massive cytokine storm induced pneumonia caused by SARS-CoV-2 (severe acute respiratory syndrome coronavirus-2). The antiviral effect of an older antimalarial drug, chloroquine (used as phosphate salt) against SARS-CoV-2 infection has also been investigated worldwide. Studies suggest that chloroquine may be beneficial in preventing coronavirus induced pneumonia in COVID-19. As per recent reports from NIH (National Institutes of Health, US), the clinical trial of a combination of hydroxychloroquine/azithromycin for the treatment of COVID-19 patients has already been started. In this combination, both the drugs are FDA approved, where hydroxychloroquine is an antimalarial drug and azithromycin is an antibacterial antibiotic. An anti-viral drug, favipiravir intended for the treatment of influenza is currently under phase-2/phase-3 clinical trials on COVID-19 patients around the world (China, Japan, US, India). Glenmark has initiated phase-3 trial on favipiravir for the treatment of COVID-19 patients in India. An investigational anti-retroviral drug called remdesivir (originally developed by Gilead Sciences Inc. for the treatment of Ebola, but failed in clinical trial) is also under clinical trial for treating COVOD-19 patients in several countries like China, US, UK and India. In India, clinical trials on favipiravir, remdesivir and colchicine are currently underway by CSIR (Council of Scientific & Industrial Research) laboratories. A fixed dose drug combination called lopinavir/ritonavir earlier approved

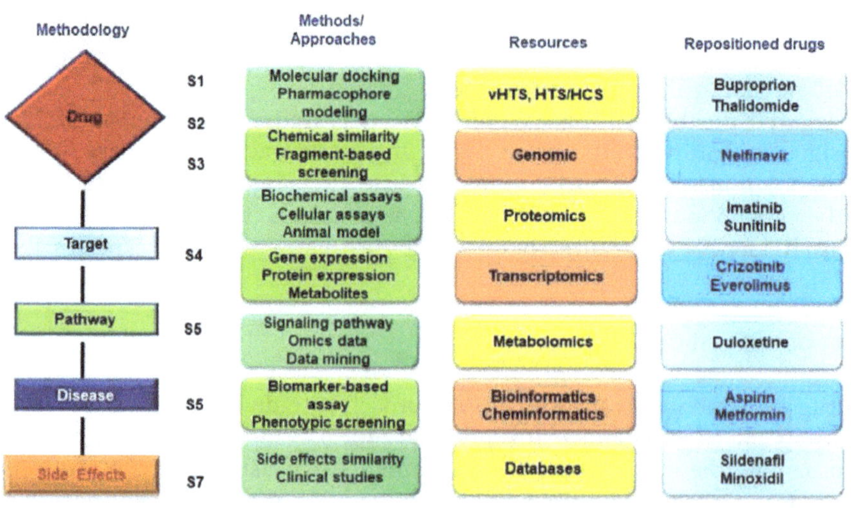

Figure 5.
Strategies of drug repositioning with examples. vHTS: virtual high-throughput screening; HTS/HCS: high-throughput and/or high-content screening; Strategy 1 (S1): serendipitous observation; Strategy 2 (S2): observance of novel activity (specific disease phenotype, rational approach); Strategy 3 (S3): new drug-target interaction; Strategy 4 (S4): new roles for existing protein target; Strategy 5 (S5): new biochemical pathways; Strategy 6 (S6): disease-specific repositioning; Strategy 7 (S7): unexpected side effects.

to treat HIV/AIDS under the brand name *Kaletra* is currently being studied to treat COVID-19 patients in several countries. This drug combination was investigated along with the flu drug, oseltamivir (Tamiflu) to cure infection caused by SARS-CoV-2 in Thailand. The clinical trial of an anti-parasitic drug called ivermectin (used traditionally as an approved treatment in worm infestations) for the treatment of COVID-19 is being undertaken in several parts of the world after a successful *in vitro* effectiveness against SARS-CoV-2 infection at Monash University in Melbourne, Australia. The clinical trial of toclizumab, an IL-6 receptor antagonist (marketed under the brand name *Actemra*) used for the treatment of inflammatory illness such as rheumatoid arthritis is also being conducted for the treatment of patients with COVID-19 [25, 26].

Drug, pharmacological category	Original indication	New indication	Status of development
Amphotericin B (AMB), Anti-fungal antibiotic	Fungal infections	Leishmaniasis	Already developed*
Aspirin, NSAID	Pain and inflammation	CVDs (Anti-platelet)	Already developed*
		Prostate cancer	Under development*
Amantadine, Anti-viral	Influenza	PD	Already developed*
Astemizole, Anti-histaminic	Allergic illness such as urticaria	Malaria	Under development*
Atomoxetine, Anti-depressant	Depression	Attention deficit, Hyperactivity disorder	Already developed*
Avermectin, Anthelmintic	River blindness, Elephantiasis	Tuberculosis	Under development*
Azithromycin, Anti-bacterial antibiotic	Bacterial infections	COVID-19	Under development*
Bromocriptine, Dopamine receptor antagonist	PD	DM (type 2)	Under development*
Bupropion, SSRI, Anti-depressant	Depression	Smoking cessation	Already developed*
Celecoxib, COX-2 inhibitor, NSAID	Inflammation	Breast and colon cancer	Under development*
Chloroquine, Anti-malarial	Malaria	COVID-19	Under development*
Cimetidine, H2 receptor antagonist	Gastric ulcer	Breast, lung and prostate cancer	Under development*
Crizotinib, ALK inhibitor	Lymphoma (under clinical trial for ALCL)	NSCLC	Already developed#
Colchicine, Anti-inflammatory agent	Gout (Gouty arthritis)	Pericarditis	Already developed*
		COVID-19	Under development*
Daunorubicin, Antibiotic		Breast cancer	Already developed*
Digoxin, Cardiotonic	CVDs such as heart failure	Prostate Cancer	Under development*
Dimethyl fumarate, Anti-allergic	Psoriasis	Multiple sclerosis (MS)	Already developed*
Disulfiram, Acetaldehyde dehydrogenase inhibitor	Chronic alcoholism	Cancer	Under development*

Drug, pharmacological category	Original indication	New indication	Status of development
Duloxetine, SSNRI	Depression	Generalized anxiety disorder, fibromyalgia, chronic musculoskeletal pain, neuropathic pain	Already developed*
Everolimus, Immune suppressant	Immune suppressant	Pancreatic neuroendocrine tumors	Already developed*
Favipiravir, Anti-viral	Influenza	COVID-19	Under development*
Fluorouracil, Antimetabolite, Anti-cancer	Cancer	Breast cancer	Already developed*
Fluoxetine, Anti-depressant	Depression	Premenstrual dysphoria	Already developed*
Gabapentin, Anti-epileptic	Epilepsy	Neuropathic pain	Already developed*
Galantamine, AChE inhibitor	Neuromuscular paralysis	AD	Already developed*
Hydroxychloroquine, Anti-malarial	Malaria, RA	COVID-19	Under development*
Ibudilast, PDE inhibitor (Anti-asthmatic)	Asthma	Neuropathic pain	Already developed*
Imatinib, TKI (Anti-cancer)	CML, ALL	GIST	Already developed*
Isoniazid, Anti-tubercular	Tuberculosis	Certain types of tumor	Already developed*
Itraconazole, Anti-fungal	Fungal infections	Cancer like NSCLC (Anti-angiogenic)	Under development*
Ivermectin, Anthelmintic (Anti-parasitic)	Scabies, river blindness, helminthiasis	COVID-19	Under development*
Lopinavir/Ritonavir, Anti-viral	HIV/AIDS	COVID-19	Under development*
Metformin, Anti-diabetic	DM (type 2)	Breast and colon Cancer, CVDs	Under development*
Methotrexate, Anti-metabolite (Anti-cancer)	Cancer	Psoriasis, RA	Already developed*
Milnacipram, Anti-depressant	Depression	Fibromyalgia	Already developed*
Miltefosine, Anti-leishmanial	Cancer	Leishmaniasis, Amoeba infection	Already developed*
Mifepristone, Antiprogestin	Termination of pregnancy in combination with misoprostol	Cushing's syndrome	Already developed*
Minoxidil, Vasodilator (Anti-hypertensive)	Hypertension	Androgenic alopecia	Already developed*
Nelfinavir, Anti-viral	HIV/AIDS	Breast cancer, NSCLC (under clinical trials)	Under development*
Nitroxoline, Anti-bacterial	UTI	Breast, bladder and pancreatic cancers	Under development*

Drug, pharmacological category	Original indication	New indication	Status of development
Orlistat, Anti-obesity agent	Obesity	Cancer	Already developed*
Penfluridol/Pimozide, Anti-psychotics	Psychiatric illness	Breast cancer	Under development*
Propranolol, β-Blocker	Hypertension	Migraine	Already developed*
Remdesivir, Anti-viral	Influenza, Ebola (failed in clinical trial)	COVID-19	Under development#
Retinoic acid	Acne	Acute leukemia	Already developed*
Ribavirin, Anti-viral	Viral infection such as RSV, hepatitis C infections	Cancers like leukemias and lymphomas	Under development*
Ritoximab			
Ropinirole, Anti-Parkinsonian drug	PD	Restless leg syndrome	Already developed*
Sildenafil, PDE inhibitor	Angina pectoris, Pulmonary arterial hypertension	Erectile dysfunction	Already developed*
Simvastatin, Hypolipidemic	CVDs	Lung cancer	Already developed*
Sunitinib, TKI (Anti-cancer)	Imatinib-resistant GIST, RCC	Pancreatic neuroendocrine tumors	Already developed*
Tamoxifen, Anti-estrogen (Anti-cancer)	Breast cancer, Anticancer	Systemic lupus erythematosus	Already developed*
		NTDs like Leishmaniasis (in combination with miltefosine)	Under development*
Thalidomide, Immune modulator	Immunomodulation, Morning sickness (withdrawn)	Multiple myeloma, Leprosy	Already developed#
Tocilizumab, IL-6 inhibitor (Immune modulator)	RA	COVID-19	Under development*
Topiramate	Fungal infections	IBD	Already developed*
Valproic acid, Anti-epileptic	Epilepsy	Manic depression (bipolar disorder), migraine headache	Already developed*
Valsartan, ARB (Anti-hypertensive)	Hypertension, Heart attack	AD	Already developed*
Zidovudine, Anti-viral	Cancer (failed clinical trial)	HIV/AIDS	Already developed#

**Indicates successful repositioning from FDA approved drug.*
#Indicates successful repositioning from investigational new drug (IND).
AD: Alzheimer's disease; AChE: acetylcholine esterase inhibitor; ALCL: anaplastic large cell lymphoma; ALL: acute lymphocytic leukemia; ALK: anaplastic lymphoma kinase; ARB: angiotensin-receptor blocker; CML: chronic myeloid leukemia; COVID-19: coronavirus diseases-19; COX: cyclooxygenase; CVDs: cardiovascular diseases; DM: diabetes mellitus; GIST: gastrointestinal stromal tumor; HIV/AIDS: human immunodeficiency virus/acquired immunodeficiency syndrome; IBD: inflammatory bowel disease; IL: interleukin; NSAID: non-steroidal anti-inflammatory drug; NSCLC: non-small cell lung carcinoma; NTD: neglected tropical diseases; PD: Parkinson's diseases; PDE: phosphodiesterase; RA: rheumatoid arthritis; RCC: renal cell carcinoma; RSV: respiratory syncytial virus; SSNRI: selective serotonin and norepinephrine reuptake inhibitor; SSRI: selective serotonin reuptake inhibitor; TKI: tyrosine kinase inhibitor; UTI: urinary tract infections.

Table 3.
Examples of some repositioned drugs from approved and investigational drugs [24–29].

7. Opportunities and challenges

On contrary to traditional drug discovery program (a complex and time consuming process with high cost of development and risk of failure), drug repositioning, reduces the time and cost of drug development. Drug repositioning is also a low-risk strategy. Computational or machine learning approach has significantly improved the performance of drug repositioning. In comparison to computational approaches, using experimental approaches (such as target protein-based screening, cell-based assay, testing in animal model, and clinical testing) that provide direct evidence-based understanding of links between drugs and diseases are more reliable and credible. However, in recent years computational approaches are usually combined with the experimental approaches to identify new indications for old drugs, called mixed approaches. In this approach, computational methods are validated by biological experiments and clinical tests. Mixed approach of repositioning offers a rational and exhaustive exploration of all possible repositioning opportunities, taking into consideration improved access to available databases and technological advances. Furthermore, the R&D investment required for drug repositioning is lower than that for traditional drug discovery. Thus, drug repositioning offers an opportunity for many pharmaceutical companies to develop drugs with lower investments [27, 28]. Mixed approach of DR offers opportunities for developing repositioned drugs more effectively and rapidly. From the market perspective, a large number of diseases require new drugs to be treated with a potential market demand and economic impacts. For example, the discovery of drugs for rare/neglected diseases has a large potential market to explore. There is, therefore, an opportunity for repurposing of drugs for the treatment of rare, neglected, orphan diseases or difficult to treat diseases. There are over 6000 rare diseases that lack proper treatment. About 5% of them are being researched. Rare diseases have a large potential market to explore. Given the high attrition rates, substantial costs and slow pace of drug discovery and development, repurposing of old drugs to treat both common and rare diseases is increasingly becoming an attractive area of research because it involves the use of drug molecules with reduced risk of failure at shorter time and lower cost development [30–33].

With the advent of technologies such as genomics, proteomics, transcriptomics, metabolomics, etc., and availability of huge databases resources including drug omics data, disease omics data, etc., there are a plenty of opportunities to discover drugs by drug repositioning in a collective and integrated effort of all the above methods/approaches mentioned above. Researchers are currently equipped with the latest reliable tools and data to explore the novel unknown mechanism of actions/pathways based upon disease-specific target proteins/genes and/or specific bio-markers associated with the progression of the disease [34, 35].

Various databases and software are available publicly for genomics, proteomics, metabolomics and pathway analysis. Several computational strategies are already developed to increase the speed and ease of the repurposing process. Some important databases used in drug repositioning studies are outlined in **Table 4**.

However, opportunities come often with many challenges in drug repositioning. The identification of a new therapeutic indication for an existing drug poses a major challenge in repositioning. However, drug repositioning is a complex process involving multiple factors such as technology, commercial models, patents, and investment and market demands. Some multiple challenges which include choosing the right therapeutic area for the drug under investigation, issues related to clinical trials such as need to run new trials from start if the data from clinical or preclinical trials for the original drug or drug product are outdated or are not satisfactory [34, 35].

Information available about	Database	Website
Chemical structure	PubChem	http://pubchem.ncbi.nlm.nih.gov
	Drugbank	http://www.drugbank.ca/
	Chemspider	http://www.chemspider.com
	ChemDB	http://www.chemdb.com
	Therapeutic Target Database (TTD)	http://bidd.nus.edu.sg/group/cjttd/
Target 3D structure	RCSB Protein Data Bank (PDB)	http://www.rcsb.org
	OCA	http://oca.weizmann.ac.il/oca-bin/ocamain
	Proteopedia	http://proteopedia.org
Drug-target information	Drugbank	http://www.drugbank.ca/
	Therapeutic Target Database (TTD)	http://bidd.nus.edu.sg/group/cjttd/
	Pharmacogenetics Knowledge Base (PharmGKB)	http://www.pharmgkb.org/
	DrugMap Central (DMC)	http://r2d2drug.org/index.html
Protein interaction information	Human Protein Reference Database (HPRD)	http://www.hprd.org/
	Biological General Repository for Interaction	http://thebiogrid.org/
	Database of Interacting Proteins (DIP)	http://dip.doe-mbi.ucla.edu/dip/Main.cgi
	STRING	http://string-db.org/
Pathway information	NCI Pathway Interaction Database (NCI-PID)	http://pid.nci.nih.gov/
	Kyoto Encyclopedia of Genes and Genomes (KEGG)	http://www.genome.jp/kegg/
	PathwayCommons	http://www.pathwaycommons.org/about/
Clinical trial information and adverse effects	Clinicaltrial.gov	http://clinicaltrials.gov
	Adverse Reaction Database (Canada)	http://www.fda.gov/Drugs/
	SIDER	http://sideeffects.embl.de/
FDA label information	FDALABEL (US FDA)	http://www.fda.gov/ScienceResearch/
	DailyMed (US FDA)	http://dailymed.nlm.nih.gov/dailymed/about.cfm
	Structured Product Labeling (SPL)	http://www.fda.gov/ForIndustry/DataStandards/
Omics data (Target/Drug)	NCBI-GEO	http://www.ncbi.nlm.nih.gov/geo/
	Sequence Read Archive (SRA)	http://www.ncbi.nlm.nih.gov/Traces/sra/
	ArrayExpress	http://www.ebi.ac.uk/arrayexpress/
	Cancer Cell Line Encyclopedia (CCLE)	http://www.broadinstitute.org/ccle/home
	Sequence Read Archive (SRA)	http://www.ncbi.nlm.nih.gov/Traces/sra/

Table 4.
Databases used in repositioning studies [34–36].

8. Regulatory and intellectual property issues

Traditional drug development strategies are costly, failure prone and expensive ventures. Therefore, drug repositioning has recently drawn considerable attention to discover drugs with new therapeutic uses with the goal to bring drugs out at comparatively faster rate for clinical use. Some regulatory issues that are commonly encountered in drug repositioning are described as follows [37, 38]. As per regulatory guidelines, new preclinical and/or clinical trials may be required to be carried out if the available data are not satisfactory and do not comply with the requirements of regulatory agencies such as FDA or EMA. Another important issue is related to patent application and intellectual property rights (IPR). There are no provisions of IP protection of drug discovery by repositioning approach as per the IP and patent laws. For repositioned drugs, IP protection is limited. For repositioning drugs, IP protection is limited. For example, some novel drug-target disease associations found by repositioning researchers were confirmed by publications or online databases; however, it is difficult to seek IP protection for such associations because of the law. The IP issue prevents some repositioned drugs from entering even into the market [39, 40]. Moreover, some repositioning projects are forced to be abandoned, which is a waste of time, money and lot of efforts. Although many omics data and medical databases have been established, selecting the appropriate approach for repositioning is still a challenge due to the regulatory issues because massive amounts of data may not be valid if not obtained from reliable sources. It is, therefore, necessary that researchers or manufacturers must strictly adhere with standard regulatory guidelines for drug discovery by repositioning approaches [2, 41–43].

9. Conclusion

Traditionally, the dug repurposing has a long recorded history discovery of drug molecules particularly through serendipitous observations. In recent years, it has embarked a new avenue in the development of new therapies based upon existing/approved medicines. The strategic drug repositioning in a more systematic and rational way has brought innovation with the discovery of drug molecules with unknown therapeutic indications. As drug repositioning approach offers significant reduction in R&D costs, greater chances of success, shorter research time and lower investment risk, it has gained increasing market demands. Because these advantages are beneficial for discovery scientists, drug researchers, consumers and pharmaceutical companies, enabling the application of novel approaches of repositioning strategy in the drug discovery program for almost all human diseases. Moreover, the use of *in silico* techniques along with the application of structure-based drug design (SBDD) and pharmacophore modeling strategies and artificial intelligence (AI) technology can further accelerate the process of drug purposing in the drug discov-ery program. In the era of precision medicine, the drug repositioning strategy has become very much useful to establish the unknown mechanism of action of drugs through exploration of novel disease/metabolic/signaling pathways, or off-targets and target-specific mechanisms/genetic expression profile for even genetic disor-ders. Advancement in genomics have provided us with genomic and transcriptomic data in huge quantities using technologies like next generation sequencing, microarray data and transcriptomics, etc. Network biology and systems biology approaches may add additional benefits to unveil such novel mechanisms of actions with through insights into drug-target interaction profile at molecular/genetic level. For better drug repositioning, more in-depth understanding are required to be executed with integrated approaches between computational and experimental methods to ensure high success rates of repositioned drugs. However, drug repurposing can be successfully utilized in the discovery and development of new drugs with novel and effective therapeutic indications for human diseases.

Author details

Mithun Rudrapal*, Shubham J. Khairnar and Anil G. Jadhav Sandip Institute of Pharmaceutical Sciences, Sandip Foundation, Mahiravani, Nashik, India

*Address all correspondence to: rsmrpal@gmail.com

References

[1] Ashburn TT, Thor KB. Drug repositioning: Identifying and developing new uses for existing drugs. Nature Reviews. Drug Discovery. 2014;**3**:673-683

[2] Dey G. An overview of drug repurposing: Review article. Journal of Medical Science and Clinical Research. 2019;7(2):3-5

[3] Deotarse PP, Jain AS, Baile MB, Kolhe NS, Kulkarni AA. Drug repositioning: A review. International Journal of Pharmaceutical Sciences Review and Research. 2015;**4**(8):51-58

[4] Chong CR, Sullivan DJ Jr. New uses for old drugs. Nature. 2007;**448**(7154):645-646

[5] Xue H, Li J, Xie H, Wang Y. Review of drug repositioning approaches and resources. International Journal of Biological Sciences. 2018;**14**(10):1232-1244

[6] Cha Y, Erez T, Reynolds IJ, Kumar D, Ross J, Koytiger G, et al. Drug repurposing from the perspective of pharmaceutical companies. British Journal of Pharmacology. 2018;**175**(2):168-180

[7] Aggarwal S, Verma SS, Aggarwal S, Gupta SC. Drug repurposing for breast cancer therapy: Old weapon for new battle. Seminars in Cancer Biology. 2020. DOI: 10.1016/j.semcancer.2019.09.012

[8] Hughes JP, Rees S, Kalindjian SB, Philpott KL. Principles of early drug discovery. British Journal of Pharmacology. 2011;**162**(6):1239-1249

[9] Rudrapal M, Chetia D. Endoperoxide antimalarials: Development, structural diversity and pharmacodynamic aspects with reference to 1,2,4-trioxane-based structural scaffold. Drug Design, Development and Therapy. 2016;**10**:3575-3590

[10] Kalita J, Chetia D, Rudrapal M. Design, synthesis, antimalarial activity and docking study of 7-chloro-4-(2-(substituted benzylidene)hydrazineyl) quinolines. Medicinal Chemistry. 2020. DOI: 10.2174/15734064156661908061 54722

[11] Agrawal P. Artificial intelligence in drug discovery and development. Journal of Pharmacovigilance. 2018;**6**:2

[12] Ferreira LG, Andricopulo AD. Drug repositioning approaches to parasitic diseases: A medicinal chemistry perspective. Drug Discovery Today. 2016;**21**(10):1699-1710

[13] Allarakhia M. Open-source approaches for the repurposing of existing or failed candidate drugs: Learning from and applying the lessons across diseases. Drug Design, Development and Therapy. 2013;7:753-766

[14] Jin G, Wong STC. Towards better drug repositioning: Prioritizing and integrating existing methods into efficient pipelines. Drug Discovery Today. 2014;**19**(5):637-644

[15] Oprea TI, Overington JP. Computational and practical aspects of drug repositioning. Assay and Drug Development Technologies. 2015;**13**:299-306

[16] Lionta E, Spyrou G, Vassilatis DK, Cournia Z. Structure-based virtual screening for drug discovery: Principles, applications and recent advances. Current Topics in Medicinal Chemistry. 2014;**14**:1923-1938

[17] Talevi A. Drug repositioning: Current approaches and their implications in the precision medicine

era. Expert Review of Precision Medicine and Drug Development. 2018;**3**(1):49-61

[18] Kim TW. Drug repositioning approaches for the discovery of new therapeutics for Alzheimer's disease. Expert Review of Neurotherapeutics. 2015;**12**:132-142

[19] Rosa SGV, Santos WC. Clinical trials on drug repositioning for COVID-19 treatment. Revista Panamericana de Salud Pública. 2020;**44**:e40

[20] Turanli B, Grøtli M, Boren J, Nielsen J, Uhlen M, Arga KY, et al. Drug repositioning for effective prostate cancer treatment. Frontiers in Physiology. 2018;**9**:500

[21] Koch U, Hamacher M, Nussbaumer P. Cheminformatics at the interface of medicinal chemistry and proteomics. Biochimica et Biophysica Acta. 1844;**2014**:156-161

[22] Napolitano F, Zhao Y, Moreira VM, et al. Drug repositioning: A machine-learning approach through data integration. Journal of Cheminformatics. 2013;**5**(1):30

[23] Chong CR, Chen X, Shi L, Liu JO, Sullivan DJ Jr. A clinical drug library screen identifies astemizole as an antimalarial agent. Nature Chemical Biology. 2006;**2**:415-416

[24] Appleby BS, Cummings JL. Discovering new treatments for Alzheimer's disease by repurposing approved medications. Current Topics in Medicinal Chemistry. 2013;**13**:2306-2327

[25] Shah B, Modi P, Sagar SR. *In silico* studies on therapeutic agents for COVID-19: Drug repurposing approach. Life Sciences. 2020;**20**:117652

[26] Serafin MB, Bottega A, Foletto VS, da Rosa TF, Horner A, Horner R. Drug repositioning is an alternative for the treatment of coronavirus COVID-19. International Journal of Antimicrobial Agents. 2020. DOI: 10.1016/j.ijantimicag.2020.105969

[27] Shivaprasad C, Kalra S. Bromocriptine in type 2 diabetes mellitus. Indian Journal of Endocrinology and Metabolism. 2011;**15**(1):S17–S24

[28] Matthews H, Usman-Idris M, Khan F, Read M, Nirmalan N. Drug repositioning as a route to anti-malarial drug discovery: Preliminary investigation of the *in vitro* anti-malarial efficacy of emetine dihydrochloride hydrate. Malaria Journal. 2013;**12**(359):1-11

[29] Shim JS, Liu JO. Recent advances in drug repositioning for the discovery of new anticancer drugs. International Journal of Biological Sciences. 2014;**10**(7):654-663

[30] Talevi A, Bellera CL. Challenges and opportunities with drug repurposing: Finding strategies to find alternative uses of therapeutics. Expert Opinion on Drug Discovery. 2020;**15**(4):397-401

[31] Pushpakom S, Iorio F, Eyers PA, Escott KJ, Hopper S, Wells A, et al. Drug repurposing: Progress, challenges and recommendations. Nature Reviews. Drug Discovery. 2019;**18**(1):41-58

[32] de Oliveira EAM, Lang KL. Drug repositioning: Concept, classification, methodology, and importance in rare/orphans and neglected diseases. Journal of Applied Pharmaceutical Science. 2018;**8**(8):157-165

[33] Ekins S, Williams AJ, Krasowski MD, Freundlich JS. In silico repositioning of approved drugs for rare and neglected diseases. Drug Discovery Today. 2011;**16**(7-8):298-310

[34] Naylor S, Kauppi DM, Schonfeld JM. Therapeutic drug

repurposing, repositioning and rescue. Part II: Business review. Drug Discovery World. 2015;**16**:57-72

[35] Naylor S, Schonfeld JM. Therapeutic drug repurposing, repositioning and rescue: Part I—Overview. Drug Discovery World. 2014;**16**:49-62

[36] Jin G, Wong STC. Toward better drug repositioning: Prioritizing and integrating existing methods into efficient pipelines. Drug Discovery Today. 2014;**19**:637-644

[37] Naylor S, Kauppi DM, Schonfeld JM. Therapeutic drug repurposing, repositioning and rescue. Part III: Market exclusivity using intellectual property and regulatory pathways. Drug Discovery World. 2015;**16**:62-69

[38] Jourdan JP, Bureau R, Rochais C, Dallemagne P. Drug repositioning: A brief overview. The Journal of Pharmacy and Pharmacology. 2020. DOI: 10.1111/jphp.13273

[39] Li YY, Jones SJ, Smith M. The importance of drug repositioning in the era of genomic medicine drug repositioning for personalized medicine. Review. Genome Medicine. 2012;**4**:27

[40] Hernandez JJ, Pryszlak M, Smith L, et al. Giving drugs a second chance: Overcoming regulatory and financial hurdles in repurposing approved drugs as cancer therapeutics. Frontiers in Oncology. 2017;7:1-8

[41] Boguski MS, Mandl KD, Sukhatme VP. Repurposing with a difference. Science. 2019;**324**:1394-1395

[42] Simsek M, Meijer B, van Bodegraven AA, et al. Finding hidden treasures in old drugs: The challenges and importance of licensing generics. Drug Discovery Today. 2018;**23**:17-21

[43] GNS HS, GR S, Murahari M, Krishnamurthy M. An update on drug repurposing: Re-written saga of the drug's fate. Biomedicine & Pharmacotherapy. 2019;**110**:700-716

4

Repurposing Fumaric Acid Esters to Treat Conditions of Oxidative Stress and Inflammation: A Promising Emerging Approach with Broad Potential

Ravirajsinh N. Jadeja, Folami L. Powell and Pamela M. Martin

Abstract

The medicinal benefit of salts of fumaric acid and its esters (FAE), known as fumarates (mono and dimethyl fumarate), was realized many years ago. Early on, FAE were derived from plants and mushrooms (e.g., *Fumaria officinalis, Boletus fomentarius var. pseudo-igniarius*). The FAE containing formulation Fumaderm® was licensed in Germany for the treatment of psoriasis in 1994. Recently, a clinical formulation of dimethyl fumarate known as BG12 (Tecfidera) was approved for use in the United States, New Zealand, Australia, European Union, Switzerland, and Canada for the treatment of multiple sclerosis. Others and we have assessed the potential benefit of FAE in a number of disease condi-tions that are diverse with respect to etiology but unified with regard to the involvement of inflammation and oxidative stress. Hence, a FAE-based drug with robust anti-oxidative and anti-inflammatory effects that is already US-FDA approved is a perfect contender for repurposing and rapid clinical implementation for their management. There is a burgeoning literature on the use of FAE in the prevention and treatment of diseases, other than psoriasis and MS, in which oxidative stress and/or inflammation are prominent. This chapter highlights critical information gleaned from these studies, exposes lacunae of potential importance, and provides related perspectives.

Keywords: fumaric acid esters, oxidative stress, Nrf2, antioxidant

1. Introduction

The salts of fumaric acid (known as fumarates) occur naturally in some plants (*Fumaria officinalis*) and mushrooms. Traditionally, aerial parts of *Fumaria officinalis* (common fumitory, drug fumitory or earth smoke) have been utilized for the treatment of various skin diseases [1]. Because of its utilization as an herbal remedy for skin ailments, German chemist W. Schweckendiek, who was suffering from psoriasis, developed an interest in and isolated fumaric acid esters (FAE) from the plant extract. Excited about the positive effects of the FAE mixture on his own psoriatic lesions, he began offering it also to other psoriasis patients. Schweckendiek later published his findings on the beneficial effects of FAE in psoriasis [2], effects that he believed to be attributed to the improvements of this fumarate therapy on dysregulation of the citric acid cycle, the potential underlying cause of psoriasis. Nonetheless, with advancements in the understanding of psoriasis, his hypothesis was found to be incorrect. However, his preliminary observations laid the foundation for the successful development of a drug to treat psoriasis and interestingly, multiple sclerosis.

In 1994, some three decades following Schweckendiek's initial report, a fumaric acid mixture composed in large (60%) of dimethyl fumarate (DMF) and ethyl hydrogen fumarates was authorized for the treatment of psoriasis in Germany under the brand name Fumaderm® [3]. In the clinical setting, Fumaderm® proved effective against moderate to severe forms of psoriasis. To date, it remains to be the most widely used oral compound for psoriasis therapy in Germany. However, Fumaderm® was not licensed and currently remains unlicensed for use in the UK and US [4]. Despite this, results establishing DMF to be the major active principle in the Fumaderm® led to numerous clinical and experimental studies worldwide on the immunomodulatory potential of Fumaderm® and DMF in other immune-mediated diseases [5, 6]. The extremely positive results that emanated from these studies led to DMF being tested clinically for the treatment of relapsing-remitting multiple sclerosis (RRMS). Like the original discovery of FAEs, the exploratory clinical trial of FAE for MS was performed in Germany [7]. In this trial, Fumaderm® was given to 10 patients with highly active RRMS; six patients completed the 70-week trial. Magnetic resonance imaging (MRI)-based results showed that Fumaderm® significantly reduced the number of gadolinium-enhanced lesions as well as lesion volumes without further worsening of any clinical parameters [7]. Although the overall safety profile of Fumaderm® was found to be favorable in this study, the associated unwanted gastrointestinal discomforts were a major concern. Although this initial study was a small, single-center, MRI-based and open-label clinical trial, it set the stage for a number of subsequent MS trials with DMF.

After Fumaderm® was licensed to be used in Germany, efforts to develop an improved formulation with better tolerability began. This culminated ultimately in the introduction of BG12 (brand name Tecfidera) a modified FAE formulation [8–10]. Indeed BG-12, comprised only of DMF made available in enteric-coated micro tablets, showed better gastrointestinal tolerability compared to Fumaderm® and following several clinical trials, this gastro-resistant, delayed-release formulation of DMF was ultimately approved for use in the United States, New Zealand and Australia for the treatment of relapsing forms and relapsing MS, respectively, and in the European Union, Switzerland and Canada for the treatment of RRMS [11]. A plethora of additional information exists on the use of DMF in the treatment of MS and psoriasis. For further reading on DMF and MS, please refer to the following referenced excellent reviews [12–17].

Drug repurposing is a highly appreciated strategy in the pharmaceutical industry [18]. The fact that agents have been previously tested prior testing of in humans and therefore a wealth of detailed information is already available regarding pharmacology, formulation and safety profile is a huge advantage! Such new candidate therapies can often be fast-tracked for clinical trials and related approval by the U.S. Food and Drug Administration. There is a burgeoning literature on the use of FAE in the prevention and treatment of diseases, other than psoriasis and MS, in which oxidative stress and/or inflammation are prominent. The present review highlights critical information gleaned from these studies and exposes and provides perspectives on lacunae of potential importance.

2. Pharmacokinetics of fumaric acid esters

Dimethyl fumarate (PubChem CID: 637568), described as a "white crystalline compound with a fruit-like taste" [19], is a dimethyl ester of fumaric acid with the official chemical name of trans-1,2-ethylene carboxylic acid dimethyl ester [20]. Because of its rapid degradation by intestinal esterase, DMF does not cross the intestinal wall in significant amounts [21]. Thus, because of its short-lived activity, evidence of direct, sustained anti-inflammatory or antioxidant effects derived directly from DMF is limited [22]. Instead, monomethyl fumarate (MMF; PubChem CID: 21721168), the product of DMF metabolism by intestinal esterase, is said to be the main active metabolite [23]. This is confirmed by pharmacokinetic studies that demonstrate following oral DMF intake, serum concentrations of MMF peak within 2–2.5 h and its half-life is approximately 1 h [24]. Further, the ingestion of DMF along with a high fat/high-calorie diet was found to interfere with intestinal absorption, delaying the systemic peak of MMF significantly [16, 17]. Following doses of delayed-release DMF of up to 240 mg, the mean C_{max} of MMF in healthy human subjects was 1.43 μg/ml with a corresponding MMF area under the curve of 2.41 μg h/ml. There was no evidence of accumulation after multiple doses (e.g. 240 mg delayed-release DMF three times daily for 2 days) as MMF concentrations fell below detectable limits at the end of day 1 and day 2 [24]. MMF is eliminated primarily through breathing; negligible amounts of intact MMF are excreted through urine or feces. Additionally, there is no evidence of cytochrome P450-dependent metabolism of the compound in the liver [25]. Because of the lack of cytochrome P 450 involvement, DMF has very limited drug–drug interactions. Congruent with the above, both DMF and MMF have been popularly used for various pre-clinical pharmacological studies aimed at the testing and development of new therapeutics for various indications. The intestinal metabolism of DMF and diroximel fumarate (DRF), two current clinical FAE formulations is shown in **Figure 1**.

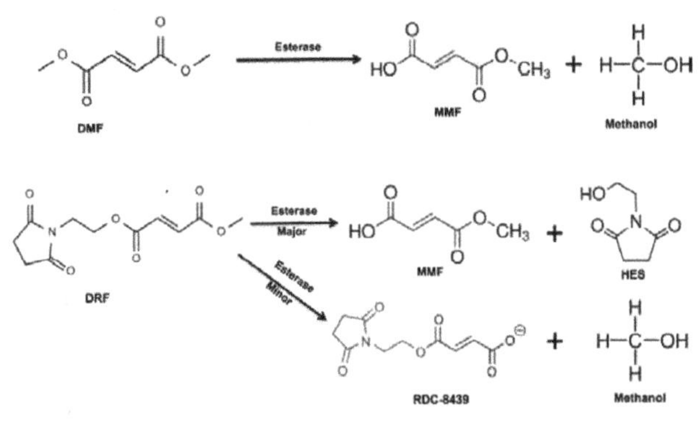

Figure 1.
Metabolism of fumaric acid esters. Clinical formulations of FAE are composed of dimethyl fumarate (DMF) or diroximel fumarate (DRF). Following oral administration, intestinal esterase metabolizes both DMF and DRF into the major bioactive ingredient MMF (monomethyl fumarate). Methanol, hydroxyethyl succinimide (HES) and RDC-8439 are also produced but only as minor metabolites (< 10%).

3. Mechanism of action: fumaric acid esters

Despite the numerous *in vitro* and *in vivo* studies that have been conducted over the years, the mechanism of action of FAE is still not fully understood and novel aspects continue to emerge. The generic hypothesis to explain the benefits of FAE is that DMF/MMF interferes with the cellular redox system by inducing a strong antioxidant response. Indeed, the robust induction of Nrf2 (nuclear factor E2 (erythroid-derived 2)-related factor) by DMF/MMF has been well described (**Figure 2**). In cells, DMF/MMF leads to the nuclear translocation of Nrf2, a phenomenon that is known to in turn, enhance the expression of antioxidant enzymes [26]. Specifically, it has been shown that MMF induces alkylation of a critical reactive thiol, Cys151, on Keap1 (Kelch-like ECH associated protein 1) which results in the release of Nrf2 [26, 27]. Once dissociated from Keap-1, Nrf2 translocates to the

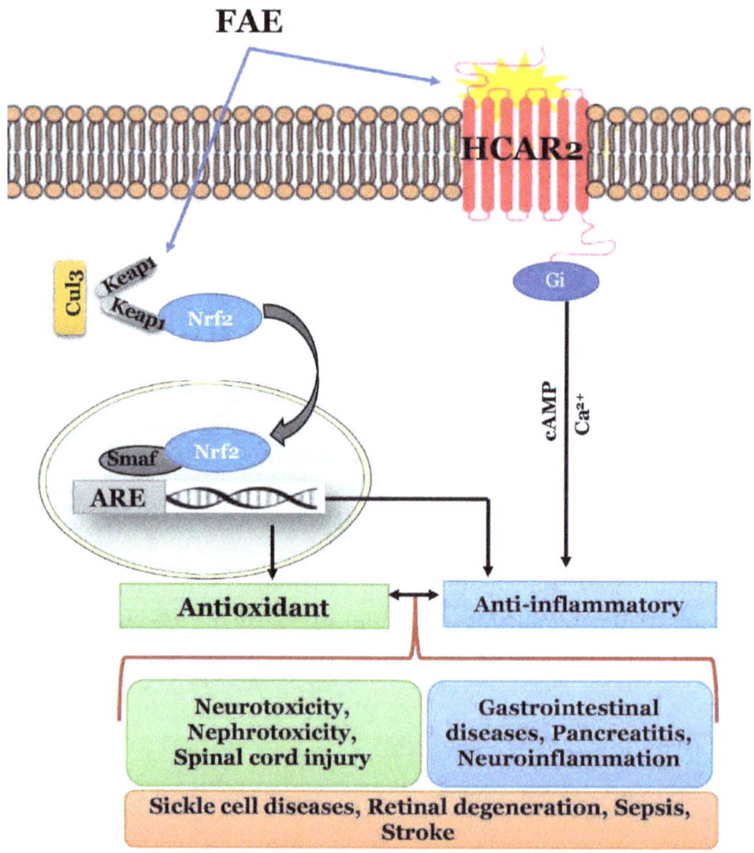

Figure 2.
Involvement of Nrf2-dependent and independent mechanisms in FAE-mediated antioxidant and anti-inflammatory effects. Fumaric acid esters (DMF/MMF) disrupt Keap1-Nrf2 binding to induce nuclear translocation of Nrf2 which in turn, activates a number of downstream antioxidant response genes. This mode of action of FAE is well known and is purported to be responsible for the positive actions of FAE in neurotoxicity, nephrotoxicity, and spinal cord injury. Additionally, however, MMF, the major bioactive ingredient of FAE, is an agonist of HCAR2, a G_i-protein coupled membrane receptor that potentiates robust anti-inflammatory signaling. Various studies have shown that while FAE-mediated Nrf2 signaling elicits both antioxidant and anti-inflammatory responses, HCAR2-dependent signaling predominantly provides an anti-inflammatory effect. The HCAR2-mediated actions of FAE have been implicated its protective effects in gastrointestinal diseases, pancreatitis and neuroinflammation. Importantly however, the combined actions (Nrf2- and HCAR2-mediated) have been demonstrated in several pathologic conditions (sickle cell disease, retinal degeneration, sepsis and stroke). FAE, fumaric acid esters; HCAR2 or HCA2, hydroxycarboxylic acid receptor 2; DMF, dimethyl fumarate; MMF, monomethyl fumarate; Keap1; kelch-like ECH associated protein 1; Nrf2, nuclear factor erythroid 2-related factor 2; ARE; antioxidant responsive element.

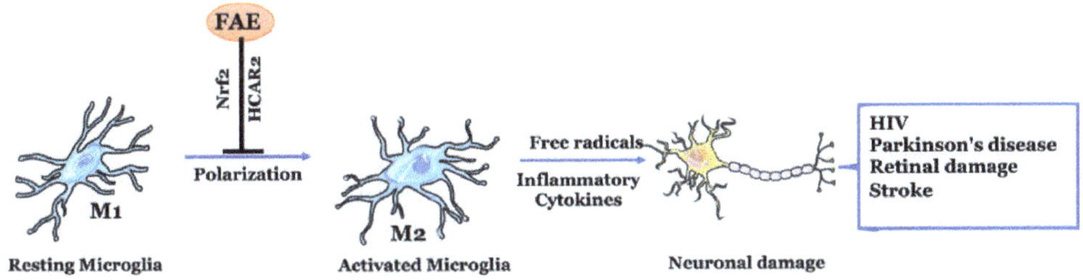

Figure 3.
The role of FAE in regulating microglia activation. FAE (DMF/MMF) are known to induce Nrf2 and to activate HCAR2. Various studies have shown that via these mechanisms, FAE prevent the polarization of microglia from the M1 (resting) phenotype to the M2 (active and thereby pro-inflammatory) phenotype, the consequences of which are reduced free radical and pro-inflammatory cytokine production. This action of FAE is thought to underlie the neuroprotective effects of the drug in conditions like HIV-induced neuroinflammation, Parkinson's disease, retinal degeneration, and stroke. FAE, fumaric acid esters, HCAR2, hydroxycarboxylic acid receptor 2; DMF, dimethyl fumarate; MMF, monomethyl fumarate; Nrf2, nuclear factor erythroid 2-related factor 2; HIV, human immunodeficiency virus.

nucleus and therein, binds to the antioxidant response element (ARE) of an array of antioxidant target genes thereby upregulating their expression and related activity. This effect was corroborated in Nrf2-deficient cells in which the antioxidant effects of DMF/MMF were lost [27].

The majority of preclinical studies of DMF/MMF, highlight the Nrf2-mediated mechanism of the drug as the principal factor underlying its therapeutic effects. However, DMF/MMF has also been shown to elicit a robust anti-inflammatory response. This additional desirable effect is thought to be accomplished via the inhibition of NF-kB translocation into the nucleus, an action that impacts negatively the expression of a plethora of inflammatory cytokine, chemokine, and adhesion molecule genes. Relevant also to the anti-inflammatory effects of DMF/MMF, is hydroxycarboxylic acid receptor 2 (HCAR2; GPR109A)-dependent signaling (**Figure 2**). MMF is a strong agonist of HCAR2. DMF activates the receptor as well although with a comparably lower affinity [28]. In a study by Chen et al. 2014 it was shown that DMF treatment reduced pathological features of experimental autoimmune encephalomyelitis in WT mice, but not in *Hcar2*$^{-/-}$ mice, indicating the importance of HCAR2-mediated signaling by DMF [29]. In another study, Parodi et al. [30] demonstrated the importance of HCAR2 to the anti-inflammatory effects of MMF in microglia. Specifically, it was reported that MMF could modulate microglia activation through inhibition of the NF-κB pathway via the AMPK/SIRT-1 axis. MMF treatment to microglia cells resulted in the activation of the HCAR2 receptor via enhanced intracellular calcium levels, an effect that prevents microglial polarization into an inflammatory phenotype (**Figure 3**). Downstream, it induced CAMKK (Calcium/calmodulin-dependent protein kinase kinase 2) dependent activation of AMPK/SIRT-1 axis which also contributes to reduced inflammation. Several other studies have also reported on the HCAR2 receptor-dependent and independent anti-inflammatory effects of FAE in additional cell types including keratinocytes [31–33] and epithelial cells of the retina [34, 35].

4. Role of FAE in inflammatory and oxidative stress conditions

Herein we highlight the findings of preclinical studies on the use of DMF/MMF to counter inflammation and oxidative stress associated with the pathogenesis of pathological conditions other than psoriasis and MS (**Figure 2**). A summary is provided in **Table 1**.

Disease condition	Experimental model	Effective dose	Outcomes	References
Cerebral ischemia–	Middle cerebral artery occlusion in rats	25 and 50 mg/kg DMF (i.g.)	DMF protected against experimental stroke by inducing immunomodulatory and antioxidant response	[36]
	Middle cerebral artery occlusion in mice	30 and 45 mg/kg DMF and MMF (i.p.)	DMF and MMF suppressed glial activation via increasing the expression of Nrf2	[37]
Experimental colitis	a. Mice treated with DNBS. b. IL-$10^{-/-}$ mice.	30 and 100 mg/kg DMF (i.g.)	DMF induced antioxidant response by regulating SOD-2 and inflammation by Nf-kB signaling to reduce colitis.	[38]
	Mice treated with 3% (w/v) DSS drinking water	30 and 60 mg/kg DMF (i.g.)	DMF alleviated DSS-induced colitis by regulating Nrf2-mediated inhibition of NLRP3 inflammasome	[39]
Intracerebral hemorrhage	Intra-striatal injection of autologous blood in rats and mice	15 mg/kg DMF (i.g.)	DMF can ameliorate ICH-mediated injury with a therapeutic window of at least 24 h	[40]
	Mice using either the collagenase injection model (cICH) or the autologous blood (bICH)	100 mg/kg (i.p.)	DMF-induced dissociation of Nrf2 from Keap1, and the consequent casein kinase 2 phosphorylation of Nrf2, resulted in neuroprotection after ICH	[41]
Nephrotoxicity	Rats treated with 20 mg/kg Cyclosporin A for 28 days	50 mg / kg DMF (i.g.)	DMF reduced nephrotoxicity by inhibiting oxidative stress and inflammation	[42]
Neurotoxicity	Mice treated with 10 nmol sodium nitroprusside	60 and 200 mg/kg DMF (i.g.)	DMF reduced neurotoxicity by activating HO-1.	[43]
Pancreatitis	Rats treated with 2.5 g/kg L-arginine	25 mg/kg DMF (i.g.)	DMF was effective in ameliorating the histological lesions and biochemical abnormalities and improving beta-cell function	[44, 45]
	Rats treated with 3 g/Kg L-arginine	25 mg/Kg DMF (i.g.)	DMF treated rats showed reductions in the severity of inflammatory cell infiltration, acinar damage, perilobar edema, and cell necrosis	[46]
Parkinson's disease	6-OHDA-induced neurotoxicity in mice	50 mg/kg DMF (i.g.)	DMF reduced neurotoxicity by Nrf2 mediated antioxidant response.	[47]
	Mice treated with MPTP	100 mg/kg MMF/DMF (i.g.)	DMF and MMF exhibit neuroprotective effects via Nrf2-mediated antioxidant, anti-inflammatory, and mitochondrial functional/biogenetic effects.	[48]
	Mice treated with a viral vector expressing human α-SYN	100 and 300 mg/kg DMF (i.g.)	DMF prevented Synucleinopathy in a mouse model of PD by activating Nrf2 signaling	[49]
	MPTP-treated mice	10, 30, and 100 mg/kg DMF (i.g.)	DMF protected against experimental PD via regulation of the NF-κB/Nrf-2 pathway	[50]

Disease condition	Experimental model	Effective dose	Outcomes	References
Retinal degeneration	I/R injury in mice	50 mg/kg MMF (i.p.)	MMF reduced retinal I/R injury in mice via induction of Nrf2 signaling	[51]
	Light-induced retinal damage in mice	100 mg/kg MMF (i.p.)	MMF-mediated HCAR2 signaling provided neuroprotection via reduced microglial activation, inflammation, and oxidative stress.	[52]
Sepsis	Rats subjected to cecal ligation and puncture procedure	15 mg/kg of DMF (i.g.)	DMF reduced inflammation and oxidative stress in heart, liver, lung, kidney, and brain, and improved cognitive function	[53, 54]
		50 mg/kg MMF (i.p.)	MMF alleviated sepsis-induced hepatic dysfunction by reducing oxidative and inflammatory via the inhibition of the TLR-4/NF-κB signaling pathway.	[55]
Sickle cell disease	HbSS-Townes and NY1DD mice	30 mg/kg DMF (i.g.)	DMF increased expression of nuclear Nrf2 in the liver and kidney to decreases oxidative stress and inflammation	[56]
Sickle cell retinopathy	HbSS-Townes mice	1 mM (intravitreal) and 15 mg/ml MMF (in drinking water)	MMF treatment-induced fetal hemoglobin production and reduced oxidative stress and inflammation via Nrf2 activation	[34, 35]
Spinal cord injury	SCI injury in mice using aneurysm clip	30 mg/kg (i.g.)	DMF and MMF improved SCI injury in mice.	[57]
Ulcer	Rats exposed to chronic foot-shock stress	2.5 and 5 mg/kg MMF (i.p.)	MMF restored monoamine, corticosterone, and cytokine homeostasis by regulating neuroendocrine-immune systems	[39]

Table 1.
Some important in vivo *studies showing the use of fumaric acid esters for the treatment of oxidative stress and inflammation.*

4.1 Gastrointestinal diseases

Inflammatory bowel disease (IBD) is a group of inflammatory conditions of the colon and small intestine that includes Crohn's disease and ulcerative colitis [58, 59]. Treatments for IBD range from symptomatic treatment with anti-diarrheal medica-tions, anti-inflammatory agents or immunosuppressive drugs to more radical surgical interventive strategies (e.g. partial or complete colectomy). These strategies are effective in a number of patients however given the complex etiology of IBD, the need for new and/or improved therapeutic strategies remains high. Given the well-established link between inflammation and IBD development and progression, it is not surprising that several groups have sought to test the efficacy of FAE in this condition. For the most part, these studies have been conducted using experimental models of colitis; rodents treated with dinitrobenzene sulfuric acid (DNBS) or dextran sodium sulfate (DSS), etc. [60, 61]. Casili et al. induced colitis in mice via intrarectal administration of DNBS (4 mg/mouse). DMF (10, 30 or 100 mg/kg) was then administered orally every 24 h, starting 3 h after the administration of DNBS and continuing over the course of 4 days. DMF treatment to DNBS treated mice significantly improved colon injury and histological score. Further DMF also reduced lipid peroxidation by regulating the expression of SOD2 (superoxide dismutase 2, mitochondrial) and Nrf2. The anti-inflammatory effect of DMF was evident by a reduction in the expression of TNF-α (tumor necrosis factor- α), IL-1β (Interleukin 1 beta) and ICAM-1 (intercellular adhesion molecule 1) and P- selectin. This effect was thought to be a result of reduced IκB-α degradation to prevent nuclear translocation of p65 NF-κB (Nuclear factor-κB). Moreover, *in vitro* DMF treatment improved hydrogen peroxide-induced barrier dysfunction of human intestinal epithelial cells. The authors also confirmed the protective effect of DMF on experimental colitis using another model (9-week-old IL-10KO mice). Collectively, this study demonstrated that DMF could reduce experimental colitis by regulating inflammation and oxidative stress [38]. In another study, Liu et al., 2016 evaluated the efficacy of DMF in reducing DSS-induced murine colitis. Wild-type and *Nrf2*$^{-/-}$ mice received either vehicle or 3% (w/v) DSS in drinking water for 7 days and thereafter provided with only drinking water for another 3 days. Groups of mice were also given 30 or 60 mg/kg DMF (i.g.) from day 1 to 10. DMF treatment significantly reduced oxidative stress and inflammation and thereby improved signs/symptoms of colitis in DSS-treated mice. However, these effects were lost in *Nrf2*$^{-/-}$ mice, highlighting the importance of the Nrf2-mediated mechanism of action of the drug. This was supported by additional *in vitro* studies in which the authors showed that DMF-mediated Nrf2 activation reduces NLRP3 (NLR family pyrin domain containing 3) inflammasome activation to control intestinal inflammation.

Consistent with the above gastrointestinal benefits derived from DMF/MMF treatment, the efficacy of MMF treatment in improving stomach ulcers in rats has also been described. Although the detailed mechanism of action was not evaluated, the authors attributed the protective effect of the compound in this condition to be due primarily to the anti-inflammatory activity of MMF [39]. Collectively, these studies indicate that DMF/MMF therapy may be of benefit the clinical management of inflammatory gastrointestinal disorders. This is interesting given that gastrointestinal (GI) side effects (e.g., nausea, vomiting, diarrhea, and upper abdominal pain) are one of the most commonly reported complaints in patients receiving DMF therapy [62, 63]. Indeed, during phase 3 clinical trials for multiple sclerosis, adverse events (AEs) involving the GI system were reported in 40% of patients treated with DMF compared with 30% of patients treated with placebo [64, 65]. Though the adverse GI events are generally mild in severity and typically resolve within the first 2 months of treatment, these issues may impact patient quality of life and ultimately medication adherence. Thus, while a number of experimental studies have reported gastroprotective effects of DMF, there is some concern as to whether such therapy could reliably be extrapolated to clinical management of gastrointestinal disorders in human patients. However, the increasing number of additional reports of DMF/MMF benefit in the digestive system that continue to arise in the scientific literature suggests that perhaps efforts to implement DMF/MMF therapy for use in this regard should not be dismissed completely. For example, Rao and Mishra [66] performed a preliminary study demonstrating the hepatoprotective effects of MMF isolated from *Fumaria Indica* extract in various models of hepatotoxicity. Although the study was preliminary and had some limitations, it does introduce a possible hepatoprotective effect of MMF. This is supported also by a recent study by Abdelrahman et al. [67] that reported the protective effects of DMF treatment on acetaminophen-induced hepatic injury in mice. Acetaminophen-treated mice receiving a single or double dose of DMF (100 mg/kg) showed reduced oxidative stress, inflammation, and associated liver damage compared to non-DMF treated animals. Hence, additional studies in larger animal models and at some point, in humans, to test, develop and/or refine DMF/MMF formulations to improve potential suitability for use in the treatment of gastrointestinal or liver diseases are warranted.

4.2 HIV-induced neuroinflammation and neurotoxicity

With improvements in treatments for HIV (human immunodeficiency virus), lifespan has increased significantly affected persons. However, neuroinflamma-tion and/or toxicity remain major concerns in this disease. The critical relevance of neuroinflammation to the etiology of MS, a disease for which DMF/MMF therapy is already approved, is undeniable [68]. Further, patients with MS are at considerably higher risk for neurotoxicity than are patients without the demyelinating disease [69]. Given these commonalities between MS and HIV-induced neurologic disease, preclinical testing of DMF/MMF in the latter is of interest. Using an *in vitro* model of HIV-mediated neurotoxicity, Cross et al. 2011 [70] showed that HIV infection dysregulates macrophage antioxidant response and reduces the expression of heme oxygenase-1 (HO-1). Importantly, DMF and MMF (5–30 μM) dose-dependently suppressed HIV replication, improved antioxidant response and reduced neuro-toxin release, effects that the authors proposed to be mediated via a two-way action of DMF: (1) inhibition of NF-kB nuclear translocation and consequent suppression of HIV replication, and (2) decreased neurotoxin release stemming from HO-1 induction. Further, they also found that DMF reduces CCL2 (C-C Motif Chemokine Ligand 2)-induced monocyte chemotaxis, suggesting that DMF additionally decreased the recruitment of activated monocytes to the CNS (central nervous system) in response to inflammatory mediators. Based on the above, the authors concluded that dysregulation of the antioxidant response during HIV infection drives macrophage-mediated neurotoxicity and DMF could serve as an adjunctive neuro-protectant. In a separate study, Ambrosius et al. [71] evaluated the effect of MMF on microglia activation and subsequent neurotoxicity. MMF treatment (10–30 μM) significantly reduced HIV-mediated neurotoxicity in microglia cells (**Figure 3**). A similar but prior study by a different group showed MMF to be capable of inducing a phenotypic shift from pro-inflammatory to anti-inflammatory macrophages [72] however, Ambrosius et al. did not observe such effects. These differences could be model-dependent or related to methodological differences in the two studies and therefore require further investigation since the authors did not comprehensively evaluate the possible mechanism of action in these short reports. Notwithstanding, however, the opposing effects of DMF/MMF on microglial responses, particularly those of an inflammatory nature, appear to be solidly supported by several other studies [30] which in turn, collectively support additional effort to advance DMF/MMF therapy for potential use in HIV-associated neuroinflammation and toxicity.

4.3 Nephrotoxicity

Very little information exists on the protective effect of FAEs on renal function. A study by Takasu et al. [42] evaluated the effect of DMF treatment on CsA (calcineurin inhibitor)-induced nephrotoxicity. Male *Sprague–Dawley* rats were treated with 20 mg/kg CsA or CsA + 50 mg/kg DMF (i.g.) for 28 days. At the end of the treatment schedule, renal function, histopathology, malondialdehyde (MDA), myeloperoxidase levels, and antioxidant enzyme expression were determined. DMF co-treatment ameliorated CsA-induced renal dysfunction as evidenced by a significant decrease in serum creatinine and urea levels, as well as improvement of creatinine clearance. DMF also significantly decreased serum and renal MDA and myeloperoxidase contents whereas, protein expression of NQO-1 (NAD (P) H quinone oxidoreductase-1), a major cellular antioxidant and the detoxifying enzyme, was significantly enhanced by DMF administration. Although evidence is limited, the above study supports the protective potential of DMF/MMF therapy in a clinically relevant model of nephrotoxicity, an effect that is afforded in part via DMF's robust ability to enhance the cellular antioxidant capacity and thereby, inhibit oxidative stress and inflammation [42] as described in other cell and tissue systems. Thus, while much remains to be learned about the possible use of DMF/ MMF in the treatment of renal diseases, initial results are encouraging.

4.4 Non-HIV related neurotoxicity

Prior discussion (subSection 4.2) of neurotoxicity in this chapter was related specifically to that occurring in HIV. Irrespective, however, of the mitigating disease or pathologic process, the brain is indisputably sensitive to pro-inflammatory and/or oxidative insult. Hence, neurotoxicity can emanate from multiple variable causes. Kume et al. [43] evaluated the ability of DMF to protect against *in vitro* and *in vivo* oxidative stress in the central nervous system induced via pro-oxidant agents like sodium nitroprusside and hydrogen peroxide (H_2O_2). DMF pretreatment (60–200 mg/kg) for 24 h dose-dependently protected against 10 nM sodium nitroprusside-induced brain damage and in rat primary striatal cell cultures, 10 μM DMF markedly prevented cytotoxicity stemming from exposure of cells to H_2O_2 (1 mM). Interestingly, the protective effects of DMF against *in vitro* oxidative stress were countered by the HO-1 inhibitor zinc protoporphyrin IX however, buthionine sulfoximine, an inhibitor of glutathione synthesis, did not interfere with the protection afforded by DMF. Collectively, these results support the potential of DMF/MMF therapy in conditions of neurotoxicity and suggest that its ability to activate HO-1 may be critical. Neural stem/progenitor cells (NPCs) are a heterogeneous population of self-renewing and multi-potent cells that can differentiate into neurons, astrocytes, or oligodendrocytes (post-mitotic daughter cells) [73, 74]. Hence, the survival of these cells could greatly impact various forms of neurodegenerative diseases. Wang et al. [75] reported on the neuroprotective effects of DMF on mouse and rat neural stem/progenitor cells (NPCs) and neurons. DMF treatment reduced reactive oxygen species (ROS) production, increased the frequency of the multi-potent neurospheres and enhanced the survival of NPCs following H_2O_2-mediated oxidative stress. DMF also decreased oxidative stress-induced apoptosis and promoted the survival of motor neurons, effects that this group demonstrated to be mediated via the Nrf2-ERK1/2 MAPK pathway. These studies provide additional support of the overwhelmingly protective effects of FAE in multiple brain cell types and therefore, of the potential feasibility of this therapy in the prevention and treatment of neurodegenerative diseases.

4.5 Pancreatitis

Chronic pancreatitis (CP) is a progressive inflammatory disorder that results in the destruction and fibrosis of the pancreatic parenchyma and its endocrine and exocrine dysfunctions [76]. Various research groups have evaluated the effect of DMF treatment on acute and chronic pancreatitis. In one of the studies, chronic pancreatitis in rats was induced by five injections of 250 mg/100 g L-Arginine and sacrificed 7 weeks later. In another group 25 mg/kg DMF was given orally 24 before L-arginine treatment and continued thereafter until the end of the study. DMF treatment significantly improved glucose tolerance, pancreas histology, biochemical parameters (MDA and MPO; myeloperoxidase), and induced HO-1 expression [44].

However, this study did not evaluate the mechanism of action for DMF-induced protection. Another study by Robles et al. [45] evaluated the efficacy of DMF in an acute model of pancreatitis. Acute pancreatitis was induced by two injections of 3 g/kg L-Arginine (1 hr. apart) to rats and sacrificed later at 24 and 72 hr. DMF (25 mg/kg) was orally administered to rats 24 h before L-arginine and continued until sacrifice. The histology of the pancreas was significantly improved in DMF-treated animals possibly due to decreased cleaved caspase-3 (apoptosis) and MDA levels. This group additionally stimulated splenocytes with 1 μg/ml for 24 h with or without DMF 20 μM. *In vitro* DMF treatment significantly reduced proinflammatory cytokine secretion in rat splenocytes, although a definitive mechanism for this DMF-mediated action was not put forward. Recently, however, Zhang and colleagues [46] too evaluated the effect of DMF on L-arginine induced chronic pancreatitis. In brief, this group treated *Wistar* rats intraperitoneally with L-arginine 5 times (250 mg/100 kg, twice per time, each interval of 1 h) to induce chronic pancreatitis (CP). One group of rats was treated with 20 mg/kg DMF. Compared with control (untreated) group, the weight of rats in CP group was significantly reduced at weeks 2, 4 and 6; blood glucose levels were significantly increased, the histopathological scores of pancreatic atrophy, acinar injury, edema, and cellular infiltration increased, levels of MDA and MPO increased, and the islet equivalent and islet activity decreased at 0, 30, 60, 120 and 180 min., parameters that were all prevented or reversed in the DMF-treated CP group. Thus, DMF treatment can protect against CP induced by L-arginine and islet function in rats. Although these three studies support the potential of DMF/MMF therapy in pancreatitis, the exact mechanism (s) to explain the benefits attained remains unknown. Because therapies to impact pancreatitis are extremely limited at present, additional detailed studies to test the efficacy of FAE in this condition would certainly be worthwhile in hopes that findings emanating therefrom could be carried forward to use in a clinical setting.

4.6 Parkinson's disease

Again, the brain is especially sensitive to perturbations caused by oxidative and/or inflammatory stress. In fact, these factors, particularly oxidative stress, are central to the pathology of several neurodegenerative diseases, including Parkinson's disease (PD) [77, 78] therefore, therapies designed to enhance antioxi-dant potential and counter this stress may be of clinical value [79, 80]. Scientific studies published within the last couple of years highlight the high clinical potential the repurposing of DMF/MMF for the treatment of PD holds. Using various *in vitro* and *in vivo* studies it has been demonstrated that DMF/MMF induced Nrf2 signaling can protect against oxidative stress and inflammatory conditions related to PD. In an initial study by Jing et al. [47], DMF (2–4 μM) pre-treatment significantly reduced hydroxydopamine (6-OHDA) induced generation of ROS and subsequent cytotoxicity in SH-SY5Y cells. The increase in ROS production caused by 6-OHDA treatment was also attenuated by DMF. Further, siNrf2 treatment blocked DMF's protection against 6-OHDA-induced neurotoxicity. *In vivo*, oral administration of DMF (50 mg/kg) to C57BL/6 mice up-regulated expression of Nrf2 and Nrf2-dependent cytoprotective genes. Taken together, this study provided initial evidence for the protective role of DMF in PD. This was followed by three different studies focusing on the mechanism of action for DMF and its metabolite, MMF in mediated protection against PD. Ahuja et al. [48] compared the effects of DMF and MMF on Nrf2 signaling by evaluating its ability to block 1-methyl-4-phenyl-1,2,3,6-tetrahydropyridine (MPTP)-induced experimental PD. Their results showed that Nrf2 activation by DMF was associated with depletion of glutathione, decreased cell viability, and inhibition of mitochondrial oxygen consumption and glycolysis rates in a dose-dependent manner. Contrary to this, MMF increased these activities *in vitro*. However, both DMF and MMF activated the Nrf2 pathway via S-alkylation of the Nrf2 inhibitor Keap1 which promoted the nuclear exit of the Nrf2 repressor Bach1 to improve mitochondrial biogenesis. Despite the *in vitro* differences, both DMF and MMF exerted similar neuroprotective effects and blocked MPTP neurotoxicity in wild type but not in *Nrf2*$^{-/-}$ mice. It was concluded that DMF and MMF exhibit neuroprotective effects because of their distinct Nrf2-mediated antioxidant, anti-inflammatory, and mitochondrial functional/biogenetic effects, but MMF does so without depleting glutathione and inhibiting mitochondrial and glycolytic functions. Therefore, the authors advocated for the possible development of MMF rather than DMF as a novel therapy for PD. Synucleinopathies (also called α-synucleinopathies; α-SYN) are neurodegenerative diseases characterized by the abnormal accumulation of aggregates of alpha-synuclein protein in neurons, nerve fibers or glial cells [81]. Lastres-Becker et al. [49] conducted a study in which they focused primarily on the role of DMF in regulating synucleinopathies associated with oxidative stress and inflammation. In brief, an adeno-associated pseudotype 6 (rAAV6) viral vector was used to express human α-SYN under the neuron-specific human synapsin 1 promoter to create conditions of PD and animals were treated daily with DMF (100–300 mg/kg) via oral gavage. DMF protected nigral dopaminergic neurons against α-SYN toxicity and decreased astrocytosis and microgliosis. However, this protective effect was not observed in *Nrf2*$^{-/-}$ mice. Additionally, *in vitro* studies indicated that the neuroprotective effect was correlated with altered regulation of autophagy markers and with a shift in microglial dynamics toward a less pro-inflammatory and a more wound-healing phenotype (**Figure 3**). These experiments provide a compelling rationale for targeting Nrf2 with DMF as a therapeutic strategy to reinforce endogenous brain defense mechanisms against PD-associated synucleinopathy. These findings are supported by another study in which daily oral administration of DMF (10, 30, and 100 mg/kg) significantly reduced neuronal cell degeneration of the dopaminergic tract and behavioral impairments induced by four injections of the dopaminergic neurotoxin MPTP. Moreover, treatment with DMF prevented dopamine depletion, increased tyrosine hydroxylase, and dopamine transporter activities, and also reduced the number of α-synuclein-positive neurons. Furthermore, DMF treatment up-regulated Nrf2 as evidenced by the increased activation of SOD2 and HO-1 and elevated levels of glutathione, and increased NeuN$^+$/Nrf2$^+$ cell number in the striatum. Moreover, DMF reduced IL-1β levels, cyclooxygenase 2 activities, and neuronal nitrite oxide synthase expression. This treatment also modulated microglial activation (**Figure 3**), restored nerve growth factor levels, and preserved microtubule-associated protein 2 alterations. Using the Nrf2 inhibitor trigonelline, the authors were able to confirm the Nrf2 dependency of the protective mechanism. Collectively, these results demonstrated that DMF protects against experimental PD via NF-κB/Nrf2 pathway [50]. Several other antioxidants have shown potential as therapeutic options for PD, however, because DMF/MMF is already FDA-approved, the potential viability of this candidate therapy for PD is enhanced.

4.7 Retinal degenerative diseases

In recent years, others and we have investigated the potential of MMF in the treatment of degenerative retinal diseases. In an early study, we showed MMF to be protective against reactive gliosis, a characteristic response of Muller glial cells to an environment rich in pro-oxidant and inflammatory factors in retinal disease. Folate uptake by Muller cells is considered a key event in this process [82]. MMF treatment significantly reduced folate uptake by Muller cells by decreasing the expression and activity of proton-coupled folate transporter (PCFT), a transporter integral to the uptake of folate. This was the first report demonstrating that MMF could regulate folate transport in retinal glial cells and therefore, be potentially useful in the treatment of degenerative retinal diseases. To determine whether, in addition to down-regulating pro-inflammatory mechanisms, MMF affects counteractive or protective signaling, in a subsequent study we evaluated also the effect of the compound on the expression and activity of the cysteine/glutamate exchanger SLC7A11 (system x_c^-), a transport system critical for the intracellular entry of the amino acid cysteine which is required for glutathione synthesis [28]. Glutathione is the most abundant endogenous antioxidant in the retina and is therefore essential for the protection of retinal cells against oxidative stress. Further, retinal pigment epithelial (RPE) cells are one of the highest producers of glutathione of any cell type in the body. As such, we exposed human retinal pigment epithelial (ARPE-19) cells to MMF in the presence or absence of pro-oxidant stimuli and evaluated the dose- and time-dependent effects on system x_c^- mRNA, protein, and activity levels. MMF was found to up-regulate each of these parameters and additionally, up-regulate hypoxia-inducible factor 1-alpha (Hif-1α), nuclear factor erythroid 2-related factor 2 (Nrf2) expression and increase total reduced glutathione (GSH) content. Collectively, our early *in vitro* studies demonstrated that MMF affects multiple pathways in multiple retinal cell types in a manner that is overall protective against oxidative damage.

We sought next to determine whether our findings extrapolate to the *in vivo* condition, therefore, we evaluated the efficacy of MMF in a living animal model of retinal disease. Retinopathy is a major cause of vision loss in sickle cell disease (SCD) and therapies to prevent and treat sickle retinopathy (SR) are very limited. Therapeutic induction of γ-globin expression and subsequent induction of fetal hemoglobin (HbF) production can alleviate some SCD-associated complications. Interestingly, Nrf2 inducers have been demonstrated to be effective γ-globin inducers [83]. The robust inductive properties of MMF on Nrf2 translocation and activity have been long recognized therefore, it was logical to explore the effects of MMF in SCD. Not only did we confirm that RPE cells, cells integral to retinal health and function, produce HbF but that MMF treatment of Townes humanized SCD mice of SCD resulted in reductions in the expression of pro-oxidant and inflammatory factors and turn, preserved retinal morphology [35]. Shortly after this study, Cho et al. [51] too reported on the potential benefit of MMF in the treatment of retinal disease in a mouse model of retinal ischemia-reperfusion. Specifically, they showed that MMF promotes Nrf2-neuroprotection in this model. MMF treatment was associated with significant increases in the expression of Nrf2-responsive antioxidant genes and a suppression of inflammatory responses as evidenced by increased expression of NAD (P) H quinone dehydrogenase 1, thioredoxin reductase 1 and heme oxygenase-1 along with decrease in interleukin-1β, chemokine (C-C motif) ligands (2, 7 and 12), expressions. Collectively, these molecular improvements interpreted to improved retinal function as evidenced by electroretinogram recordings performed on live mice and were heavily dependent upon the expression and activity of Nrf2.

Because these initial reports of MMF's potential efficacy in protecting against retinal degeneration were conducted acutely, we decided to evaluate the effect of long-term administration of the compound (5 months administration of 15 mg/ml MMF in drinking water) in the humanized SCD model [34]. Importantly we found via high-pressure liquid chromatography (HPLC) and hematological analyses of peripheral blood that MMF treatment reduced sickle hemoglobin (HbS) content and white blood cell counts, and improved hematocrit, red blood cell number, and hemoglobin concentrations significantly in SCD mice. In retina specifically, the mRNA and protein expression of well-established markers of inflammation and oxidative stress (i.e., vascular endothelial growth factor, intercellular adhesion molecule-1, interleukin-1β, dihydroethidium labeling) was reduced and the development and progression of SCD-like retinal pathology in these mice were ameliorated. Additional related *in vitro* studies performed toward elucidating the molecular mechanisms responsible for the MMF-induced improvements that were observed implicate Nrf2 and Bcl11A (B-cell lymphoma/leukemia 11A) as key players. This study was of extreme significance because not only did it support strongly the notion that fumaric acid ester therapy may be of benefit for the treatment of retinal pathology, especially in SCD, but for SCD in general, a concept that we have since patented [84]. Perhaps equally as astounding is the fact that MMF delivered systemically induced such robust effects in retina, meaning that MMF must be capable of crossing in significant quantities or otherwise inducing signaling across the blood-retinal barriers. Given the known difficulties with non-invasive yet efficacious drug delivery to the posterior segment of the eye (retina) and the commonality of oxidative stress and inflammation as key causative factors in the development and progression of numerous retinal diseases, the clinical relevance and therefore potential impact of the above findings is extremely high. Indeed, new reports of potential benefit derived from MMF in animal models of the degenerative retinal disease continue to surface, such as the recent study by Jiang et al. [52] demonstrating that MMF treatment protects against light-induced retinal damage on BALB/C mice and effect due potentially to HCAR2-dependent signaling in retinal microglia cells (**Figure 3**). Eventually, data emanating from these preclinical reports may spur increased interest in moving toward clinical testing and implementation of FAE therapy in the near future.

4.8 Sepsis

Sepsis is a potentially fatal illness that can lead to the damage of multiple organs [85]. The condition is deeply associated with oxidative stress and inflammation. Firstly, a study by Giustina et al. [53] reported the protective effects of DMF against multi-organ sepsis by modulating oxidative stress and inflammation. It was reported that oral administration of 15 mg/kg of DMF provides significant protection against sepsis-induced multi-organ (heart, liver, and lung) damage in rats. Later, the same research group reported the protective effects of DMF treatment on sepsis-associated inflammation and oxidative stress and cognitive impairment in the brain [54]. Although both these studies were descriptive in nature as neither evaluated in detail the underlying mode of action, they provide evidence that DMF might be used successfully for the clinical management of sepsis. This is supported by a study by Shalmani et al. [55] in which it was reported that 50 mg/kg (i.p.) MMF treatment improved sepsis-induced liver dysfunction by regulating the TLR-4/NF-κB signaling pathway. Collectively, these preclinical studies provide a great foundation for future clinical evaluations of the utility of FAE in the manage-ment of organ damage in sepsis.

4.9 Sickle cell disease-associated oxidative stress and inflammation

Uncontrolled hemolysis and subsequent release of hemoglobin (Hb) and heme into the vasculature is a hallmark of sickle cell disease (SCD) [86, 87]. Heme, a damage-associated molecular pattern, is highly pro-oxidative and proinflammatory and induces vaso-occlusion in murine models of sickle cell disease (SCD) [88]. A study by Belcher et al. evaluated the protective effect of DMF treatment on SCD associated oxidative stress and inflammation in the liver and kidneys [56]. DMF (30 mg/kg/day) or vehicle (0.08% methylcellulose) was administered for 3–7 days to NY1DD and HbSS-Townes SCD mice. DMF had a significant reductive impact on vaso-occlusion in SCD mice. It increased the nuclear translocation of Nrf2 and cellular mRNA of Nrf2-responsive genes in livers and kidneys, and increased heme defenses, including HO-1, haptoglobin, hemopexin, and ferritin heavy chain, without altering plasma Hb and heme levels. Markers of inflammation were also reduced. Interestingly, much of the DMF-induced benefit was blunted by the HO-1 inhibitor, protoporphyrin. Chronic treatment (24 weeks) of SCD with DMF decreased hepatic necrosis, inflammatory cytokines, and irregularly shaped erythrocytes, and increased HbF but did not alter hematocrit, reticulocyte counts, lactate dehydrogenase or plasma heme levels or, spleen weights. These results [56] together with our previously highlighted findings in SCD (subSection 4.7) [34, 35], are supportive of the multiple beneficial effects of DMF/MMF on the pathogenesis of SCD and the need for further clinical evaluation of the drug for this indication.

4.10 Spinal cord injury

Patients with spinal cord injury (SCI) usually have permanent and often devastating neurologic deficits and disabilities. The currently available therapeutic options include surgical decompression, methylprednisolone and hemodynamic control [89, 90]. Hence, the development of a new therapy for SCI holds great merits. Recent work by Cordaro et al. [57] evaluated the beneficial effects of DMF and MMF in a mouse model of traumatic SCI. Using an aneurysm clip, SCI was induced by extradural compression of the spinal cord at T6-T7 for 1 min. Mice were then treated with 30 mg/kg (i.g) DMF or MMF one and 6 h post-SCI. To evaluate the locomotor activity, study mice were treated with DMF/MMF once daily for 10 days. It was observed that mice treated with DMF exhibited a significant and sustained recovery of motor function. DMF/MMF significantly reduced the severity of inflammation by modulation of pro-inflammatory cytokines and apoptosis factors and increased neurotrophic factors. The authors concluded that the observed results were attributable to reduced secondary inflammation and tissue injury and therefore, DMF may constitute a promising target for future SCI therapies [57]. This study provided the first scientific evidence for the protective role of DMF in the treatment of SCI, however, additional detailed experimental and preclinical studies are needed to identify the potential mechanism(s) of action and enhance the likelihood that this therapy could be advanced to clinical testing and implementation.

4.11 Stroke

Over the past 2 years, researchers worldwide have published several articles on the role of FAE in the treatment of stroke. In one of the early studies on intracerebral hemorrhage (ICH), male rats and mice (including *Nrf2*-deficient animals) were subjected to intracerebral injection of blood and then treated with DMF [40]. In rats, 5 mg/kg DMF was administered at 2 h post-ICH and again orally twice a day on days 1–3, whereas in mice, the same dose of DMF was injected (i.p.) 24 h post-ICH and then at days 2 and 3. Treatment with DMF induced Nrf2-target genes, improved hematoma resolution, reduced brain edema and eventually enhanced neurological recovery in rats and wild type mice, but not in $Nrf2^{-/-}$ mice. Based on these findings, the authors proposed that DMF may offer an impressive 24 h therapeutic window of opportunity in which to treat ICH, a concept certainly worthy of further evaluation. The potential of DMF/MMF therapy in ICH is supported further by work by Iniaghe et al. [41] in which male CD-1 mice were subjected to intrastriatal infusion of bacterial collagenase, autologous blood or sham surgery. After ICH, animals either received vehicle, DMF (10 mg or 100 mg/kg) or casein kinase 2 inhibitor (E)-3-(2,3,4,5-tetrabromophenyl) acrylic acid (TBCA). Some mice also received scrambled siRNA or MAFG siRNA 24 h before ICH. DMF treatment reduced Evans blue dye extravasation, decreased brain water content, microglia activation (**Figure 3**), ICAM-1 expression and, improved neurological deficits and casein kinase 2 levels. Interestingly, TBCA and MAFG siRNA blunted protection afforded by DMF. Hence, it was concluded that DMF reduced inflammation, blood-brain barrier permeability, and improved neurological outcomes via casein kinase 2 and Nrf2 signaling pathways in mice.

Similar to other neurodegenerative disorders, oxidative stress is common also to the pathogenesis of ischemic stroke, potentiating the neuronal malfunction and cell death characteristic of this disease [91]. Given that the up-regulation of antioxidant genes through activation of the Nrf2 is one of the key mechanisms of cellular defense against oxidative stress [92], it is logical to explore the efficacy of FAE therapy in this condition. Congruent with this, three additional groups used experimental models of ischemic stroke to evaluate the efficacy of FAEs. In 2016, Lin et al. [36] observed that MMF (25–100 μM) rescued cultured cortical neurons from oxygen–glucose deprivation (OGD) and suppressed pro-inflammatory cytokines produced by primary mixed neuron/glia cultures subjected to OGD. In rats, DMF treatment (25 or 50 mg/kg twice daily) significantly decreased infarction volume by nearly 40% and significantly improved neurobehavioral deficits after middle cerebral artery occlusion (MCAO). In the acute early phase (72 h after MCAO), DMF induced Nrf2 expression and its downstream mediator HO-1. In addition to its antioxidant role, DMF also acted as a potent immunomodulator, reducing the infiltration of neutrophils and T-cells as well as the number of activated microglia/ macrophages in the infarct region. Concomitantly, levels of pro-inflammatory cytokines were greatly reduced in the plasma and brain and oxygen–glucose deprived neuron/glia cultures. Further, using a mouse model of transient focal brain ischemia, Yao et al. [37] showed that DMF and MMF (30 mg/kg i.p.) significantly reduced neurological deficits, infarct volume, brain edema, and cell death. Additionally, DMF and MMF suppress glial activation following brain ischemia. Importantly, the protection of DMF and MMF was most evident during the sub-acute stage and was abolished in *Nrf2*$^{-/-}$ mice, indicating that the Nrf2 pathway is required for the beneficial effects of DMF and MMF [37]. In another study, murine organotypic hippocampal slice cultures, and two neuronal cell lines were treated with DMF and MMF [93]. The ischemic condition was generated by exposing cells and slice cultures to oxygen-glucose deprivation. Treatment with both DMF and MMF (30–100 μM) immediately upon reoxygenation strongly reduced cell death in hippocampal cultures *ex vivo*. Both DMF and MMF promoted neuronal survival in HT-22 and SH-SY5Y cell lines exposed to ischemic stress. However, interestingly, DMF but not MMF activated the anti-oxidative Nrf2 pathway in neurons. Accordingly, the protective effect of DMF but not MMF was abrogated in the neurons of Nrf2-deficient mice. These results provide the basis for a new therapeutic approach to treat ischemic pathologies such as stroke using a drug that is already approved by US-FDA for clinical use.

5. Safety profile

By and large, the short-term safety profile for DMF in patients with RMS is highly favorable [64, 65] and long-term safety analyses from the ENDORSE study sustains a favorable benefit: risk ratio [94]. The most common adverse events observed in patients receiving DMF include flushing, gastrointestinal (GI) events (e.g., diarrhea, nausea, abdominal pain, and vomiting), proteinuria, and pruritus [64, 65]. Aspirin pretreatment has been shown to reduce DMF induced adverse GI events [95]. Additionally, the leukotriene-receptor antagonist montelukast has been shown to help as well [96]. Further, it has been observed that consuming a high fat and high protein meal just before DMF administration may reduce GI and flushing side effects by delaying its intestinal absorption. Notably, the risk of lymphopenia is higher in adults older than 55 years, in those with lower baseline lymphocyte counts, and those switching from natalizumab [97]. Cases of multifocal leukoencephalopathy (PML) following DMF treatment have also been reported [98–107]. Highly worthy of mention, however, is the fact that each of the affected patients detailed above had well-known pre-existing risk factors for PML including lymphocytopenia, sarcoidosis, cancer history, and/or prior efalizumab use. Thus, the negative effects of MMF treatment on PML should be interpreted very carefully. Like other pharmacological therapies, DMF/MMF treatment is associated with some side effects importantly however, advancements toward developing improved formulations minimize these events without losing efficacy are already being realized. For example, Alkermes, Inc. has developed diroximel fumarate (DRF), also known as ALKS8700, a novel MMF prodrug. Importantly, this new formulation has been shown to yield bioequivalent levels of MMF at the cellular level when compared directly to DMF (**Figure 1**) [108] while interacting less with off-target proteins and therefore producing fewer unwanted side effects [109]. Indeed, interim findings from EVOLVE-MS-1 and EVOLVE-MS-2 which demonstrate that DRF has a favorable safety and efficacy profile and is well-tolerated in MS patients [108, 110].

6. Conclusions

Drug repurposing is a very viable therapeutic strategy [18]. Many agents approved for other uses already have been tested in humans, so detailed information is available on their pharmacology, formulation and potential side effects. Since repurposing expands upon past innovative endeavors, hopeful new treatments could be prepared for clinical trials rapidly. Historically, pharmaceutical companies have achieved a number of successes via drug repositioning (e.g., for Viagra, thalidomide, metformin, etc.). Based on the literature available, DMF/MMF has been shown to protect against a variety of diseases other than MS and psoriasis.

7. Future perspectives

FAE are perhaps most noted for the robust antioxidant effects that they elicit via Nrf2 induction. A number of additional (non-FAE based) Nrf2 inducing drugs have been developed and tested in experimental and clinical systems in recent years (e.g., resveratrol, sulforaphane, etc.) and several have been with considerable success with regard to potential for clinical development [111]. However, the multimodal actions of FAE make this emerging drug stand out among the rest. It is commonly said that oxidative stress and inflammation go hand-in-hand, meaning that one potentiates the other in somewhat of a cyclic manner. Thus, it can only be hoped that in turn, if one is suppressed then the other similarly complies. However, things are usually not that simple. In the case of FAE, there are two arms of action: one induces Nrf2 and the other interacts with the anti-inflammatory hydroxycarboxylic acid receptor (HCAR2 or HCA2; **Figure 2**). Thus, the compound has a direct impact on inflammation independent of its actions on oxidative stress. The fascinating thing about these two mechanistic arms, is that they appear to act simultaneously in many cell and tissue systems. This may explain why FAE has exceled in so many variable pathologic conditions. MMF through its interaction with HCAR2, which is expressed by primary immune cells and a multitude of accessory immune cells (i.e., those that initiate the immune response and those cells like retinal pigment epithelial cells, for example, that aren't truly "immune" cells but are capable just the same of secreting pro- and anti-inflammatory factors depending upon the stimulus), elicits a tremendous anti-inflammatory response. The combined Nrf2-inducing and immune-modulatory properties of FAE have enabled this drug to be efficacious in a broad range of body systems. The evidence provided in this chapter alone demonstrates convincingly that the benefits of FAE have been realized in the central nervous system (brain and retina), the cardiovascular system, the digestive and/or gastrointestinal system, the immune system, the integumentary system and the renal system; this list continues to grow. Thus, the potential clinical impact of FAE therapy use is high and importantly extremely broad. It is acknowledged that as with virtually all pharmacologic agents, FAE therapy is not without adverse effects. Importantly, however, the effects are relatively mild and the benefit(s) indisputably outweigh the risks. As such, there is a prompt need for additional experimental and clinical studies to translate the information gleaned from exploratory trials of FAE therapy in various cell, tissue, and disease types into clinical use.

Acknowledgements

We would like to acknowledge funding support from the National Eye Institute grants EY022704 and EY029113 to Pamela M. Martin.

Author details

Ravirajsinh N. Jadeja[1], Folami L. Powell[1,2] and Pamela M. Martin[1,2,3]*

1 Department of Biochemistry and Molecular Biology, Medical College of Georgia, Augusta University, Augusta, GA, USA

2 James and Jean Culver Vision Discovery Institute, Augusta University, Augusta, GA, USA

3 Department of Ophthalmology, Medical College of Georgia, Augusta University, Augusta, GA, USA

*Address all correspondence to: pmmartin@augusta.edu

References

[1] Amenta R, Camarda L, Di Stefano V, Lentini F, Venza F. Traditional medicine as a source of new therapeutic agents against psoriasis. Fitoterapia. 2000;**71**(Suppl 1):S13-S20

[2] Schweckendiek W. Treatment of psoriasis vulgaris. Medizinische Monatsschrift. 1959;**13**(2):103-104

[3] Roll A, Reich K, Boer A. Use of fumaric acid esters in psoriasis. Indian Journal of Dermatology, Venereology and Leprology. 2007;**73**(2):133-137

[4] Available from: http://www.voteidaneekmiller.com/tag dimethylfumarate/

[5] Reich K, Thaci D, Mrowietz U, Kamps A, Neureither M, Luger T. Efficacy and safety of fumaric acid esters in the long-term treatment of psoriasis--a retrospective study (FUTURE). Journal der Deutschen Dermatologischen Gesellschaft = Journal of the German Society of Dermatology : JDDG. 2009;**7**(7):603-611

[6] Meissner M, Valesky EM, Kippenberger S, Kaufmann R. Dimethyl fumarate - only an anti-psoriatic medication? Journal der Deutschen Dermatologischen Gesellschaft = Journal of the German Society of Dermatology: JDDG. 2012;**10**(11):793-801

[7] Schimrigk S, Brune N, Hellwig K, Lukas C, Bellenberg B, Rieks M, et al. Oral fumaric acid esters for the treatment of active multiple sclerosis: An open-label, baseline-controlled pilot study. European Journal of Neurology. 2006;**13**(6):604-610

[8] Ruggieri S, Tortorella C, Gasperini C. Pharmacology and clinical efficacy of dimethyl fumarate (BG-12) for treatment of relapsing-remitting multiple sclerosis. Therapeutics and Clinical Risk Management. 2014;**10**:229-239

[9] Fox RJ, Kita M, Cohan SL, Henson LJ, Zambrano J, Scannevin RH, et al. BG-12 (dimethyl fumarate): A review of mechanism of action, efficacy, and safety. Current Medical Research and Opinion. 2014;**30**(2):251-262

[10] Havrdova E, Hutchinson M, Kurukulasuriya NC, Raghupathi K, Sweetser MT, Dawson KT, et al. Oral BG-12 (dimethyl fumarate) for relapsing-remitting multiple sclerosis: A review of DEFINE and CONFIRM. Evaluation of: Gold R, Kappos L, Arnold D, et al. Placebo-controlled phase 3 study of oral BG-12 for relapsing multiple sclerosis. N Engl J Med 2012;367:1098-107; and Fox RJ, Miller DH, Phillips JT, et al. Placebo-controlled phase 3 study of oral BG-12 or glatiramer in multiple sclerosis. N Engl J Med 2012;367:1087-97. Expert Opinion on Pharmacotherapy. 2013;**14**(15):2145-2156

[11] Su W, Kansal A, Vicente C, Deniz B, Sarda S. The cost-effectiveness of delayed-release dimethyl fumarate for the treatment of relapsing-remitting multiple sclerosis in Canada. Journal of Medical Economics. 2016;**19**(7):718-727

[12] Linker RA, Haghikia A. Dimethyl fumarate in multiple sclerosis: Latest developments, evidence and place in therapy. Therapeutic Advances in Chronic Disease. 2016;**7**(4):198-207

[13] Prosperini L, Pontecorvo S. Dimethyl fumarate in the management of multiple sclerosis: Appropriate patient selection and special considerations. Therapeutics and Clinical Risk Management. 2016;**12**:339-350

[14] Deeks ED. Dimethyl Fumarate: A review in relapsing-remitting MS. Drugs. 2016;**76**(2):243-254

[15] Xu Z, Zhang F, Sun F, Gu K, Dong S, He D. Dimethyl fumarate for multiple sclerosis. The Cochrane Database of Systematic Reviews. 2015;**4**:CD011076

[16] Dubey D, Kieseier BC, Hartung HP, Hemmer B, Warnke C, Menge T, et al. Dimethyl fumarate in relapsing-remitting multiple sclerosis: Rationale, mechanisms of action, pharmacokinetics, efficacy and safety. Expert Review of Neurotherapeutics. 2015;**15**(4):339-346

[17] Bomprezzi R. Dimethyl fumarate in the treatment of relapsing-remitting multiple sclerosis: An overview. Therapeutic Advances in Neurological Disorders. 2015;**8**(1):20-30

[18] Cha Y, Erez T, Reynolds IJ, Kumar D, Ross J, Koytiger G, et al. Pharma Perspective on Drug Repurposing. British Journal of Pharmacology. 2017;**175**(2):168-180

[19] Gimenez-Arnau A. Dimethyl fumarate: A human health hazard. Dermatitis: Contact, Atopic, Occupational, Drug. 2011;**22**(1):47-49

[20] Available from: https://pubchem.ncbi.nlm.nih.gov/compound/Dimethyl_fumarate#section=Top

[21] Litjens NH, Burggraaf J, van Strijen E, van Gulpen C, Mattie H, Schoemaker RC, et al. Pharmacokinetics of oral fumarates in healthy subjects. British Journal of Clinical Pharmacology. 2004;**58**(4):429-432

[22] Albrecht P, Bouchachia I, Goebels N, Henke N, Hofstetter HH, Issberner A, et al. Effects of dimethyl fumarate on neuroprotection and immunomodulation. Journal of Neuroinflammation. 2012;**9**:163

[23] Werdenberg D, Joshi R, Wolffram S, Merkle HP, Langguth P. Presystemic metabolism and intestinal absorption of antipsoriatic fumaric acid esters. Biopharmaceutics & Drug Disposition. 2003;**24**(6):259-273

[24] Available from: http://www.accessdata.fda.gov/drugsatfda_docs/label/2013/204063lbl.pdf

[25] Gold R, Linker RA, Stangel M. Fumaric acid and its esters: An emerging treatment for multiple sclerosis with antioxidative mechanism of action. Clinical Immunology. 2012;**142**(1):44-48

[26] Linker RA, Lee DH, Ryan S, van Dam AM, Conrad R, Bista P, et al. Fumaric acid esters exert neuroprotective effects in neuroinflammation via activation of the Nrf2 antioxidant pathway. Brain: A Journal of Neurology. 2011;**134**(Pt 3):678-692

[27] Scannevin RH, Chollate S, Jung MY, Shackett M, Patel H, Bista P, et al. Fumarates promote cytoprotection of central nervous system cells against oxidative stress via the nuclear factor (erythroid-derived 2)-like 2 pathway. The Journal of Pharmacology and Experimental Therapeutics. 2012;**341**(1):274-284

[28] Ananth S, Babu E, Veeranan-Karmegam R, Bozard Baldowski BR, Boettger T, Martin PM. Induction of the cystine/glutamate exchanger SLC7A11 in retinal pigment epithelial cells by the antipsoriatic drug monomethylfumarate. Investigative Ophthalmology & Visual Science. 2013;**54**(3):1592-1602

[29] Chen H, Assmann JC, Krenz A, Rahman M, Grimm M, Karsten CM, et al. Hydroxycarboxylic acid receptor 2 mediates dimethyl fumarate's protective effect in EAE. The Journal of Clinical Investigation. 2014;**124**(5):2188-2192

[30] Parodi B, Rossi S, Morando S, Cordano C, Bragoni A, Motta C, et al. Fumarates modulate microglia activation through a novel HCAR2

signaling pathway and rescue synaptic dysregulation in inflamed CNS. Acta Neuropathologica. 2015;**130**(2):279-295

[31] Hanson J, Gille A, Offermanns S. Role of HCA(2) (GPR109A) in nicotinic acid and fumaric acid ester-induced effects on the skin. Pharmacology & Therapeutics. 2012;**136**(1):1-7

[32] Hanson J, Gille A, Zwykiel S, Lukasova M, Clausen BE, Ahmed K, et al. Nicotinic acid- and monomethyl fumarate-induced flushing involves GPR109A expressed by keratinocytes and COX-2-dependent prostanoid formation in mice. The Journal of Clinical Investigation. 2010;**120**(8):2910-2919

[33] Tang H, Lu JY, Zheng X, Yang Y, Reagan JD. The psoriasis drug monomethylfumarate is a potent nicotinic acid receptor agonist. Biochemical and Biophysical Research Communications. 2008; **375**(4):562-565

[34] Promsote W, Powell FL, Veean S, Thounaojam M, Markand S, Saul A, et al. Oral Monomethyl Fumarate therapy ameliorates retinopathy in a humanized mouse model of sickle cell disease. Antioxidants & Redox Signaling. 2016;**25**(17):921-935

[35] Promsote W, Makala L, Li B, Smith SB, Singh N, Ganapathy V, et al. Monomethylfumarate induces gamma-globin expression and fetal hemoglobin production in cultured human retinal pigment epithelial (RPE) and erythroid cells, and in intact retina. Investigative Ophthalmology & Visual Science. 2014;**55**(8):5382-5393

[36] Lin R, Cai J, Kostuk EW, Rosenwasser R, Iacovitti L. Fumarate modulates the immune/inflammatory response and rescues nerve cells and neurological function after stroke in rats. Journal of Neuroinflammation. 2016;**13**(1):269

[37] Yao Y, Miao W, Liu Z, Han W, Shi K, Shen Y, et al. Dimethyl fumarate and monomethyl fumarate promote post-ischemic recovery in mice. Translational Stroke Research. 2016;**7**(6):535-547

[38] Casili G, Cordaro M, Impellizzeri D, Bruschetta G, Paterniti I, Cuzzocrea S, et al. Dimethyl Fumarate reduces inflammatory responses in experimental colitis. Journal of Crohn's & Colitis. 2016;**10**(4):472-483

[39] Shakya A, Soni UK, Rai G, Chatterjee SS, Kumar V. Gastro-protective and anti-stress efficacies of Monomethyl Fumarate and a Fumaria indica extract in chronically stressed rats. Cellular and Molecular Neurobiology. 2016;**36**(4):621-635

[40] Zhao X, Sun G, Zhang J, Ting SM, Gonzales N, Aronowski J. Dimethyl fumarate protects brain from damage produced by intracerebral hemorrhage by mechanism involving Nrf2. Stroke. 2015;**46**(7):1923-1928

[41] Iniaghe LO, Krafft PR, Klebe DW, Omogbai EK, Zhang JH, Tang J. Dimethyl fumarate confers neuroprotection by casein kinase 2 phosphorylation of Nrf2 in murine intracerebral hemorrhage. Neurobiology of Disease. 2015;**82**:349-358

[42] Takasu C, Vaziri ND, Li S, Robles L, Vo K, Takasu M, et al. Treatment with dimethyl Fumarate attenuates Calcineurin inhibitor-induced nephrotoxicity. Transplantation. 2015;**99**(6):1144-1150

[43] Kume T, Suenaga A, Izumi Y, Akaike A. Protective effect of dimethyl Fumarate on an oxidative stress model induced by sodium Nitroprusside in mice. Biological & Pharmaceutical Bulletin. 2016;**39**(6):1055-1059

[44] Robles L, Vaziri ND, Li S, Masuda Y, Takasu C, Takasu M, et al. Dimethyl fumarate protects pancreatic islet cells

and non-endocrine tissue in L-arginine-induced chronic pancreatitis. PLoS One. 2014;**9**(9):e107111

[45] Robles L, Vaziri ND, Li S, Takasu C, Masuda Y, Vo K, et al. Dimethyl fumarate ameliorates acute pancreatitis in rodent. Pancreas. 2015;**44**(3):441-447

[46] Zhang WX, Zhao JH, Ping FM, Liu ZJ, Gu JX, Lu XQ. Effect of dimethyl fumarate on rats with chronic pancreatitis. Asian Pacific Journal of Tropical Medicine. 2016;**9**(3):261-264

[47] Jing X, Shi H, Zhang C, Ren M, Han M, Wei X, et al. Dimethyl fumarate attenuates 6-OHDA-induced neurotoxicity in SH-SY5Y cells and in animal model of Parkinson's disease by enhancing Nrf2 activity. Neuroscience. 2015;**286**:131-140

[48] Ahuja M, Ammal Kaidery N, Yang L, Calingasan N, Smirnova N, Gaisin A, et al. Distinct Nrf2 Signaling mechanisms of fumaric acid esters and their role in neuroprotection against 1-Methyl-4-Phenyl-1,2,3,6-tetrahydropyridine-induced experimental Parkinson's-like disease. The Journal of Neuroscience. 2016;**36**(23):6332-6351

[49] Lastres-Becker I, Garcia-Yague AJ, Scannevin RH, Casarejos MJ, Kugler S, Rabano A, et al. Repurposing the NRF2 activator dimethyl fumarate as therapy against Synucleinopathy in Parkinson's disease. Antioxidants & Redox Signaling. 2016;**25**(2):61-77

[50] Campolo M, Casili G, Biundo F, Crupi R, Cordaro M, Cuzzocrea S, et al. The neuroprotective effect of dimethyl Fumarate in an MPTP-mouse model of Parkinson's disease: Involvement of reactive oxygen species/nuclear factor-kappaB/nuclear transcription factor related to NF-E2. Antioxidants & Redox Signaling. 2017

[51] Cho H, Hartsock MJ, Xu Z, He M, Duh EJ. Monomethyl fumarate promotes Nrf2-dependent neuroprotection in retinal ischemia-reperfusion. Journal of Neuroinflammation. 2015;**12**:239

[52] Jiang D, Ryals RC, Huang SJ, Weller KK, Titus HE, Robb BM, et al. Monomethyl fumarate protects the retina from light-induced retinopathy. Investigative Ophthalmology & Visual Science. 2019;**60**(4):1275-1285

[53] Giustina AD, Bonfante S, Zarbato GF, Danielski LG, Mathias K, de Oliveira AN Jr, et al. Dimethyl Fumarate modulates oxidative stress and inflammation in organs after Sepsis in rats. Inflammation. 2018;**41**(1):315-327

[54] Zarbato GF, de Souza Goldim MP, Giustina AD, Danielski LG, Mathias K, Florentino D, et al. Dimethyl fumarate limits neuroinflammation and oxidative stress and improves cognitive impairment after polymicrobial sepsis. Neurotoxicity Research. 2018;**34**(3):418-430

[55] Shalmani AA, Ghahremani MH, Jeivad F, Shadboorestan A, Hassanzadeh G, Beh-Pajooh A, et al. Monomethyl fumarate alleviates sepsis-induced hepatic dysfunction by regulating TLR-4/NF-kappaB signalling pathway. Life Sciences. 2018;**215**:152-158

[56] Belcher JD, Chen C, Nguyen J, Zhang P, Abdulla F, Nguyen P, et al. Control of oxidative stress and inflammation in sickle cell disease with the Nrf2 activator dimethyl Fumarate. Antioxidants & Redox Signaling. 2016

[57] Cordaro M, Casili G, Paterniti I, Cuzzocrea S, Esposito E. Fumaric acid esters attenuate secondary degeneration following spinal cord injury. Journal of Neurotrauma. 2016;**34**(21):3027-3040

[58] Kim DH, Cheon JH. Pathogenesis of inflammatory bowel disease and recent

advances in biologic therapies. Immune Network. 2017;**17**(1):25-40

[59] Bettenworth D, Rieder F. Pathogenesis of intestinal fibrosis in inflammatory bowel disease and perspectives for therapeutic implication. Digestive Diseases. 2017;**35**(1-2):25-31

[60] Kim HS, Berstad A. Experimental colitis in animal models. Scandinavian Journal of Gastroenterology. 1992;**27**(7):529-537

[61] Low D, Nguyen DD, Mizoguchi E. Animal models of ulcerative colitis and their application in drug research. Drug Design, Development and Therapy. 2013;**7**:1341-1357

[62] Mrowietz U, Morrison PJ, Suhrkamp I, Kumanova M, Clement B. The pharmacokinetics of Fumaric acid esters reveal their In vivo effects. Trends in Pharmacological Sciences. 2018;**39**(1):1-12

[63] Fox EJ, Vasquez A, Grainger W, Ma TS, von Hehn C, Walsh J, et al. Gastrointestinal tolerability of delayed-release dimethyl Fumarate in a Multicenter, open-label study of patients with relapsing forms of multiple sclerosis (MANAGE). International Journal of MS Care. 2016;**18**(1):9-18

[64] Fox RJ, Miller DH, Phillips JT, Hutchinson M, Havrdova E, Kita M, et al. Placebo-controlled phase 3 study of oral BG-12 or glatiramer in multiple sclerosis. The New England Journal of Medicine. 2012;**367**(12):1087-1097

[65] Gold R, Kappos L, Arnold DL, Bar-Or A, Giovannoni G, Selmaj K, et al. Placebo-controlled phase 3 study of oral BG-12 for relapsing multiple sclerosis. The New England Journal of Medicine. 2012;**367**(12):1098-1107

[66] Rao KS, Mishra SH. Antihepatotoxic activity of monomethyl fumarate isolated from Fumaria indica. Journal of Ethnopharmacology. 1998;**60**(3):207-213

[67] Abdelrahman RS, Abdel-Rahman N. Dimethyl fumarate ameliorates acetaminophen-induced hepatic injury in mice dependent of Nrf-2/HO-1 pathway. Life Sciences. 2019;**217**:251-260

[68] Bjelobaba I, Savic D, Lavrnja I. Multiple sclerosis and Neuroinflammation: The overview of current and prospective therapies. Current Pharmaceutical Design. 2017;**23**(5):693-730

[69] Gupta N, Shyamasundar S, Patnala R, Karthikeyan A, Arumugam TV, Ling EA, et al. Recent progress in therapeutic strategies for microglia-mediated neuroinflammation in neuropathologies. Expert Opinion on Therapeutic Targets. 2018;**22**(9):765-781

[70] Cross SA, Cook DR, Chi AW, Vance PJ, Kolson LL, Wong BJ, et al. Dimethyl fumarate, an immune modulator and inducer of the antioxidant response, suppresses HIV replication and macrophage-mediated neurotoxicity: A novel candidate for HIV neuroprotection. Journal of Immunology. 2011;**187**(10):5015-5025

[71] Ambrosius B, Faissner S, Guse K, von Lehe M, Grunwald T, Gold R, et al. Teriflunomide and monomethylfumarate target HIV-induced neuroinflammation and neurotoxicity. Journal of Neuroinflammation. 2017;**14**(1):51

[72] Han RR, Xiao JT, Zhai H, Hao JW. Dimethyl fumarate attenuates experimental autoimmune neuritis through the nuclear factor erythroid-derived 2-related factor 2/ hemoxygenase-1 pathway by altering the balance of M1/M2 macrophages. Journal of Neuroinflammation. 2016;**13**

[73] Namba T, Huttner WB. Neural progenitor cells and their role in the development and evolutionary expansion of the neocortex. Wiley Interdisciplinary Reviews: Developmental Biology. 2017;**6**(1)

[74] Tang Y, Illes P. Regulation of adult neural progenitor cell functions by purinergic signaling. Glia. 2017;**65**(2):213-230

[75] Wang Q , Chuikov S, Taitano S, Wu Q , Rastogi A, Tuck SJ, et al. Dimethyl fumarate protects neural stem/progenitor cells and neurons from oxidative damage through Nrf2-ERK1/2 MAPK pathway. International Journal of Molecular Sciences. 2015;**16**(6):13885-13907

[76] Manohar M, Verma AK, Venkateshaiah SU, Sanders NL, Mishra A. Pathogenic mechanisms of pancreatitis. World Journal of Gastrointestinal Pharmacology and Therapeutics. 2017;**8**(1):10-25

[77] Uttara B, Singh AV, Zamboni P, Mahajan RT. Oxidative stress and neurodegenerative diseases: A review of upstream and downstream antioxidant therapeutic options. Current Neuropharmacology. 2009;**7**(1):65-74

[78] Kim GH, Kim JE, Rhie SJ, Yoon S. The role of oxidative stress in neurodegenerative diseases. Experimental Neurobiology. 2015;**24**(4):325-340

[79] Albarracin SL, Stab B, Casas Z, Sutachan JJ, Samudio I, Gonzalez J, et al. Effects of natural antioxidants in neurodegenerative disease. Nutritional Neuroscience. 2012;**15**(1):1-9

[80] Feng Y, Wang X. Antioxidant therapies for Alzheimer's disease. Oxidative Medicine and Cellular Longevity. 2012;**2012**:472932

[81] Fellner L, Jellinger KA, Wenning GK, Stefanova N. Glial dysfunction in the pathogenesis of alpha-synucleinopathies: Emerging concepts. Acta Neuropathologica. 2011;**121**(6):675-693

[82] Bozard BR, Chothe PP, Tawfik A, Williams C, Fulzele S, Prasad PD, et al. Regulation of proton-coupled folate transporter in retinal Muller cells by the antipsoriatic drug monomethylfumarate. Glia. 2012;**60**(3):333-342

[83] Macari ER, Lowrey CH. Induction of human fetal hemoglobin via the NRF2 antioxidant response signaling pathway. Blood. 2011;**117**(22):5987-5997

[84] Ganapathy V, Martin PM. Inventor. Augusta University Research Institute Inc, Assignee. Methods of Treating Sickle Cell Disease and Related Disorders Using Fumaric Acid Esters. United States; 2017

[85] Gotts JE, Matthay MA. Sepsis: Pathophysiology and clinical management. BMJ. 2016;**353**:i1585

[86] Kato GJ, Hebbel RP, Steinberg MH, Gladwin MT. Vasculopathy in sickle cell disease: Biology, pathophysiology, genetics, translational medicine, and new research directions. American Journal of Hematology. 2009;**84**(9):618-625

[87] Schaer DJ, Buehler PW, Alayash AI, Belcher JD, Vercellotti GM. Hemolysis and free hemoglobin revisited: Exploring hemoglobin and hemin scavengers as a novel class of therapeutic proteins. Blood. 2013;**121**(8):1276-1284

[88] Belcher JD, Chen C, Nguyen J, Milbauer L, Abdulla F, Alayash AI, et al. Heme triggers TLR4 signaling leading to endothelial cell activation and vaso-occlusion in murine sickle cell disease. Blood. 2014;**123**(3):377-390

[89] Chen S, Levi AD. Restorative treatments for spinal cord injury. Neurosurgery Clinics of North America. 2017;**28**(1):63-71

[90] Karsy M, Hawryluk G. Pharmacologic Management of Acute Spinal Cord Injury. Neurosurgery Clinics of North America. 2017;**28**(1): 49-62

[91] Facecchia K, Fochesato LA, Ray SD, Stohs SJ, Pandey S. Oxidative toxicity in neurodegenerative diseases: Role of mitochondrial dysfunction and therapeutic strategies. Journal of Toxicology. 2011;**2011**:683728

[92] Johnson JA, Johnson DA, Kraft AD, Calkins MJ, Jakel RJ, Vargas MR, et al. The Nrf2-ARE pathway: An indicator and modulator of oxidative stress in neurodegeneration. Annals of the New York Academy of Sciences. 2008;**1147**:61-69

[93] Lin-Holderer J, Li L, Gruneberg D, Marti HH, Kunze R. Fumaric acid esters promote neuronal survival upon ischemic stress through activation of the Nrf2 but not HIF-1 signaling pathway. Neuropharmacology. 2016;**105**:228-240

[94] Gold R, Giovannoni G, Phillips JT, Fox RJ, Zhang A, Marantz JL. Sustained effect of delayed-release dimethyl Fumarate in newly diagnosed patients with relapsing-remitting multiple sclerosis: 6-year interim results from an extension of the DEFINE and CONFIRM studies. Neurology and Therapy. 2016;**5**(1):45-57

[95] O'Gorman J, Russell HK, Li J, Phillips G, Kurukulasuriya NC, Viglietta V. Effect of aspirin Pretreatment or slow dose titration on flushing and gastrointestinal events in healthy volunteers receiving delayed-release dimethyl Fumarate. Clinical Therapeutics. 2015;**37**(7):1402-1419 e5

[96] Carlo Tornatore JW, Mann M, Li J, Von Hehn C. Effect of montelukast on gastrointestinal tolerability in patients with relapsing forms of multiple sclerosis receiving delayed-release dimethyl fumarate: A multicenter, randomized, double-blind, placebo-controlled study (MITIGATE). Neurology. 2015;**84**(14 Supplement P1127)

[97] Longbrake EE, Naismith RT, Parks BJ, Wu GF, Cross AH. Dimethyl fumarate-associated lymphopenia: Risk factors and clinical significance. Multiple Sclerosis Journal - Experimental, Translational and Clinical. 2015;**1**:1-8

[98] Buttmann M, Stoll G. Case reports of PML in patients treated for psoriasis. The New England journal of medicine. 2013;**369**(11):1081

[99] Ermis U, Weis J, Schulz JB. PML in a patient treated with fumaric acid. The New England journal of medicine. 2013;**368**(17):1657-1658

[100] van Oosten BW, Killestein J, Barkhof F, Polman CH, Wattjes MP. PML in a patient treated with dimethyl fumarate from a compounding pharmacy. The New England journal of medicine. 2013;**368**(17):1658-1659

[101] Stoppe M, Thoma E, Liebert UG, Major EO, Hoffmann KT, Classen J, et al. Cerebellar manifestation of PML under fumarate and after efalizumab treatment of psoriasis. Journal of Neurology. 2014;**261**(5):1021-1024

[102] Dammeier N, Schubert V, Hauser TK, Bornemann A, Bischof F. Case report of a patient with progressive multifocal leukoencephalopathy under treatment with dimethyl fumarate. BMC Neurology. 2015;**15**:108

[103] Nieuwkamp DJ, Murk JL, van Oosten BW, Cremers CH, Killestein J, Viveen MC, et al. PML in a patient without severe lymphocytopenia

receiving dimethyl fumarate. The New England journal of medicine. 2015;**372**(15):1474-1476

[104] Baharnoori M, Lyons J, Dastagir A, Koralnik I, Stankiewicz JM. Nonfatal PML in a patient with multiple sclerosis treated with dimethyl fumarate. Neurology(R) neuroimmunology & neuroinflammation. 2016;**3**(5):e274

[105] Lehmann-Horn K, Penkert H, Grein P, Leppmeier U, Teuber-Hanselmann S, Hemmer B, et al. PML during dimethyl fumarate treatment of multiple sclerosis: How does lymphopenia matter? Neurology. 2016;**87**(4):440-441

[106] Nieuwkamp DJ, Murk JL, van Oosten BW. PML in patients treated with dimethyl Fumarate. The New England journal of medicine. 2015;**373**(6):584

[107] Carruthers RL, Healy BC. PML in DMF-treated patients with normal lymphocytes: Worried well or well to be worried? Multiple Sclerosis. 2016;**22**(3):394-395

[108] Naismith RT, Wolinsky JS, Wundes A, LaGanke C, Arnold DL, Obradovic D, et al. Diroximel fumarate (DRF) in patients with relapsing-remitting multiple sclerosis: Interim safety and efficacy results from the phase 3 EVOLVE-MS-1 study. Multiple Sclerosis. 2019:1352458519881761

[109] Palte MJ, Wehr A, Tawa M, Perkin K, Leigh-Pemberton R, Hanna J, et al. Improving the gastrointestinal tolerability of Fumaric acid esters: Early findings on gastrointestinal events with Diroximel Fumarate in patients with relapsing-remitting multiple sclerosis from the phase 3, open-label EVOLVE-MS-1 study. Advances in Therapy. 2019;**36**(11):3154-3165

[110] Naismith RT, Wundes A, Ziemssen T, Jasinska E, Freedman MS, Lembo AJ, et al. Diroximel fumarate demonstrates an improved gastrointestinal tolerability profile compared with dimethyl fumarate in patients with relapsing-remitting multiple sclerosis: Results from the randomized, double-blind, phase III EVOLVE-MS-2 study. CNS Drugs. 2020;**34**(2):185-196

[111] Robledinos-Antón N, Fernández-Ginés R, Manda G, Cuadrado A. Activators and inhibitors of NRF2: A review of their potential for clinical development. Oxidative Medicine and Cellular Longevity. 2019;**2019**:9372182

5

Repurposing Infectious Pathogen Vaccines in Cancer Immunotherapy

Matteo Conti

Abstract

Reports in the literature show that certain vaccines against infectious pathogens, can be effective in eliciting antitumor immune response when injected intratumorally. In mouse tumor models, intratumoral delivery of rotavirus, yellow fever, and influenza vaccines have been shown to also synergize with checkpoint inhibitors, in the leading immunotherapy in the clinical practice today. The combined approach can thus become a very promising novel strategy for anti-cancer immunotherapy. In humans, an attenuated poliomyelitis virus vaccine, a peptide-based vaccines against papilloma and one based on detoxified diphtheria protein have already been tested as intratumoral treatments readily. In those studies, the role of available anti-pathogen immunity appears an important element in mediating the activity of the repurposed vaccines against cancer. We therefore suggest how evaluating or eventually developing anti-pathogen immunity before intratumoral delivery could be helpful in repurposing infectious pathogen vaccines in cancer immunotherapy.
Keywords: cancer immunotherapy, cancer vaccines, repurposed vaccines, infectious agents vaccines, intratumoral delivery

1. Introduction

The immune system is physiologically able to detect and destroy abnormal cells and to curb the growth of clinically meaningful cancers [1]. However, during carcinogenesis, immune tolerance and immunosuppression mechanisms become more and more prevalent and critically detectable tumor masses start to appear in patients [2]. Recognized mechanisms are for instance: (1) genetic changes that make cancer cells less visible to the immune system [3], (2) release of specific molecular factors that subvert normal mesenchymal cells and certain immune cells into alleys [3, 4], (3) expression and/or overexpression of specific cancer cell surface proteins, such as checkpoint regulators, that directly inhibit immune cell activation [5].

Figure 1 provides an overview of the immunosuppressive interplay between a cancerous cell and the immune system into the tumor microenvironment. Cancer cells modulate their expression of receptors, release specific molecules and microvesicles in order not only to avoid destruction but to also recruit immune system components in their favor.

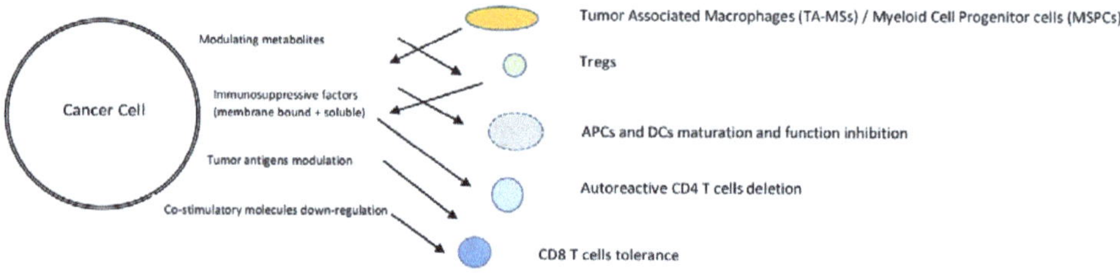

Figure 1.
Immune regulation within the tumor microenvironment.

Only quite recently scientists have started to learn how to interfere with such mechanisms and several types of immunotherapies (**Table 1**) have become available to clinicians [6, 7].

One main area of anticancer immunotherapy is that of adoptive cell transfer (ACT) therapy, which has shown remarkable activity against blood malignancies and even solid tumors [8–10]. In this therapy, immune cells are taken from patients' blood, selected, cultured, genetically modified and multiplied in the laboratory, before being reinfused to patients. Chimeric antigen receptor (CAR) T cells, in particular, are genetically modified in order to express specific very efficient receptors able to target cancer cells. These techniques actually require very special laboratories and expensive resources to be performed. Therefore, they are still out of reach for most of the patients worldwide.

Figure 2 is a schematic representation of chimeric antigen receptor (CAR) constructs delivered by retroviral transfection in T cell collected from patients and grown in culture. First-generation constructs employ a single-chain variable fragment (SCvf) connected by a linker to a transmembrane domain and an intracellular signaling domain. In second-generation constructs, one co-stimulatory domain (such as 4-1BB) has been added. In third-generation constructs, two co-stimulatory domains (such as 4-1BB or CD 134) have been employed. In fourth-generation constructs, a transgene protein for cytokines or chemokines has also been added. Despite this elaborated design, much research is still needed in order to improve CAR T cells efficacy and limit or control their toxicity.

Approved drug	Immunotherapeutic category
Nivolumab, pembrolizumab	Anti-PD-1 monoclonal antibodies
Atezolizumab, darvalumab, avelumab	Anti-PDL-1 monoclonal antibodies
Ipilimumab	Anti-CTLA-4 monoclonal antibodies
Sipuleucel-T	Dendritic cell-based vaccines
Tisagenlecleucel, axicabtagene ciloleucel (CD19 targeting)	CAR T cells
Talimogene laherparepvec	Oncolytic viruses
recombinant IL-2 and INFa	Immunostimulants
Imiquimod (TLR7 agonist)	Toll-like receptor agonists

Recently FDA-approved immunotherapies (left column) with indication of respective immunotherapeutic categories (right column).

Table 1.
Recent milestone drugs approved for immune oncology.

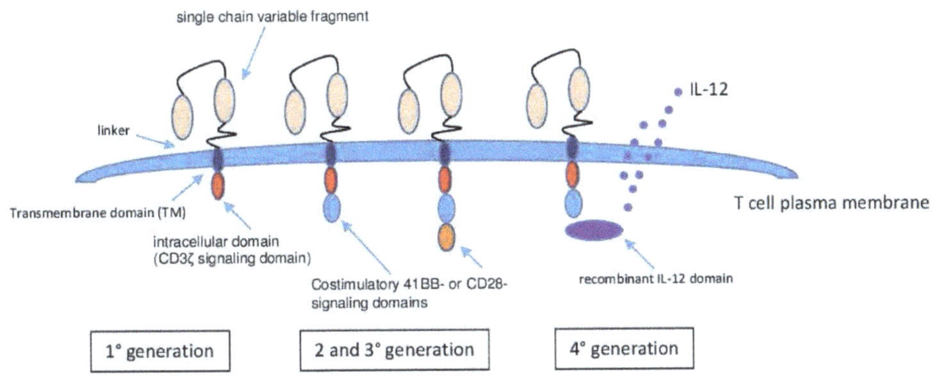

Figure 2.
Chimeric antigen receptor (CAR) constructs.

Checkpoint inhibitors (CIs) are monoclonal antibodies developed to specifically target checkpoint regulators that are responsible of immunosuppression by cancer cells in many cases. They are arguably becoming the most successful agents in the clinical practice. Some of them are already approved by regulatory agencies and broadly used in oncology practice (cf. **Table 1**). They show considerable efficacy, albeit still in a small percentage of patients, and much research is needed in order to improve their efficacy, avoid resistance development by cancer cells, and, also, reduce their systemic toxicity [10–12].

According to various reports, CIs efficacy is very much dependent on the presence and the number of tumor-infiltrating lymphocytes (TILs) in tumor lesions [5] and so various strategies in clinical trials try to increase tumor recognition by the immune system, to turn cold turn cold (immunosuppressed) tumors into hot (immunoactive) ones [11, 13].

CIs are combined with chemotherapy which, inducing cytolysis and release of neoan tigens, can trigger an activation of the immune system. The problem with this approach is that most chemotherapies are myelotoxic and immunosuppressive in nature, to the point that the immune system can become so weakened and impaired to effectively fight against left-over cancer cells. Chemotherapeutic agents, such as cyclophosphamide and gemcitabine, having relatively lower myelotoxic effects, appear among the best candidates for this approach [14–16].

Radiotherapy is also employed because it is able to cause immunogenic cell death, cytolysis, and neoantigen release [14, 17–19]. In principle, it should induce lesser systemic immunosuppression than chemotherapy. In addition, the so-called abscopal effect enable extending immunotherapeutic effects to nonirradiated lesions [20].

Other physics-based techniques, such as cryotherapy, radiofrequency, electrochemotherapy, phototherapy, chemoembolization, and others, can synergize with CIs as well, by causing release of neoantigens secondary to induced cancer cell death [20–22].

Another interesting area of combination therapy with CIs is that with intratumoral delivery of pathogen-associated molecules, which could be used to activate the immune system inside the tumor microenvironment. This approach is the focus of the next sections of this writing. It must be pointed out that it heavily relies on the possibility of delivering molecules directly into tumor lesions by interventional radiology/oncology techniques, because if delivered systemically these molecules would be neutralised by the immune system before they could even reach their target [23–25].

2. Intratumoral delivery of pathogen-associated molecules

Probably the most famous historical account on the use of pathogens to treat tumors is that of William Coley. He was the first to report the observation that soft tissue sarcoma could naturally regress after bacterial infections. Facing cases in his clinical practice, he then proceeded to cause such risky infections on purpose, using bacterial-derived material (Coley's toxins) to locally inject tumor masses, observing successful tumor regression in some case [26–28].

Another well-known example of an infectious pathogen used for local tumor treatment is that of Calmette-Guerrin bacillus for transurethral instillation in urothelial carcinoma [29].

We are today able to deliver much better defined preparations of engineered recombinant viruses and bacteria into tumors, as well as of a variety of pathogen-derived molecules to trigger the immune response. In general, the presence of pathogens is sensed by specialized immune cell receptors [30].

Main families of these receptors are: toll-like receptors (TLRs) on the plasma membrane and in endosomal compartments, cytoplasmic receptors for viral nucleic acids, such as retinoic acid-induced gene 1 (RIG-I), melanoma differentiation-associated protein 5 (MDA-5), stimulator of interferon genes (STING), and the intracellular nucleotide-binding oligomerization domain-like receptors (NOD) family of receptors. They are also entangled and shared by those that detect stressful cell death (DAMPs) secondary to infectious conditions. Therefore, many types of PAMP and DAMP agonists are under study alone and/or in combination with other immune system activators, such as CIs but also immune cell direct activators and growth stimulators.

Pharmaceutical formulations of polyinosinic: polycytosinic acids (poly I:C) can mimic double-stranded RNA molecules of viral origin sensed by the endosomal TLR3 receptors and by the intracellular RIG-I and MDA-5 sensors, and have been studied in transplantable mouse tumors, yielding good results in combination with checkpoint inhibitors [31]. Stabilized poly I:C formulation (poly ICLC, Hiltonol) has been employed for intratumoral delivery as monotherapy and/or in combination, in a few clinical trials [31–33].

TLR7/8 natural agonists imiquimod and resiquimod have been used against basal cell carcinoma [34, 35], melanoma, and other skin neoplasms [36] as well as against common warts [37, 38]. Local imiquimod has also been used in combination with radiotherapy for breast cancer in the clinic [39]. Intratumoral administration of TLR7/8 agonist NKTR-262 is being studied in patients with locally advanced or metastatic solid tumors (NCT03435640). Preliminary results from the phase I/II REVEAL trial noted a disease control rate of about 50% [40].

Intratumoral delivery of TLR9 agonists CpG oligonucleotides has been employed very successfully in mouse models and seen to be able to even determine cancer eradication by the immune system [41]; but, it failed to provide clear benefits in clinical trials [42, 43]. A combination of a CpG oligonucleotide with an agonistic anti-OX40 antibody intratumorally administered both in syngeneic transplanted and genetically determined tumor models was able to induce complete tumor eradication in mice [44] and the combination of these two agents (namely SD-101 and BMS 986178) is now under testing in ongoing trial against a variety of tumors (NCT03831295).

Intratumoral injection of STING-agonist dinucleotides can be another way to unleash the curative tumor response against transplantable mouse models [45]. Human STING agonist adu-s100, for instance, is undergoing clinical development (NCT 02675439).

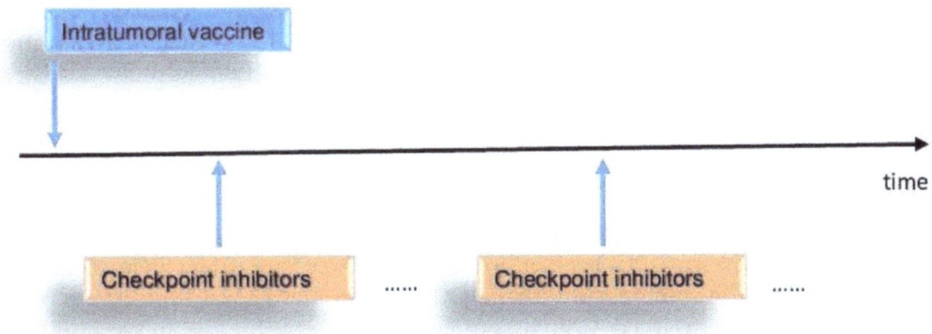

Figure 3.
Schematic diagram of the neoadjuvant intratumoral delivery of a therapeutic vaccine.

All these immune activators should be delivered intratumorally, ideally in a neoadjuvant setting, in order to synergize with current systemic immunotherapies (**Figure 3**).

3. Intratumoral delivery of pathogens

Entire pathogens, in particular recombinant oncolytic viruses, have been engineered to sustain selective replication into malignant cells [46, 47]. However, experience with the use of these oncolytic viruses, originally thought as cytolytic agents, has shown that antitumor immune response against viral-infected cells is a fundamental factor for their anticancer efficacy [48]. Therefore, modern viral vectors are genetically engineered to also express cytokines and other immune stimulating factors [49].

Vaccinia and herpes viruses have proven most effective when engineered to encode for immune-promoting genes such as interleukin 12 (IL-12) and granulocyte macrophage colony-stimulating factor (GM-CSF) [49, 50]. These agents are dramatically enhanced in their therapeutic performances by concomitant administration of PD-1/PDL-1 and CTLA-4 blocking Abs [51] as well as anti-CD137 or anti-OX40 agonist Abs [52–54]. Vectors based on vaccinia virus encoding GM-CSF (JX-594) are also under clinical development with promising results [55, 56].

The most successful agent so far in this category is herpes virus (HSV-1) modified to encode GM-CSF, named T-vec (talimogene). It has been granted Food and Drug Administration approval for unresectable melanoma [57]. Essentially, engineered pathogen preparations are delivered intratumorally in the neoadjuvant setting (essentially according to the scheme in **Figure 3**).

4. Clinical trials on intratumorally delivered pathogens and pathogen-associated molecules

Immunotherapies do not come without adverse effects and complications. In addition, patients have their own peculiarities and it is vital that clinicians identify the best therapeutic options for each one of them. In this light, there are various ongoing clinical trials evaluating intratumoral immunotherapies based on pathogen-associated molecules, alone or in combination with other therapies [25]. Poly-ICLC (Hiltonol) is in phase I against prostate cancer (NCT03262103); TLR7 agonist (Imiquimod) is in phase III against melanoma (NCT01720407);

TLR9 agonist (CMP-001) in combination with Anti-PD-1 (Nivolumab) is in phase II against melanoma and lymph node cancer (NCT03618641); and TLR8 agonist (VTX-2337) in combination with Anti-PD-1 (Tislelizumab) is in phase I against head and neck cancer (NCT03906526). JX-594 (Oncolytic virus) is in phase II against colorectal carcinoma (NCT01329809); and T-VEC (Oncolytic virus) is in phase II against melanoma (NCT02211131), in combination with Anti-PD-L1 (Atezolizumab) in phase I against breast cancer (NCT03802604), in combination with chemotherapy in phase I/II against breast cancer (NCT02779855), in combination with Anti-PD-1 (Pembrolizumab) in phase II against melanoma (NCT03842943), in combination with BRAF Inhibitor and MEK Inhibitor in phase II against melanoma (NCT03972046), in combination with radiotherapy in phase I/II against soft tissue sarcoma (NCT02453191), in combination with chemotherapy, radiotherapy, in phase I against rectal cancer (NCT03300544). Rilimogene gal-vacirepvec (PROSTVAC) in combination with Anti-PD-L1 (Atezolizumab) is in phase II against prostate adenocarcinoma (NCT04020094); GMCI (Adenovirus) in combination with radiotherapy, chemotherapy, is in phase II against pancreatic adenocarcinoma (NCT02446093); and HF10 (Oncolytic virus) in combination with Anti-PD-1 (Nivolumab) is in phase II against melanoma (NCT03259425). OrienX010 (Oncolytic virus) in combination with Anti-PD-1 (Treprizumab) is in phase I against melanoma (NCT04197882).

5. Intratumoral delivery of repurposed vaccines

Success with T-vec and other immune-boosting viruses have prompted various groups to search among routinely available attenuated viral vaccines to find other therapeutic options. The advantage of repurposing such approved and marketed agents is that clinical development would be much simplified, based on well-established safety records [58].

Commercially available attenuated rotavirus vaccines are preparations of double-stranded RNA attenuated strains. They are very potent stimulators of the nuclear factor kappa-light-chain-enhancer of activated B cells and type I interferon pathways. Interestingly, this stimulation is independent from the innate Toll-like immune receptors but dependent on RIG-I, which is able to detect intracytoplasmic dsRNA. Furthermore, rotavirus exerts cytocidal effects on adult and pediatric cancer cell lines in culture with features of immunogenic cell death. Intratumoral delivery to mouse bearing transplantable tumors, including pediatric syngeneic neuroblastoma models, elicited clear therapeutic effects medi-ated by natural killer (NK) cells and CD4 and CD8 T cells. In models of tumors refractory to checkpoint inhibitors, intratumoral rotavirus enabled to overcome resistance. Prevaccination of mice prior such intratumoral virotherapy did not spoil its efficacy [59].

A vaccine based on the 17D strain of the yellow fever virus, commonly used for travelers and dwellers in endemic areas, was demonstrated cytocidal for a large panel of human and mouse tumor cell lines. Its intratumoral administration was able to delay tumor progression by activating CD8 T cell-mediated immunity and some measurable effect could be observed against non-injected tumor lesions [60]. Additive effects with systemic immunostimulatory monoclonal antibodies directed to anti-PD1 or anti-CD137 were demonstrated. Very importantly, efficacy was potentiated by previous vaccination against the same virus in a manner dependent on T-cell antiviral acquired immunity [61].

Intratumoral injections of anti-influenza vaccines were also demonstrated to elicit immune-mediated antitumor activity in melanoma, in a series of experiments with syngeneic transplantable tumor model [62]. Most surprisingly, only unadjuvanted inactivated influenza vaccines were able to generate such antitumor efficacy. Indeed, squalene-based adjuvanted influenza vaccines were losing their antitumor activity because adjuvants were recruiting interleukin-10-secreting B regulatory cells [62]. The detrimental role of adjuvants was observed in another seminal study when analyzing the cause of a lack of therapeutic enhancement of anti–CTLA-4 monotherapy by concurrent vaccination with gp100 peptide in incomplete Freund's adjuvant (IFA) [63].

Genetically engineered poliovirus vaccine antitumor activity was studied in mice a few years ago [64]. It has later been moved to a phase I clinical trial for recurrent glioblastoma with interesting results [65]. In this study, patients were pre-immunized with the vaccine against poliomyelitis and then treated intratumorally with the genetically engineered virus. The role of previously developed immunity was important for successful activation of immunity against tumors treated locally [65].

In an older phase I-II trial, a recombinant nontoxic diphtheria protein (CRM197), used in many common vaccines, was used to treat a variety of accessible tumors by local delivery. Response was observed in patients that had an already developed immunization (measured both by IgG titer and delayed type hypersensi-tivity) against diphtheria [66].

Since immunosuppression mechanisms are in place in the tumor microenvironment [67], from these examples it is clear that an effective immunity developed outside tumors could enable a better response when antigens are later delivered intratumorally. The fact that developing immunity outside the tumor microenvironment is a valuable strategy has been also demonstrated in the case of a new neoantigen vaccine formulation. In fact, the biomaterial-based vaccine prevented the engraftment of AML cells when administered as a prophylactic and when combined with chemotherapy, and eradicated, established AML even in the absence of a defined vaccine antigen [67, 68].

As a last example, a recent Report in JAMA Dermatology suggested that Gardasil®9 might be employed for cancer treatment. Cutaneous basaloid squamous cell carcinoma (BSCC) was eradicated by intratumoral administration of the vaccine. Preventive systemic immunization was performed by a standard initial dose and a booster one, followed by intratumoral delivery of the same vaccine into just a few of the largest lesions, injected monthly over the next months. During this relatively long period, even tumors that had not been injected went into complete regression. Notably, no recurrence was observed in the follow-up period (18 months). This report first presents clinical evidence that a prophylactic antiviral vaccine may be used as an effective immunotherapy for cancer [69].

All mentioned studies point out to the value of a therapeutic strategy outlined in **Figure 4**.

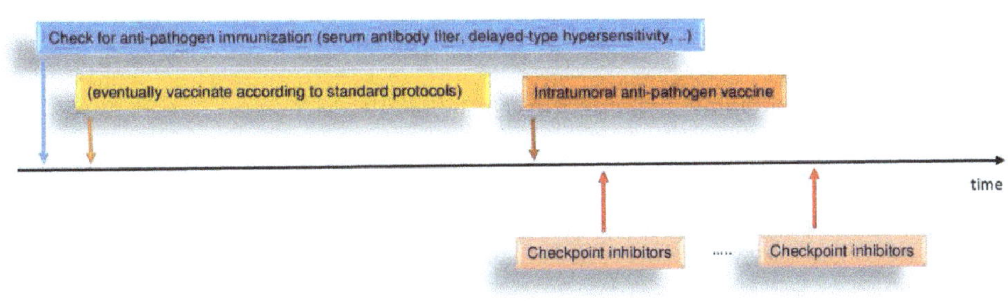

Figure 4.
Schematic diagram of the neoadjuvant intratumoral delivery of repurposed vaccines.

Available immunity against pathogen can be checked initially in patients by means of standard serological testing and/or delayed-type hypersensitivity testing. A standard vaccination protocol can be performed when required before starting intratumoral delivery of a corresponding vaccine. Afterward, timely standard delivery of other therapies (i.e., with systemic CIs) follows.

6. Future perspective

Developments in cancer immunotherapy during the last years have significantly increased our hopes for successfully treating different cancer types. However, the development of new, more effective anticancer immunotherapeutic agents and strategies urges a thorough understanding of the aspects that allow cancer cells to escape elimination by immune cells.

In addition, there are important clinical, industrial, regulatory, and economic issues that must be addressed, outside the realm of advances in cancer immunology and biology, and that would make all the difference between success or failure in real life. Under the clinical perspective, for instance, there is a strong need to develop a community of trained interventional radiologists/oncologists able to actually translate the presented approaches into practice. This is an issue basically in the hands of training centers and schools of medicine abroad. Of foremost relevance is also the involvement of the industry for all new approaches to actually become available to patients worldwide.

7. Conclusion

Designing of novel immunotherapies would require personalized approaches, tailored not only on patient's genetic profiles but also on immunologic tumor characterization. To overcome specific immune inactivation, vaccines against pathogens could become a usable tool in optimized combo-therapies, particularly with checkpoint inhibitors. The role of preexisting immunity on their efficacy has been observed in a few presented studies. In fact, immunization from previous vaccination or previous infections, developed outside the tumor microenvironment, can promote activity of intratumorally delivered preparations. In this light, we warrant future research on available and commercial vaccine preparations to be repurposed as anticancer therapeutic vaccines.

Author details

Matteo Conti
Public Health Department, Ausl Imola, Imola, Italy

*Address all correspondence to: mttconti@gmail.com

References

[1] Upadhyay S, Sharma N, Gupta KB, Dhiman M. Role of immune system in tumor progression and carcinogenesis. Journal of Cellular Biochemistry. 2018;**119**(7):5028-5042

[2] Wilczynski JR, Nowak M. Cancer immunoediting: Elimination, equilibrium, and immune escape in solid tumors. In: Interaction of Immune and Cancer Cells. Springer Verlag, Wien; 2014. pp. 143-205

[3] Pruitt K. Molecular and cellular changes during cancer progression resulting from genetic and epigenetic alterations. Progress in Molecular Biology and Translational Science. 2016;**144**:3-47

[4] Xie M, Xiong W, She Z, Wen Z, Abdirahman AS, Wan W, et al. Immunoregulatory effects of stem cell-derived extracellular vesicles on immune cells. Frontiers in Immunology. 2020;**11**:13

[5] Dundr P, Němejcová K, Bártů M, Matěj R, Rohan Z, Tichá I. Evaluation of inflammatory cells (tumor infiltrating lymphocytes) in solid tumors. Klinická Onkologie. 2017;**30**(Supplementum 3): 10-21

[6] Williams JR, DABR. The Immunotherapy Revolution: The Best New Hope for Saving Cancer Patients' Lives. Grove City, OH: Gatekeeper Press; 2019

[7] Pan C, Liu H, Robins E, Song W, Liu D, Li Z, et al. Next-generation immuno-oncology agents: Current momentum shifts in cancer immunotherapy. Journal of Hematology & Oncology. 2020;**13**(1):29

[8] Wang H, Liu P, Mi J, Chen J, Liu Y. A preliminary study of adoptive T-cell transfer therapy for patients with non-small-cell lung adenocarcinoma with brain metastasis: A case report of 3 patients. Clinical Lung Cancer. 2020;**S1525-7304**(20):30040-1

[9] Chruściel E, Urban-Wójciuk Z, Arcimowicz Ł, Kurkowiak M, Kowalski J, Gliwiński M, et al. Adoptive cell therapy-harnessing antigen-specific T cells to target solid tumours. Cancers. 2020;**12**(3):683

[10] Liu D. CAR-T "the living drugs", immune checkpoint inhibitors, and precision medicine: A new era of cancer therapy. Journal of Hematology & Oncology. 2019;**12**(1):113

[11] Wilson RAM, Evans TRJ, Fraser AR, Nibbs RJB. Immune checkpoint inhibitors: New strategies to checkmate cancer. Clinical and Experimental Immunology. 2018;**191**(2):133-148

[12] Maawy AA, Ito F. Future of immune checkpoint inhibitors. In: Immune Checkpoint Inhibitors in Cancer. Elsevier, St. Louis (MO); 2019. pp. 227-243

[13] Haanen JBAG, John BA. Converting cold into hot tumors by combining immunotherapies. Cell. 2017;**170**(6):1055-1056

[14] Newton JM, Hanoteau A, Liu H-C, Gaspero A, Parikh F, Gartrell-Corrado RD, et al. Immune microenvironment modulation unmasks therapeutic benefit of radiotherapy and checkpoint inhibition. Journal for Immunotherapy of Cancer. 2019;**7**(1):216

[15] Douchet G, Aspeslagh S. What is the place of the combinations for immunotherapy with chemotherapy or with other immune checkpoint inhibitors? Bulletin du Cancer. 2017;**104**(5):485-493

[16] Andersson P, Ostheimer C. Combinatorial approaches to enhance anti-tumor immunity: Focus on immune checkpoint blockade therapy. Frontiers in Immunology. 2019;**10**:2083

[17] Ko EC, Formenti SC. Radiotherapy and checkpoint inhibitors: A winning new combination? Therapeutic Advances in Medical Oncology. 2018;**10**:175883591876824

[18] Ruysscher DD, De Ruysscher D, Reynders K, Van Limbergen E, Lambrecht M. Radiotherapy in combination with immune checkpoint inhibitors. Current Opinion in Oncology. 2017;**29**(2):105-111

[19] Romano G, Gawlinski A. New frontiers in oncology: Immune checkpoint inhibitors in combination therapy. Drugs of Today. 2017;**53**(2):103

[20] Demaria S, Formenti SC. The abscopal effect 67 years later: From a side story to center stage. The British Journal of Radiology. 2020;**93**:20200042

[21] Symonds PR, Mills JA, Duxbury A. Walter and Miller's Textbook of Radiotherapy: Radiation Physics, Therapy and Oncology - E-Book. St. Loius (OH): Elsevier Health Sciences; 2019

[22] Younus Baba M, Saleem M, Noman M, Raheem A. A mixed therapy minimal model: Some strategies for eradication or minimization of cancer. Computer Methods and Programs in Biomedicine. 2020;**192**:105433

[23] Abdou P, Wang Z, Chen Q, Chan A, Zhou DR, Gunadhi V, et al. Advances in engineering local drug delivery systems for cancer immunotherapy. Wiley Interdisciplinary Reviews. Nanomedicine and Nanobiotechnology. 2020:e1632

[24] Liu X, Feng Z, Wang C, Su Q, Song H, Zhang C, et al. Co-localized delivery of nanomedicine and nanovaccine augments the postoperative cancer immunotherapy by amplifying T-cell responses. Biomaterials. 2020;**230**:119649

[25] Hong WX, Haebe S, Lee AS, Westphalen B, Norton JA, Jiang W, et al. Intratumoral immunotherapy for early stage solid tumors. Clinical Cancer Research. 2020. DOI: 10.1158/1078-0432. CCR-19-3642. [Epub ahead of print]

[26] Coley WB. The treatment of malignant tumors by repeated inoculations of erysipelas. With a report of ten original cases. 1893. Clinical Orthopaedics and Related Research. 1991;**262**:3-11

[27] Coley WB. End results in Hodgkin's disease and lymphosarcoma treated by the mixed toxins of erysipelas and *Bacillus prodigiosus*, alone or combined with radiation. Annals of Surgery. 1928;**88**(4):641-667

[28] Coley WB. The treatment of malignant disease by the injection of toxins of erysipelas. BMJ. 1897;**1**(1888):625-625

[29] D'Andrea D, Witjes F, Soria F, Shariat SF. Urothelial Carcinoma in Situ and Treatment of Bacillus Calmette-Guérin Failures. Springer, Cham: Urologic Oncology. 2018. pp. 1-13

[30] Nrnberger T, Kemmerling B. Pathogen-associated molecular patterns (PAMP) and PAMP-triggered immunity. In: Molecular Aspects of Plant Disease Resistance. 2008;**34**:16-47

[31] Charlebois R, Allard B, Allard D, Buisseret L, Turcotte M, Pommey S, et al. PolyI:C and CpG synergize with anti-ErbB2 mAb for treatment of breast tumors resistant to immune checkpoint inhibitors. Cancer Research. 2017;**77**(2):312-319

[32] Hartman LLR, Crawford JR, Makale MT, Milburn M, Joshi S, Salazar AM, et al. Pediatric phase

II trials of poly-ICLC in the management of newly diagnosed and recurrent brain tumors. Journal of Pediatric Hematology/Oncology. 2014;**36**(6):451-457

[33] Holloway R, Nicodemus CF. 302 A phase IB study of indirect immunization with oregovomab and TLR3 stimulation with hiltonol® (H) in patients with recurrent platinum resistant ovarian cancer (PROC). International Journal of Gynecological Cancer. 2019;**29**(3):A126

[34] Ozolins M, Williams HC, Armstrong SJ, Bath-Hextall FJ. The SINS trial: A randomised controlled trial of excisional surgery versus imiquimod 5% cream for nodular and superficial basal cell carcinoma. Trials. 2010;**11**(1):42

[35] Olabi B, Tasker F, Williams HC. "Efficacy and safety of imiquimod 5% cream for basal cell carcinoma: A meta-analysis of randomized controlled trial": A critical appraisal. The British Journal of Dermatology. 2020. DOI: 10.1111/bjd.18891. [Epub ahead of print]

[36] Meyer T, Surber C, French LE, Stockfleth E. Resiquimod, a topical drug for viral skin lesions and skin cancer. Expert Opinion on Investigational Drugs. 2013;**22**(1):149-159

[37] Beutner K, Edwards L, Owens M, Fox T. Comparison of two vehicle-controlled trials of imiquimod 5% cream for the treatment of external genital warts. Journal of Dermatological Science. 1998;**16**:S210

[38] Bertolotti A, Ferdynus C, Milpied B, Dupin N, Huiart L, Derancourt C. Local management of anogenital warts in non-immunocompromised adults: A network meta-analysis of randomized controlled trials. Dermatologic Therapy. 2020;**10**(2):249-262

[39] Higgins DM, Childs J, Parker S, Disis ML, Salazar LG. OT3-01-19: Phase II study of topical imiquimod and weekly abraxane for the treatment of breast cancer cutaneous metastases. Ongoing Clinical Trials Poster Session Abstracts. Cancer Research 2011. **71**(24 Suppl):Abstract nr OT3-01-19

[40] Diab A, Marcondes M, Tagliaferri MA, Hoch U, Zhang J, Rubas W, et al. REVEAL: A phase I/II, open-label, multicenter, dose escalation and dose expansion study of NKTR- 262 [TLR 7/8 agonist] plus NKTR-214 [CD122-biased agonist] with or without nivolumab (nivo) in patients (pts) with locally advanced or metastatic solid tumor malignancies. Annals of Oncology. 2018;**29**:viii146-viii147

[41] Krieg AM. Development of TLR9 agonists for cancer therapy. Journal of Clinical Investigation. 2007;**117**(5):1184-1194

[42] Ribas A, Medina T, Kummar S, Amin A, Kalbasi A, Drabick JJ, et al. SD-101 in combination with pembrolizumab in advanced melanoma: Results of a phase Ib, multicenter study. Cancer Discovery. 2018;**8**(10):1250-1257

[43] Cohen EEW, Bell RB, Bifulco CB, et al. The society for immunotherapy of cancer consensus statement on immunotherapy for the treatment of squamous cell carcinoma of the head and neck (HNSCC). Journal for Immunotherapy of Cancer. 2019;**7**(1):184

[44] Sagiv-Barfi I, Czerwinski DK, Levy S, Alam IS, Mayer AT, Gambhir SS, et al. Eradication of spontaneous malignancy by local immunotherapy. Science Translational Medicine. 2018;**10**(426)

[45] Sivick KE, Desbien AL, Glickman LH, Reiner GL, Corrales L, Surh NH, et al. Magnitude of therapeutic STING activation determines CD8 T cell-mediated anti-tumor immunity. Cell Reports. 2018;**25**(11):3074-3085.e5

[46] Mondal M, Guo J, He P, Zhou D. Recent advances of oncolytic virus in cancer therapy. Human Vaccines & Immunotherapeutics. 2020;**1**:1-14

[47] Aurelian L. Oncolytic virotherapy: The questions and the promise. Oncolytic virotherapy. 2013;**2**:19-29

[48] Yokoda R, Nagalo B, Vernon B, Oklu R, Albadawi H, DeLeon T, et al. Oncolytic virus delivery: From nano-pharmacodynamics to enhanced oncolytic effect. Oncolytic virotherapy. 2017;**6**:39-49

[49] Mehta R, Puzanov I. Oncolytic viruses: T-VEC and others. Oncoimmunology. Cham: Springer International Publishing; 2018. pp. 387-403

[50] Thomas S, Kuncheria L, Roulstone V, Kyula JN, Mansfield D, Bommareddy PK, et al. Development of a new fusion-enhanced oncolytic immunotherapy platform based on herpes simplex virus type 1. Journal for Immunotherapy of Cancer. 2019;**7**(1):214

[51] Babacan NA, Eroglu Z. Treatment options for advanced melanoma after anti-PD-1 therapy. Current Oncology Reports. 2020;**22**(4):38

[52] Chiu M, Armstrong EJL, Jennings V, Foo S, Crespo-Rodriguez E, Bozhanova G, et al. Combination therapy with oncolytic viruses and immune checkpoint inhibitors. Expert Opinion on Biological Therapy. 2020;**20**:1-18

[53] Gellrich FF, Schmitz M, Beissert S, Meier F. Anti-PD-1 and novel combinations in the treatment of melanoma—An update. Journal of Clinical Medical Research. 2020;**9**(1):223

[54] Broman KK, Zager JS. An evaluation of talimogene laherparepvec for the treatment of melanoma. Expert Opinion on Biological Therapy. 2020;**20**(1):9-14

[55] Breitbach CJ, Thorne SH, Bell JC, Kirn DH. Targeted and armed oncolytic poxviruses for Cancer: The Lead example of JX-594. Current Pharmaceutical Biotechnology. 2012;**13**(9):1768-1772

[56] Moehler M, Heo J, Lee HC, et al. Vaccinia-based oncolytic immunotherapy Pexastimogene Devacirepvec in patients with advanced hepatocellular carcinoma after sorafenib failure: A randomized multicenter Phase IIb trial (TRAVERSE). Oncoimmunology. 2019;**8**(8):1615817

[57] Trager MH, Geskin LJ, Saenger YM. Oncolytic viruses for the treatment of metastatic melanoma. Current Treatment Options in Oncology. 2020;**21**(4):26

[58] Melero I, Gato M, Shekarian T, Aznar A, Valsesia-Wittmann S, Caux C, et al. Repurposing infectious disease vaccines for intratumoral immunotherapy. Journal for Immunotherapy of Cancer. 2020;**8**(1):e000443

[59] Shekarian T, Sivado E, Jallas A-C, Depil S, Kielbassa J, Janoueix-Lerosey I, et al. Repurposing rotavirus vaccines for intratumoral immunotherapy can overcome resistance to immune checkpoint blockade. Science Translational Medicine. 2019;**11**(515):eaat5025

[60] Mastrangelo G, Pavanello S, Fadda E, Buja A, Fedeli U. Yellow fever

vaccine 17D administered to healthy women aged between 40 and 54 years halves breast cancer risk: An observational study. European Journal of Cancer Prevention. 2018;**27**(4):303-309

[61] Aznar MA, Molina C, Teijeira A, Rodriguez I, Azpilikueta A, Garasa S, et al. Repurposing the yellow fever vaccine for intratumoral immunotherapy. EMBO Molecular Medicine. 2020;**12**(1):e10375

[62] Newman JH, Chesson CB, Herzog NL, Bommareddy PK, Aspromonte SM, Pepe R, et al. Intratumoral injection of the seasonal flu shot converts immunologically cold tumors to hot and serves as an immunotherapy for cancer. Proceedings of the National Academy of Sciences of the United States of America. 2020;**117**(2):1119-1128

[63] Hailemichael Y, Woods A, Fu T, He Q, Nielsen MC, Hasan F, et al. Cancer vaccine formulation dictates synergy with CTLA-4 and PD-L1 checkpoint blockade therapy. Journal of Clinical Investigation. 2018;**128**(4):1338-1354

[64] Matthias Gromeier SKN. Recombinant poliovirus for cancer immunotherapy. Annual Review of Medicine. 2018;**69**:289

[65] Desjardins A, Gromeier M, Herndon JE 2nd, Beaubier N, Bolognesi DP, Friedman AH, et al. Recurrent glioblastoma treated with recombinant poliovirus. The New England Journal of Medicine. 2018;**379**(2):150-161

[66] Buzzi S, Rubboli D, Buzzi G, Buzzi AM, Morisi C, Pironi F. CRM197 and cancer: Effects of intratumoral administration. Therapy. 2004;**1**(1):61-66

[67] Umansky V. Immunosuppression in the tumor microenvironment: Where are we standing? Seminars in Cancer Biology. 2012;**22**(4):273-274

[68] Shah NJ, Najibi AJ, Shih T-Y, Mao AS, Sharda A, Scadden DT, et al. A biomaterial-based vaccine eliciting durable tumour-specific responses against acute myeloid leukaemia. Nature Biomedical Engineering. 2020;**4**(1):40-51

[69] Nichols AJ, Gonzalez A, Clark ES, Khan WN, Rosen AC, Guzman W, et al. Combined systemic and intratumoral administration of human papillomavirus vaccine to treat multiple cutaneous basaloid squamous cell carcinomas. JAMA Dermatology. 2018;**154**(8):927-930

6

Drug Repurposing in Oncotherapeutics

Alkeshkumar Patel

Abstract

Repurposing or repositioning means validating and application of previously approved drugs in the treatment of another disease that might be relevant or irrelevant to existing use in disease based on the principle of polypharmacology. Repurposed drugs are already well documented for pharmacokinetic, pharmacodynamic, drug interaction, and toxicity parameters. In 1962, thalidomide treatment in pregnant women led to phocomelia in their newborn but while repurposed based on anti-angiogenesis property, it showed efficacy in hematologic malignancies like multiple myeloma. The repurposing is becoming an essential tool in the anti-cancer drug development due to existing drugs are not effective, high cost of treatment, therapy may degrade the quality of life, improvement of survival after treatment is not guaranteed, relapse may occur, and drug resistance may develop due to tumor heterogeneity. Repurposing can be addressed well with the help of literature-based discovery, high throughput technology, bioinformatics multi-omics approaches, side effects, and phenotypes. Many regulatory bodies like EML, NIH, and FDA promote repurposing programs that support the identification of alternative uses of existing medicines. Cancer becomes the major health issue, and the need to discover promising anti-cancer drugs through repurposing remains very high due to decline in FDA approval since 1990, huge expenses incurred in the drug development and prediction of dangerous future burden.

Keywords: repurposing, cancer, bioinformatics, multi-omics, thalidomide tragedy, metformin

1. Introduction

1.1 What are the problems?

Cancer is the second deadliest disease after cardiovascular diseases, causing loss of billions of lives across the world. Although human kind has developed so many anti-cancer medicines, none of them are able to cure the disease. After spending of around $650 million for the development in research and development of New Chemical Entity (NCE) during time periods of 12–17 years, successful outcome compared to standard drugs is less [1]. The success ratio for this NCE in clinical trial is less than 10%. Many times, the effects on outcomes like disease free survival, quality of life treatment related side effects and complications are discouraging. According to ESMO 2019 press release, there was no link between drug cost and clinical benefit measured by ESMO-MCBS and the American Society of Clinical Oncology Value Framework (ASCO-VF) for various drugs approved for adult solid tumor in four European countries and the USA from 2009 to 2017. So, it would add extra treatment cost to patient therapy. According to Prof. Kerstin Vokinger, University of Zurich, Switzerland, and affiliated with the Program on Regulation, Therapeutics, and Law (Harvard Medical School, USA), drug pricing should be aligned with clinical value [2]. There was drastic decline in average number of FDA approved drug since the 1990, but the number of cancer cases rising every year for each cancer. So, this imbalance of demand and supply of effective anti-cancer drugs can be balanced by implication of drug repurposing [3]. In the oncology medicine, the US FDA approved 4 new drugs in 2016 while it was 14 drugs in 2015 and 9 drugs in 2014 and 2013 that indicate decrease in anti-cancer drug discovery [4].

1.2 How repurposing can help?

To overcome the problems linked to high expenditures, lengthy and tedious research for every NCE with low success in clinical trial, repurposing can help where scientists are trying to investigate new therapeutic indication for existing approved drugs. Drug repurposing has many advantages in terms of efficient utilization of time and money for drug discovery and development processes. The proposed medicines for repurposing already have approved pharmaceutical data related to its formulation, Pharmacokinetic (absorption, distribution, metabolism and excretion) and pharmacodynamic profile that collected during preclinical and clinical trial. The proposed medicine also passed through much toxicity, side effects testing and passed the phase 4 of post marketing surveillance so the safety is already established and that reduce the chances of drug failure at the end screening process of drug discovery [5]. The repurposing can drastically reduce drug discovery time line from 12–17 years to 3–12 years due to availability of drug's pharmacology and pharmaceuticals data [6]. The concept of Drug Repurposing is based on validating and application of previously approved drug by FDA in the treatment of another disease that might be relevant or irrelevant to existing use in disease. The principle of polypharmacology and pleiotropy was working behind drug repurposing. The anti-cancer drugs receive FDA approval are very costliest in recent years that significantly affect pharmacoeconomics of patients. For consideration, the cost for a combination-targeted therapy of monoclonal antibodies ipilimumab and nivolumab in treatment of metastatic melanoma has been estimated to per responder is around $400,000 US [7, 8]. So, all these problems can be targeted by drug repurposing where it improves the chances of success, shortens the testing time, and reduces the huge investment in cancer drug design and development.

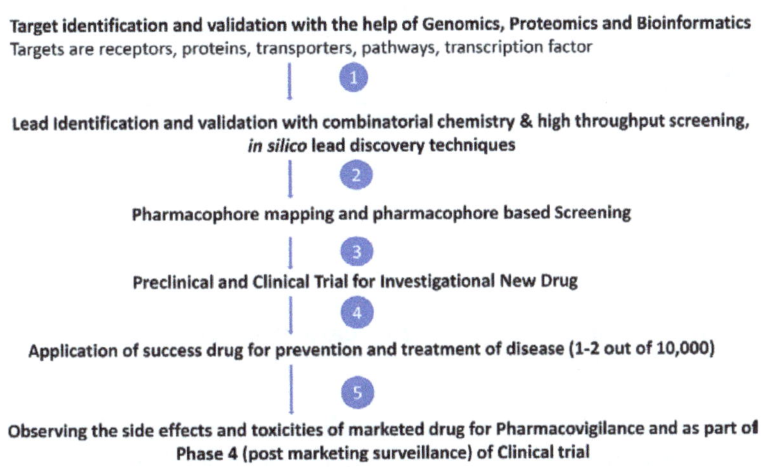

Figure 1.
Drug discovery and development with potential windows for drug repurposing.

1.3 Opportunities for drug repositioning comes from path of drug discovery and development

The process of new drug designing and development involve many steps as mentioned in **Figure 1**. It may happen that Drug is serendipitously screened and found positive result for another disease. Gills et al. tested few anti-HIV drugs against many cancer cell lines using cytotoxicity assays. He found that nelfinavir has potent broad-spectrum antitumor activity [9]. Repurposing can also possible if new role discovered for an existing target. In case of metformin, the similar pathway of is found to be important in two different diseases like diabetes and cancer. It has been observed that unexpected side effects found during and after clinical trials show lead for drug repurposing like thalidomide for certain cancer.

2. Drug repositioning strategy

During preliminary screening on Drug, many possibilities of drug repurposing may arise by chance and later based on proper justification few of them have been tested for alternate application in another disease that called as shifting from bench to bedside. Oppositely, it may happen that unpredicted results of clinical trials suggest ideas for drug repurposing and later same things justified by scientific experiments that called as bedside to bench. According to FDA approved drug database, around 80–90% of drug gets failed in clinical trials due to various reasons and one of the majors is that the lack of efficacy during phase- III of clinical trial. That failure rate figures out around 30–50% and all these drugs might be good candidate for repurposing. The **Figure 2** indicate different approaches that begin with constructing hypothesis based on existing fund of knowledge to expanding its *in silico* frame work for preliminary testing and later on validating facts based on more vigorous and stringent analysis like preclinical and clinical studies [10].

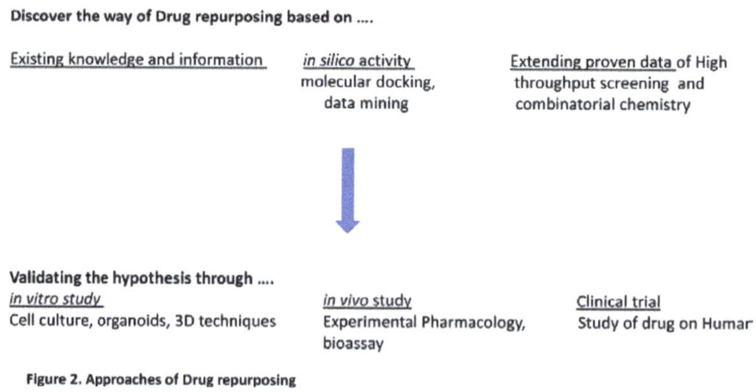

Figure 2.
Various approaches of drug repurposing.

3. Necessity for drug repurposing in cancer treatment and availability of attractive candidates

Comparing cancer with other disease that takes much time to develop and working insidiously. Every cancer begins with few mutations that suppress tumor suppression gene and promoting oncogene that leads to abnormal cell proliferation, escape of apoptosis, immune evasion, inflammation, defects in DNA damage repair mechanism,

Warburg effects, angiogenesis and lack of differentiation of cell with most of the cells remain immature. As there is progress happen the picture of tumor microenvironment become more and more complicated. At this time tumor is no more homogenous but packed with heterogeneous cells and changing itself to more resistance form. The cancer might be supported by systemic condition of the body or in the other words internal anti-cancer mechanism become compromised to eradicate the tumor. The tumor microenvironment begins to secret many immunosuppressive cytokines and inflammatory mediators that sustain the tumor growth and save this corrupted cellular structure against honest immune system that work in the form of vigilance. After dominate at local region, tumor intrude to the other favorable region. Later on, metastasis start based on seed and soil theory of Stephan Paget, where cancer cells work as "seeds" and the specific organ microenvironments work as "soil." The success interaction between these two entities determines the development of a secondary tumor [11].

After get metastasis, the most of the patients give response to first line treat-ment not more than 50% for various cancers. At advance stages of cancer, majority of patients will develop anti-cancer resistance due to drastic abnormal genetic, epigenetic changes and surviving of cancer stem cells that not killed even after the death of tumor cells [12, 13]. So, it becomes important to repurpose drugs that able to act at multiple targets in tumors in patient that display genetic heterogeneity.

The following table (**Table 1**) consists of brief reviews of available good drug candidates for drug repurposing and some of that already approved.

Drug	First approved target	Approved in disease	Repurposed in cancer (preclinical/clinical)
Thalidomide [14]	Might affect the medullary control centers (the vomiting center and the chemoreceptive trigger zone) or affect the peripheral receptors	Nausea, vomiting of pregnant woman (banned now)	Multiple myeloma by targeting TNF-α
Metformin [15]	Activate the adenosine monophosphate activated protein kinase (AMPK) signaling pathway	Type-II diabetes mellitus	Mitochondrial respiration, reducing insulin and insulin-like growth factor levels, inhibits mTOR and activate p53, AMPK pathway
Everolimus [16]	mTOR	Immuno-suppressant	In Pancreatic neuroendocrine by targeting mTOR signaling pathway
Trastuzumab [17]	HER2	HER2-positive breast cancer	For HER2-positive metastatic gastric cancer
Aspirin (low dose; 50–100 mg daily)	COX-1	Prevent Platelets aggregation in cardiovascular disease	Prostaglandin E2 (PGE2) decreased in colon cancer [18], inhibition of platelets to suppress NK cell-mediated lysis of cancer cells [19]
Propranolol [20]	β-receptor blocker	Cardiovascular diseases	Reduced 57% risk of metastasis in Breast cancer by blocking cyclic AMP (cAMP), focal adhesion kinase (FAK)
Digoxin [21, 22]	Na + -K + -ATPase	Heart failure, to reduce heart rate	Rise in intracellular Na + and Ca2+ in human prostate adenocarcinoma cells, lead to activation of calcineurin and transcriptional upregulation of Fas ligand cause apoptosis. Also, suppression nuclear factor-kappa B and inhibition of DNA topoisomerase II are well documented.

Drug	First approved target	Approved in disease	Repurposed in cancer (preclinical/clinical)
Chlorpromazine [19]	Dopamine receptor antagonist	In psychosis, bipolar disorder, schizophrenia	Increase in p21 [23], p51 expression [24]
Artemisinins	Induce formation of reactive oxygen species (ROS) within the infected red blood cells (RBC)	Anti-malarial [25]	Anti-proliferative, pro-apoptotic effects [26]
Doxycycline	Protein synthesis in bacteria	Antibiotics	Down regulation of MMP-2 and MMP-9 expression in leukemia [27] and colorectal cancer cells [28]

Table 1.
Repurposed drug for the cancer treatment.

3.1 Various anti-cancer targets that can be used for repurposing of drug

Based on global statistics, more than 20 million individuals will be detected with cancer in 2025. Certain cancer like breast cancer, colorectal, prostate is mostly remaining incurable in advanced stages with existing treatment and that leads to increase in number of cases. Thus, addressing these present and future challenges requires more effective cancer drugs [29]. Traditional anti-cancer therapy like Chemotherapy and radiation have dangerous side effects that range from bone marrow suppression, oral mucositis, arising of secondary cancer to vomiting, diarrhea and organ specific toxicity that drastically decrease the quality life and overall survival of cancer patients [30]. From this point of view, drug repositioning option is promising strategy to identify non-cancer drugs like aspirin and chlorpromazine which have anti-tumor activity with less side effects comparable to traditional anti-cancer drugs. Traditionally limited targets were identified for anti-cancer drugs that involve cell cycle inhibitors, anti-metabolites, anti-angiogenesis, growth factor inhibitors, pro-apoptotic. But today many new targets identified that work in more specific way and reduce dangerous side effects of anti-cancers. Some novel drug target mentioned in following diagram that might be work well for future drug repurposing in oncotherapeutics (**Figure 3**).

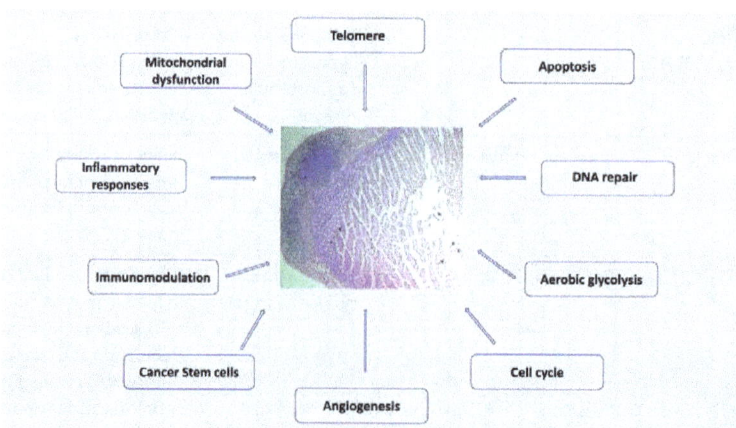

Figure 3.
Hall marks of cancer.

4. Methods for drug repurposing

It might be apparent that identifying specific drugs with pleiotropic effects is easy task but the execution is a complex. Following methods work well to repositioning of drug with the help of existing data, reducing the time of investigation, helping to reduce unnecessary animal experiments and regulatory obligations.

4.1 Computational methods

Although high through put screening (HTS) and many assay techniques available, it is difficult to predict drug and target interaction and its subsequence consequences [31]. Every drug bind with variety of targets but most of them attach with proteins that present in the form of receptors, ion channels, enzymes, antigen and transcriptional factors [32]. To screen the drugs interaction with every of this target is not possible and also it consumes lots of time and money. Certain computational approaches are available that able to screen thousands of test drug molecule with many targets within short time period. The selection of drug and its possible targets are based on similarities based on structure, its protein binding and typical side effects that drugs produce [33–35]. Many molecular docking software are available that predict binding of drug molecule within active site of the target and able to predict the three-dimensional interaction at atomic level. In this approach it is necessary to discover protein structures of both normal and disease condition to target it in proper way else binding of drug with normal protein structure may lead to side effects. Computational approach needs lots of information that can be derived from various databases and webservers like DrugBank [36], E medstore [37], KEGG: Kyoto Encyclopedia of Genes and Genomes [38], SuperTarget and Manually Annotated Targets and Drugs Online Resource (MATADOR) [39], Potential Drug Target Database (PDTD) [40], ZINC [41], CancerDR [42] and many others. Computational models broadly categorized in to network based model that working based on the principles of multiple target optimal intervention (MTOI) [43], Drug side-effect similarity-based method [35] and machine learning-based model that further categorized into supervised learning method and semi-supervised learning method [32].

4.2 Biological experimental approaches

In this method the interaction in between drug and its target is determined. To accomplish this, we may fix the drugs on certain bead and allowing reaction of washing cell lysate extracts with drugs [44]. It is also possible to carry out high-throughput screening based direct-binding assays to test drugs against certain kinases [45]. Cell based screening examine the evidence of autophagy, apoptosis or inhibition of proliferation in proper cell culture environment of different cancer cells [46–48]. Also, genetic expression study of drugs based on cell line can help in drug repurposing.

5. Drug repurposing database

Physical collection of approved drugs to carry out experimental repositioning screens is challenging task. Smaller digital libraries containing information of approved drugs or drugs with expired patents are available to serve drug repurposing like Enzi Life Sciences, Prestwick, Spectrum and many other like National Institute of Health's Chemical Genomics Center (NCGC) [49]. It may happen that drug get failed in clinical trials because of lack of effectiveness (efficacy) but not due to toxicity represent good candidate for drug repositioning. There is some web portal available that store large drug screening database based on clinical trials and can be used for repurposing.

- http://drugrepurposingportal.com
- CLUE: The Drug Repurposing Hub

Current status of drug repurposing based on drug and disease search option is available at repoDB site. This drug repositioning database contains information of about 2051 diseases, all mapped to UMLS terms for easier integration [50].

- http://apps.chiragjpgroup.org/repoDB/

6. Conclusion

The process of drug repurposing or repositioning help the Pharmaceutical companies in terms saving capital expenditure and decrease efforts of scientific community from long drug discovery and development process that pass through much experimental and regulatory task. Drug repositioning works well for those drug molecules for which disease targets are not get altered over a period of time. All the drug repositioning hypothesis will not transferred to successful outcome. It was happened with bevacizumab (Avastin), a kinase inhibitor drug that failed to prove its efficacy during phase- III of clinical trial in gastric cancer therapy although it has good efficacy against colon, rectal, brain, lung and kidney cancer by targeting vascular endothelial growth factor (VEGF) and decreasing the blood supply to the tumor that required for tumor growth and metastasis [51, 52]. Similar thing happened for sunitinib, a kinase inhibitor where it has proven its efficacy in certain cancers while unable to show same in other cancers [53]. It is significant to consider the unique drug indication during repositioning with proper justification for risk and benefits ratio. Any cytotoxic anti-cancer drug may not be an ideal drug for cardiovascular disorder in same dose, as it may kill many normal cells with high proliferation index. But it can be utilized at low doses for drug repurposing with less side effects as in the case of methotrexate at 10–20 mg per week for rheumatoid arthritis due to its anti-inflammatory property. Although, there are many obstacles present on the path of drug repurposing now, but future will bring more advancement in the technologies with the help of combinatorial chemistry, virtual screening, data mining and artificial intelligence that raise the success rates. At the last, we hope that all these scientific advancements translated into clinical setting to improve oncotherapy and reduce the burden of cancer related mortality in the world.

7. Future perspective

Tumor is heterogeneous mutated cell mass with genomic instability that acquired new forms over period of time. As time goes on, tumor heterogeneity environment become less vulnerable to chemotherapeutic and radiation agent with development of tumor resistance in multiple ways. So, every tumor shows different pathological picture in every cancer patient and even different pattern of intratumoural mutation in same patient at different time interval. Based of therapeutic modality, specific subpopulation of drug tolerant cancer cells come out as resistant cells within tumor. So, it seems personalized medicine will be future of Cancer medicines. In these regards, single cell analysis, multiple omics, research autopsy, and sampling from multiple regions can help. Based on tumor heterogeneity and evolution of drug resistance point of view, the drug repurposing might be not evolved as unjustifiable tool with time consuming approach, if not utilized for early stages of Cancer patients.

Drug repurposing involves many challenges like proper utilization of database, demand of expected repurposing drug, issues associated with intellectual property rights and patents. Although to accomplish efficient drug repurposing, there is a need to work from multiple paradigms. Many drugs get failed in third phase of clinical trials and Drug repurposing trials due to lack of efficacy, so it should be realized in well advance by combining multiple techniques. Literature belongs to applied sciences and medical fields containing important information for complementary relationship in between repositioning of drugs and its proposed targets. The vital information can be extracted with "text mining" tools like Biovista, BioWisdom, TextFlow, DrugQuest, Polysearch, etc. Based on semantic integration network approach, diverse information can be interrelated. Later, many algorithms in machine learning techniques can be developed to promote the efficacy and speed of drug repurposing. At present, multiple-omics discipline emerge out like genomics, proteomics, transcriptomics, bioinformatics, metabolomics and interactomics that consist of vast data related to biological sciences. Analyzing these multiple-omics disciplines with computational methods by integrative approach can be utilized to identify the best drug molecule that work at more than single target in different diseases. This approach may suit well with personalized medicine concept that will become inadvertent reality and demand in the case of oncotherapeutics. With these diverse but harmonizing computational with multi-omics incorporation, scientist and researcher achieve meaningful understanding of cellular physiology, Drug-receptor interaction, pathogenesis and prognosis of diseases, stages and types of same disease with acquired changes at molecular level, possible drug reactions, on-target and off-target interactions, diagnostic and prognostic biomarkers.

According to WHO, Cancer is a leading cause of death worldwide, accounting for an estimated 9.6 million deaths in 2018. The most common causes of cancer death are cancers of lung (1.76 million deaths), colorectal (862,000 deaths), stomach (783,000 deaths), liver (782,000 deaths), and breast (627,000 deaths). Definitely at present scenario priority should be given for these cancers. There are many diseases are coming under the category of orphan disease. According to U. S. FDA, an orphan disease defined as a condition that affects fewer than 200,000 people nationwide. There is good opportunity for repurposing to orphan drugs. According to Genetic and rare diseases (GARD) information center, many cancers comes under orphan diseases category like CDK4 linked melanoma (orphan drug Aldesleukin), carcinoid tumor (orphan drug Everolimus, Lutetium Lu 177 dot-atate), chronic myeloid leukemia (orphan drug Bosutinib, Omacetaxine mepesuccinate), clear cell renal cell carcinoma (orphan drug Sorafenib, Temsirolimus). These all orphan drugs that utilized for rare cancers are good candidates for Drug repurposing in other common types of cancer. Also, the drugs like thalidomide which was once withdraw from the market due to its dangerous teratogenic effects in one class of human population but later approved by FDA for myeloma and other disease treatment. The negative and positive sides of this drug are contributed by anti-angiogenesis property. But this one off-target property was proved to defame its efficacy in one situation while with Drug repurposing in other condition it has proved its anti-cancer effects. Future will become where more robust and sound techniques will be utilized to create successful Drug repurposing candidate and making drug discovery and development process beneficial to Human kind.

Acknowledgements

I personally thank CHARUSAT (Charotar University of Science and Technology, India) for providing me access to various resources to write this manuscript and encouraging me indirectly to write about this wonderful topic of Cancer Biology science. I appreciate this organization for the priority given to the research and innovation with proper nurturing.

Author details

Alkeshkumar Patel
Department of Pharmacology, Ramanbhai Patel College of Pharmacy, CHARUSAT, Anand, Gujarat, India

*Address all correspondence to: alkeshpatel.ph@charusat.ac.in

References

[1] Prasad V, Mailankody S. Research and development spending to bring a single cancer drug to market and revenues after approval. JAMA Internal Medicine. 2017;**177**(11):1569-1575. DOI: 10.1001/jamainternmed.2017.3601

[2] Kerstin NV, Thomas JH, Ariadna TM, Thomas JR, Aaron SK. Clinical benefit and prices of cancer drugs in the United States and Europe. Journal of Clinical Oncology. 2019;**37**(15):6638. DOI: 10.1200/JCO.2019.37.15_suppl.6638

[3] Sleir L, Førde HE, Netland IA, Leiss L, Skeie BS, Enger PØ. Drug repurposing in cancer. Pharmacological Research. 2017;**124**:74-91

[4] Mullard A. 2015 FDA drug approvals. Nature Reviews. Drug Discovery. 2016;**15**(2):73-76

[5] Li YY, Jones SJM. Drug repositioning for personalized medicine. Genome Medicine. 2012;**4**:27

[6] Ashburn TT, Thor KB. Drug repositioning: Identifying and developing new uses for existing drugs. Nature Reviews. Drug Discovery. 2004;**3**:673-683

[7] Kantarjian HM, Fojo T, Mathisen M, Zwelling LA. Cancer drugs in the United States: Justum pretium–the just price. Journal of Clinical Oncology. 2013;**31**(28):3600-3604

[8] Jensen IS, Zacherle E, Blanchette CM, Zhang J, Yin W. Evaluating cost benefits of combination therapies for advanced melanoma. Drugs Context. 2016;**5**:212297

[9] Gills JJ, Lopiccolo J, Tsurutani J, Shoemaker RH, Best CJ, Abu-Asab MS, et al. Nelfinavir, a lead HIV protease inhibitor, is a broad-spectrum, anticancer agent that induces endoplasmic reticulum stress, autophagy, and apoptosis in vitro and in vivo. Clinical Cancer Research. 2007;**13**:5183-5194

[10] Turanli B, Grøtli M, Boren J, Nielsen J, Uhlen M, Arga KY, et al. Drug repositioning for effective prostate cancer treatment. Frontiers in Physiology. 2018;**9**:500. DOI: 10.3389/fphys.2018.00500

[11] Paget S. The distribution of secondary growths in cancer of the breast. Lancet. 1889;**133**:571-573

[12] Ghiaur G, Gerber J, Jones RJ. Concise review: Cancer stem cells and minimal residual disease. Stem Cells. 2012;**30**(1):89-93

[13] Tournig C, Andre T, Achille E, Lledo G, Flesh M, Mery-Mignard D, et al. FOLFIRI followed by FOLFOX6 or the reverse sequence in advanced colorectal cancer: A randomized GERCOR study, Journal of Clinical Oncology. 2004;**22**(2):229-237

[14] Available from: https://www.ebi.ac.uk/chebi/searchId. do?chebiId=CHEBI:9513

[15] Leone A, Di Gennaro E, Bruzzese F, Avallone A, Budillon A. New perspective for an old antidiabetic drug: Metformin as anticancer agent. Cancer Treatment and Research. 2014;**159**:355-376. DOI: 10.1007/978-3-642-38007-5_21

[16] FDA Okays Everolimus for Rare Type of Pancreatic Cancer. Available from: http://www.medscape.com/viewarticle/742274

[17] Rose JS, Bekaii-Saab TS. New developments in the treatment of metastatic gastric cancer: Focus on trastuzumab. Oncotargets and Therapy. 2011;**4**:21-26

[18] Ruffin MT, Krishnan K, Rock CL, Normolle D, Vaerten MA, PetersGolden M, et al. Suppression of human colorectal mucosal prostaglandins: Determining the lowest effective aspirin dose. Journal of the National Cancer Institute. 1997;**89**:1152-1160

[19] Umar A, Boisseau M, Yusup A, Upur H, Begaud B, Moore N. Interactions between aspirin and COX-2 inhibitors or NSAIDs in a rat thrombosis model Fundam. The Journal of Clinical Pharmacology. 2004;**18**(5):559-563

[20] Powe DG, Voss MJ, Zänker KS, Habashy HO, Green AR, Ellis IO, et al. Beta-blocker drug therapy reduces secondary cancer formation in breast cancer and improves cancer specific survival. Oncotarget. 2010;**1**:628-638

[21] Raghavendra PB, Sreenivasan Y, Ramesh GT, Manna SK. Cardiac glycoside induces cell death via FasL by activating calcineurin and NF-AT, but apoptosis initially proceeds through activation of caspases. Apoptosis. 2007;**12**:307-318

[22] Manna SK, Sah NK, Newman RA, Cisneros A, Aggarwal BB. Oleandrin suppresses activation of nuclear transcription factor-kappaB, activator protein-1, and c-Jun NH2-terminal kinase. Cancer Research. 2000;**60**:3838-3834

[23] Shin SY, Kim CG, Kim SH, Kim YS, Lim Y, Lee YH. Chlorpromazine activates p21Waf1/Cip1 gene transcription via early growth response-1 (Egr-1) in C6 glioma cells. Experimental & Molecular Medicine. 2010;**42**(5):395-405

[24] Lee WY, Lee WT, Cheng CH, Chen KC, Chou CM, Chung CH, et al. Repositioning antipsychotic chlorpromazine for treating colorectal cancer by inhibiting sirtuin 1. Oncotarget. 2015;**6**(29):27580-27595

[25] Kundu CN, Das S, Nayak A, Satapathy SR, Das D, Siddharth S. Anti-malarials are anti-cancers and vice versa – one arrow two sparrows. Acta Tropica. 2015;**149**:113-127

[26] Holien T, Olsen OE, Misund K, Hella H, Waage A, Ro TB, et al. Lymphoma and myeloma cells are highly sensitive to growth arrest and apoptosis induced by artesunate. European Journal of Haematology. 2013;**91**(4):339-346

[27] Iwasaki H, Inoue H, Mitsuke Y, Badran A, Ikegaya S, Ueda T. Doxycycline induces apoptosis by way of caspase-3 activation with inhibition of matrix metalloproteinase in human T-lymphoblastic leukemia CCRF-CEM cells. The Journal of Laboratory and Clinical Medicine. 2002;**140**(6):382-386

[28] Onoda T, Ono T, Dhar DK, Yamanoi A, Fujii T, Nagasue N. Doxycycline inhibits cell proliferation and invasive potential: Combination therapy with cyclooxygenase-2 inhibitor in human colorectal cancer cells. The Journal of Laboratory and Clinical Medicine. 2004;**143**(4):207-216

[29] McGuire S. World Cancer Report 2014. Geneva, Switzerland: World Health Organization, International Agency for Research on Cancer, WHO Press, 2015. Advances in Nutrition. 2016;**7**(2):418-419

[30] Patel A et al. A rat model against chemotherapy plus radiation-induced oral mucositis. Saudi Pharmaceutical Journal. October 2013;**21**(4):399-403

[31] Haggarty SJ, Koeller KM, Wong JC, et al. Multidimensional chemical genetic analysis of diversity-oriented synthesis-derived deacetylase inhibitors using cell-based assays. Chemistry & Biology. 2003;**10**:383-396

[32] Chen X, Yan CC, Zhang X, Zhang X, Dai F, Yin J, et al. Drug–target interaction prediction: Databases, web servers and computational models. Briefings in Bioinformatics. 2016;**17**(4):696-712. DOI: https://doi. org/10.1093/bib/bbv066

[33] Keiser MJ, Setola V, Irwin JJ, Laggner C, Abbas AI, Hufeisen SJ, et al. Predicting new molecular targets for known drugs. Nature. 2009;**462**:175-181

[34] Kinnings SL, Liu N, Buchmeier N, Tonge PJ, Xie L, Bourne PE. Drug discovery using chemical systems biology: Repositioning the safe medicine Comtan to treat multi-drug and extensively drug resistant tuberculosis. PLoS Computational Biology. 2009;**5**:e1000423

[35] Campillos M, Kuhn M, Gavin AC, Jensen LJ, Bork P. Drug target identification using side-effect similarity. Science. 2008;**321**:263-266

[36] Available from: https://www.drugbank.ca/

[37] Available from: https://www.emedstore.in/indian-medicine-database

[38] Available from:https://www.genome.jp/kegg/

[39] Günther S, Kuhn M, Dunkel M, et al. SuperTarget and Matador: Resources for exploring drug-target relationships. Nucleic Acids Research. 2008;**36**:D919-D922

[40] Gao Z, Li H, Zhang H, et al. PDTD: A web-accessible protein database for drug target identification. BMC Bioinformatics. 2008;**9**:104

[41] Irwin JJ, Sterling T, Mysinger MM, et al. ZINC: A free tool to discover chemistry for biology. Journal of Chemical Information and Modeling. 2012;**52**:1757-1768

[42] Kumar R, Chaudhary K, Gupta S, et al. Cancer DR: Cancer drug resistance database. Scientific Reports. 2013;**3**:1445

[43] Yang K, Bai H, Ouyang Q, et al. Finding multiple target optimal intervention in disease-related molecular network. Molecular Systems Biology. 2008;**4**:228

[44] Brehmer D, Greff Z, Godl K, Blencke S, Kurtenbach A, Weber M, et al. Cellular targets of gefitinib. Cancer Research. 2005;**65**:379-382

[45] Karaman MW, Herrgard S, Treiber DK, Gallant P, Atteridge CE, Campbell BT, et al. A quantitative analysis of kinase inhibitor selectivity. Nature Biotechnology. 2008;**26**:127-132

[46] Zhang L, Yu J, Pan H, Hu P, Hao Y, Cai W, et al. Small molecule regulators of autophagy identified by an image-based high-throughput screen. Proceedings of the National Academy of Sciences of the United States of America. 2007;**104**:19023-19028

[47] Antczak C, Kloepping C, Radu C, Genski T, Muller-Kuhrt L, Siems K, et al. Revisiting old drugs as novel agents for retinoblastoma: In vitro and in vivo antitumor activity of cardenolides. Investigative Ophthalmology & Visual Science. 2009;**50**:3065-3073

[48] Iljin K, Ketola K, Vainio P, Halonen P, Kohonen P, Fey V, et al. High-throughput cell-based screening of 4910 known drugs and drug-like small molecules identifies disulfiram as an inhibitor of prostate cancer cell growth. Clinical Cancer Research. 2009;**15**:6070-6078

[49] Huang R, Southall N, Wang Y, Yasgar A, Shinn P, Jadhav A, et al. The NCGC pharmaceutical collection: A comprehensive resource of clinically approved drugs enabling repurposing and chemical genomics. Science Translational Medicine. 2011;**3**(80):ps16

[50] Brown AS, Patel CJ. A standard database for drug repositioning. Scientific Data. 2017;**4**:170029

[51] Keating GM. Bevacizumab: A review of its use in advanced cancer. Drugs. 2014;**74**:1891-1925. DOI: https://doi.org/10.1007/s40265-014-0302-9

[52] Kang H, Kauh JS. Chemotherapy in the treatment of metastatic gastric cancer: Is there a global standard? Current Treatment Options in Oncology. 2011;**12**:96-106

[53] FDA Expands Sutent Label to Include Pancreatic Neuroendocrine Tumors. GEN News Highlights 23 May 2011. Available from: http://www.genengnews.com/gen-news-highlights /fda-expands-sutent-label-to-include-pancreatic neuroendocrinetumors/81245191/

7

Salicylic Acid Sans Aspirin in Animals and Man

James Ronald Lawrence, Gwendoline Joan Baxter and John Robert Paterson

Abstract

Analyses in non-aspirin takers finding salicylic acid (SA) and hydroxylated metabolites in serum also SA and salicyluric acid (SU) in urine led to a re-evaluation of dietary sources of salicylates. Fruit and vegetable sources explained higher levels found in drug-free vegetarians, which overlapped with those from patients on low dose aspirin. That drug's chemo-protective action in cancer is, at least partially, attributable to its principal metabolite, SA—which we believe contributes to the benefits of a vegetarian diet. However, diet is unlikely to be the sole source of the circulating salicylate found in aspirin-free animals and man. We adduced evidence for its persistence in prolonged fasting and biosynthesis in vivo from labelled benzoic acid. We review the roles, defined and potential, of SA in the biosphere. Emphasis on the antiplatelet effect of aspirin in man has detracted from the likely pivotal role of SA in many potential areas of bioregulation—probably as important in animals as in plants. In this expanding field, some aspirin effects, mediated by apparently conserved receptors responding to SA, are discussed. The perspectives revealed may lead to re-evaluation of the place of salicylates in therapeutics and potentially improve formulations and drug delivery systems.

Keywords: salicylic acid, salicylic acid metabolism, dietary sources, biosynthesis, homologue receptors, conserved effects, siderophores, aspirin

1. Introduction

Salicylic acid (SA) in plants is a ubiquitous compound shown to be pivotal in initiating the response to a variety of physical, chemical and biological insults [1]. Analgesic and antipyretic properties of plant extracts, notably from willow, meadowsweet and myrtle, had been known for many centuries before isolation of SA as the active principle. Since synthesis of its acetyl ester—aspirin—investigation has focused on the properties of that compound which is rapidly hydrolysed (serum $t_{1/2}$ of 20 min) to SA which itself has a half-life of 2–4 h [2]. The demonstration that aspirin works by serine side chain acetylation of Cox-1 and Cox-2 isoforms has detracted attention from SA itself; that compound, despite weak reversible Cox 1 and absent Cox 2 inhibition, is as effective as aspirin in vivo in suppressing inflammation [3]. Inhibition of transcription of the Cox-2 gene by micromolar concentrations of SA is the likely explanation [4].

2. SA without aspirin (SA sans ASA)

Investigating the possible use of low dose aspirin as an aromatic probe to measure hydroxyl free radicals by assessing the hydroxylation of SA to form 2,3 and 2,5 dihydroxybenzoic acids (DHBAs)—**Figure 1**—required a sensitive HPLC assay with appropriate controls. That work revealed the presence of substances which had identical retention times to SA, 2,3 DHBA and 2,5 DHBA in the serum extracts of subjects not taking aspirin. The exclusion of contamination was followed by studies to determine the authenticity of these substances as SA, 2,3 DHBA and 2,5 DHBA.

2.1 SA in blood

Examination of the chromatograms of blank serum or plasma from published methods of SA analysis revealed the presence of an unknown substance with a retention time (R_t) similar to SA [5, 6]. While Ruffin et al. [7] reported SA in the plasma from 17 of 53 subjects at baseline there was no information as to how they confirmed identification of the compound.

We examined samples from drug free volunteers: extracts of acidified serum were analysed by high performance liquid chromatography (HPLC) with electrochemical detection. Chromatographic conditions were altered and the R_ts of the unknown compounds compared against authentic SA, 2,3 DHBA and 2,5 DHBA. Serum samples (some spiked with SA) were also incubated with a bacterial salicylate hydroxylase and the substance which had a R_t identical to SA disappeared. Finally the trimethylsilyl (TMS) derivative of the unknown and SA had, using gas chromatography–mass spectrometry (GC–MS), a similar retention time and total ion chromatogram [8].

2.2 SA and salicyluric acid (SU) in urine

Armstrong et al. [9] had detected, by paper chromatography, a compound with characteristics similar to those of SU in the urine of 400 people who had not taken salicylate drugs. That was in an admixture of 49 compounds of predominantly, it was suggested, dietary origin. Von Studnitz and colleagues, who also used a paper system, suggested SA might be one of the phenolic acids in the urine of subjects *on a*

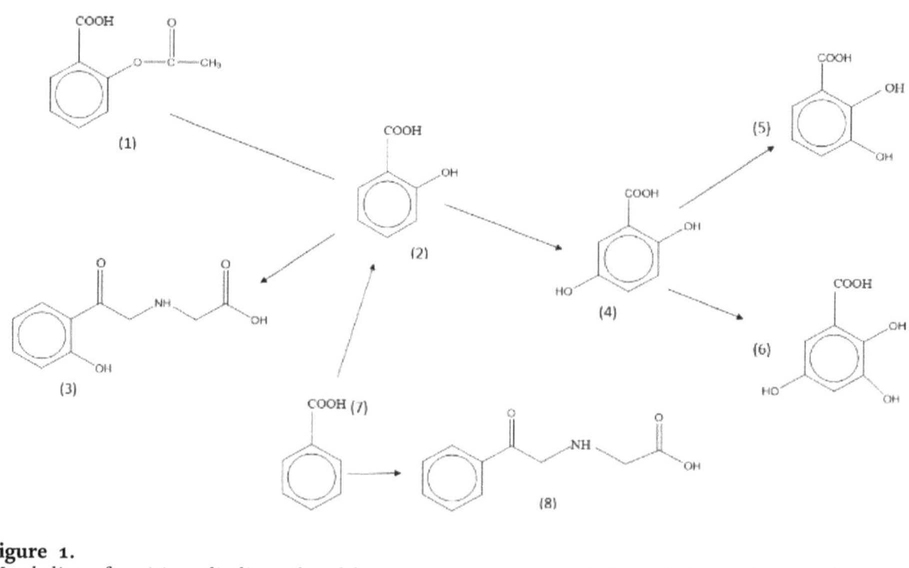

Figure 1.
Metabolism of aspirin, salicylic acid and benzoic acid. (1) acetylsalicylic acid (aspirin); (2) salicylic acid; (3) salicyluric acid; (4) 2,5 dihydroxybenzoic acid; (5) 2,3 dihydroxybenzoic acid; (6) 2,3,5 trihydroxybenzoic acid; (7) benzoic acid; and (8) hippuric acid.

diet restricted to glucose and citric acid [10]. Young reported a compound with thin layer chromatographic properties of SU [11] in a single individual on a synthetic diet, while Finnie and co-workers found a similar compound on their paper system in children not taking salicylate drugs [12]. At the time of all these earlier investigations methods for adequately characterising and quantifying the purported SA and SU were not readily available.

Other work [13] designed to assess the dietary importance of salicylates had examined acid-treated urine using HPLC with fluorescence detection but salicylates other than SA, salicylate precursors and structurally related compounds may have been included in the values reported.

We examined 24 h urine samples from 10 volunteers who had not taken any salicylate drugs during the previous 2 weeks. The acid hydrophobic compounds (=organic acids) were separated using HPLC and quantified electrochemically. The R_ts of the extracted substances and those of SA and SU were compared under two sets of chromatographic conditions and found very similar to those of authentic substances. The unknown substances, isolated by HPLC, and treated with acetyl chloride in methanol were compared with the methyl esters of SA and SU using GC–MS. After esterification the unknown compounds had mass spectra and R_ts comparable to those of methyl-SA and methyl-SU [14].

These findings in serum and urine led us on to explore, in some detail, the likely dietary sources for the salicylate compounds we found and confirmed. At the time interest was re-awakening in the potential benefits of salicylates commonly found in the diet [13]—as opposed to what were considered traditional plant medicine sources.

3. Dietary source of salicylates

3.1 Previously

The occurrence of "natural salicylates", such as SA, in strawberries and other fruits was raised in the Lancet in 1903 [15] and the matter of whether these natural salicylates were superior to synthetic salicylates was the subject of a JAMA editorial in 1913 [16]—no superiority was concluded! Interest then appeared to wane until re-invigorated by the popularity, from ~1970, in therapeutic trials—arising from the apparent cross-reactivity of tartrazine and aspirin—of exclusion diets.

3.2 Background

Many plant derived non-nutritive compounds exert, in mammalian systems, biological activities that may have an impact on health and disease risk [17] and we proposed [18] that SA might provide a link between aspirin, diet and the prevention of colorectal cancer (CRC). There is good evidence that the regular intake of aspirin decreases the risk of developing cancer [19]. A mechanism for platelet mediated CRC tumorigenesis has been proposed [20]; that would, of course not be attributable to SA itself but a more balanced view is that both constituent groups of aspirin (acetyl and SA moieties) contribute to the anti-cancer effects [21].

Assessment of the extent of the contribution of diet to SA in blood and urine cannot be easily inferred from direct analysis of its concentration therein. There is considerable variability in peak serum levels of SA in subjects receiving a standard dose [7] while urinary salicylate is influenced by urine flow, pH, the presence of other organic acids and the saturability of SU formation and/or excretion [2].

3.3 Salicylates from food

It was unclear whether sufficient salicylic acid could be obtained from dietary sources to influence health and disease with estimated daily intakes ranging from 0.4 to 200 mg/day [13, 22, 23]. That range reflected the disparate information available on the salicylate content of foods.

Comparison, in the serum of subjects not taking aspirin, of SA levels in 37 vegetarians and 39 non-vegetarians found higher concentrations in the former [24]. That study revealed median concentrations of 0.11 (range 0.04–2.47) µmol/L and 0.07 (range 0.02–0.20) µmol/L respectively: the median of the difference was 0.05 µmol/L (95% confidence interval for difference 0.03–0.08; $p < 0.0001$). The median SA level measured in serum from 14 patients on aspirin 75 mg/day was, at 10.03 (range 0.23–25.40) µmol/L, significantly higher. However there was overlap in serum SA concentrations between the vegetarians (8 higher than lowest low dose aspirin) and patients taking aspirin (6 below the highest vegetarian value). These findings should be considered in light of the inhibition of COX2 transcription that has been shown to occur at SA levels as low as 0.1 µmol/L [4].

In a further study the urinary excretion of SA and SU was assessed in 24 h samples from 27 non-vegetarians, 21 vegetarians and 40 patients taking 75 or 150 mg aspirin/day [25]. For SU, the principle urinary salicylate, vegetarians excreted significantly more than the non-vegetarians (median 11.01; range 4.98–26.60 µmol/24 h compared with 3.91; range 0.87–12.23 µmol/24 h) but these amounts were significantly lower than those excreted by patients on aspirin. Significantly more SA was excreted by the vegetarians (median 1.19; range 0.02–3.55 µmol/24 h) than by the non-vegetarians (median 0.31; range 0.01–2.01 µmol/ 24 h). The median amounts of SA excreted by the vegetarians and the patients taking aspirin were not significantly different. These values were comparable to those found earlier, using less specific methodology, in a group of drug free volunteers on a variety of diets [13].

3.3.1 The spice of life

Awareness that certain spices had been reported [22] to contain especially high concentrations of SA and the reported very low incidence of colorectal cancer in rural India [26] led to our particular assessment of spices.

Spices, Indian cooked dishes and blood and urine samples taken after ingestion of a test meal were investigated for their salicylate content. Total salicylate content determination required a preliminary alkali treatment step before our standard extraction [27] as, in plants, phenolic glycosides and carboxylic esters are present as well as the "free" phenolic acid. Our standard assay conditions for SA were then applied. All samples of spices and cooked meals examined contained SA (up to 1.5 wt%); cumin, turmeric, red chilli powder, paprika and cinnamon were especially rich sources. Our measurements were considerably higher than those previously published [22]. That was attributed to previously suboptimal extraction, chromatographic separation and detection [27]. The identity of the SA fractions (on HPLC) from cumin, paprika and turmeric was confirmed, after elution and esterification, by GC–MS of their methyl esters.

The potential bioavailability of SA derived from a prepared meal was assessed in a single aspirin free volunteer after a 10 h fast. Consumption of 545.3 g of a cooked vegetable dish (shown by aliquot assay to contain 94.03 g of total salicylates) was followed by regular blood and urine collection over 6 h. Serum SA doubled within 1.5 h and urinary SU increased ~20-fold during that time.

Native Indian volunteers, living in a rural area near Chennai, had been recruited for another study as representative of that community for health lifestyle and nutritional status. They had a diet of locally grown vegetables, grains and pulses flavoured with spices and herbs. The serum from these 21 South Indians had a median SA concentration of 0.263 μmol/L (range 0.05–0.64— significantly higher (~2.5- to 3.5-fold higher) than those found in the sera of the other groups reported above [24]; $p < 0.001$ against both vegetarians and non-vegetarians by Mann–Whitney *U* test) [27]. Summarised and compared with other results below in **Table 1**.

	Median (μmol/L)	Range (μmol/L)
Vegetarians n = 37	0.110	0.04–2.47
Non-vegetarians n = 39	0.070	0.02–2.00
Southern Indian villagers n = 21	0.263	0.05–0.64
75 mg aspirin takers n = 14	10.03	0.23–25.4

Limit of detection of the method = 0.005 μmol/L.
***Tables 1** and 2—with modification—from Ref. [28]—https://pubs.acs.org/doi/abs/10.1021/jf800974z?src=recsys: further permissions regarding use of the content should be directed to the ACS.*

Table 1.
Results in Man [24, 27].

3.4 SA in food

Given that SA is a stress hormone in plants we can anticipate that locality, varietal and growing conditions could affect total salicylate content at harvesting before any variability in processing conditions and storage effects. Wide reported ranges for different brands assayed using standard conditions are therefore not particularly surprising. For example the SA content of five brands of orange juice obtained from Scottish retailers ranged from 0.47 to 3.01 mg/kg [29].

3.4.1 Organic or not?

Usually an open question but, given the above considerations, probably not in respect of SA content. Thus the median SA contents in organic and non-organic vegetable soups were 117 ng/g (range 8–1040) and 20 ng/g (range 0–248) respectively; the median between the difference groups was 59 ng/g (95% confidence intervals 18–117 ng/g), $p = 0.032$ by Mann Whitney *U* test [30]. Consider also constraints of drought, other physical stresses and non-availability of pest control which inevitably prevail in many emergent nations.

3.4.2 A Scottish overview

Clearly sample selection and methodology will affect estimates of SA content in the diet. Using the assay methodology our group developed [27, 30] to supplement published results, Wood et al. [29] prepared a comprehensive dietary database. They filtered published results of dietary constituent total salicylate content by specific criteria. Food items had to be randomly selected and purchased from various commercial outlets at different times of the year; food samples to be prepared using standard domestic practices; optimised sample extraction and hydrolysis conditions were to be clearly described or cited, and salicylate determination to be based on modern techniques of HPLC and mass spectrometry with validation

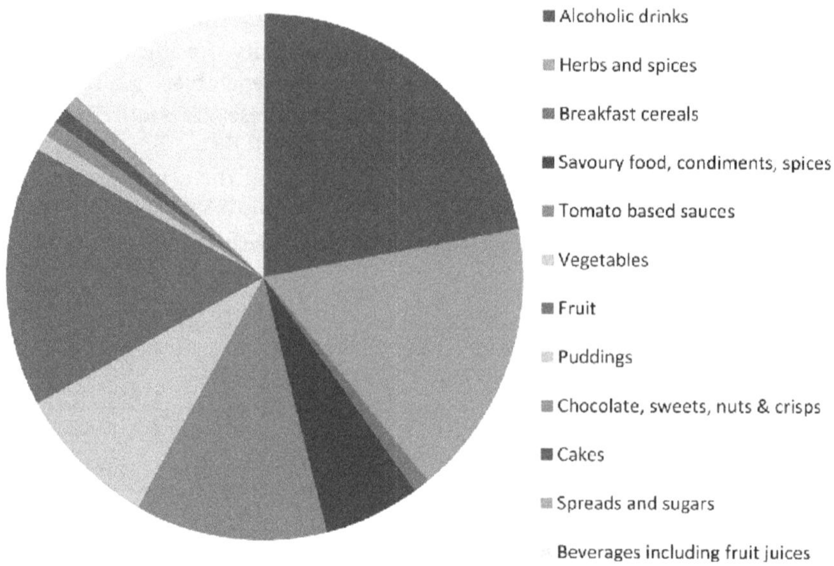

Figure 2.
Relative contributions of different food groups to total salicylate intake of a Scottish population. Source: [29].

and quality assurance methods summarised. Combination of such published data, which met these criteria, together with their in-house analyses resulted in a database of 27 types of fruit, 21 vegetables, 28 herbs, spices and condiments, 2 soups and 11 beverages—expressed as median values to reflect the non-normal distribution of the results.

Subsequently dietary intake was assessed by applying this salicylate database, using a validated questionnaire, to 237 healthy individuals age range (17–72) from Aberdeen [29]. Estimated median total salicylate intakes for men and women were 4.42 and 3.16 mg/day respectively, a gender difference not sustained when corrected for energy. Primary food sources of salicylates as shown in **Figure 2** were alcoholic beverages (22%), herbs and spices (17%), fruits (16%), non-alcoholic beverages including fruit juice (13%), tomato-based sauces (12%) and vegetables (9%). Salicylate intake was significantly ($p < 0.001$) and positively associated with intakes of fibre, potassium, vitamin C and alcohol!

4. Endogenous salicylic acid

4.1 Background

There were clear suggestions in the literature that SA and SU in urine might not all derive from diet, given their presence in the urine of subjects on restricted diets [9, 11]. In addition quantification of the contribution from fruit and vegetable consumption to circulating SA levels in man had demonstrated, using a sensitive and specific method that <20% of the variability derived from these sources [31]. So some circulating SA in aspirin-naïve or -free individuals may derive from other dietary sources or be of non-dietetic origin.

4.2 SA in animal blood

Blood samples, serum or plasma, were obtained from animals at London Zoo or the Department of Biological Services, University of Glasgow in accordance with

Animal	Phylogenetic class	SA (μmol/L)
Burrowing Owl	Aves	9.854
Ne-Ne	Aves	5.609
Indian Rhinoceros	Mammalia	4.700
Pigmy Hippopotamus	Mammalia	2.384
Agouti	Mammalia	2.116
Asian Elephant	Mammalia	1.635
Burmese Python	Reptilia	1.362
Rabbit	Mammalia	1.129
Piglet	Mammalia	1.010
Arabian Onyx	Mammalia	0.777
Sheep	Mammalia	0.715
Tiger[a]	Mammalia	0.661
Brown Trout	Pisces	0.538
Giraffe	Mammalia	0.507
Donkey	Mammalia	0.473
Sacred Ibis	Aves	0.353
Goat	Mammalia	0.310
Giant Anteater	Mammalia	0.293
Collared Peccary	Reptilia	0.237
African Lion[a]	Mammalia	0.226
Cow	Mammalia	0.216
Gelada Baboon	Mammalia	0.210
Chinese Alligator	Mammalia	0.156
Domestic Cat	Mammalia	0.144
Pond Heron	Aves	0.136
Gorilla	Mammalia	0.125
Monkey*	Mammalia	0.080
Mouse	Mammalia	0.078
Rat	Mammalia	0.069
Domestic Cat**	Mammalia	0.058
Chimpanzee	Mammalia	0.033
Crab***	Crustacea	<0.005
Prawn	Crustacea	<0.005

[a]Mean concentration in five animals.
**Red faced spider monkey.*
***Fed only meat.*
****European shore crab.*

Table 2.
Concentration of salicylic acid (SA) in the blood or body fluid of a variety of animals.

their approved codes of practice. The results (**Table 2**) showed that species regarded as primarily carnivorous had blood SA levels comparable to those measured in herbivores [28]. The highest levels detected were in the range associated with aspirin use in man and only the crustacean body fluid samples examined did not contain SA.

As some bacteria, notably *Mycobacterial*, *Yersinia* and *Pseudomonas* species, synthesise SA to enhance iron chelation (see Section 5.1) the possibility of a gastro-intestinal particularly colonic, bacterial source for SA was assessed in two animal models. Pooled serum from six mice treated with neomycin 100 mg/kg/day for 4 days had a serum SA concentration which was, at 0.309 μmol/L, slightly higher than the level of 0.268 μmol/L measured in six untreated animals. Other measurements were done on serum samples from Sprague-Dawley rats delivered by caesarean section, raised in a sterile environment and fed sterilised food. A group of 8 such germ free animals had a pooled serum SA level which was, at 0.166 μmol/L, ~2.5× greater than the level of 0.069 μmol/L in serum from a group of control animals [28].

4.3 SA in diet-restricted and fasting human subjects

A preliminary study followed serum SA and urinary SA + SU over 3 days on a water/milk diet (confirmed salicylate free on analysis) in a subject free of aspirin for at least 2 weeks. Excretion of SA + SU continued at a rate of ~2.1 μmol/24 h throughout and serum SA did not fall—over the 72 h of the study—below 0.1 μmol/L (20× the limit of detection of the assay) [28].

In six patients who had total colectomy or rectal excision following standard pre-operative bowel preparation low level serum SA (range 0.012–0.085 μmol/L) was detected and urinary SA + SU excretion persisted (median lowest level 0.613 μmol/ 24 h; range 0.184–7.607) in all subjects for up to 5 days postoperatively, rising only on refeeding [28]. These results also, of course, have some relevance to Section 4.2.

4.4 SA formation from benzoic acid

Benzoic acid (BA) is a natural constituent of plants, with high levels found in fruits and vegetables. In plants synthesis of SA derives—at least partially—from phenylalanine via cinnamic and benzoic acids. Prior work, using formula diet feed-ing, also demonstrated that hippuric acid, the main metabolite of BA, may be formed endogenously in man, while a Sprague-Dawley rat radiolabeled experiment showed phenylalanine as the likely precursor [32]. Sodium benzoate as a food preservative also contributes to human intake and very high doses have been used in hepatic encephalopathy. These considerations led us to determine whether addi-tion of BA to a very carefully standardised diet produced any change in serum or urinary salicylates—see **Figure 1**.

A preliminary study, over 4 days in two subjects, suggested that BA, 1 or 2 g/day on days 3 and 4 might be associated with a modest increase in urinary SA + SU excretion. Subsequently a labelled study was undertaken over 3 days in six individuals (4 M, 2F) who received 1 g of uniformly ring-labelled ^{13}C BA with each of their main meals on day 2. They replicated their carefully recorded day 1 diet throughout and had regular blood sampling with complete urine collections. The **total** SA + SU urinary excretion increased, but not significantly ($p = 0.052$) and only in the 8–16 h sample after the first dose of BA. While no ^{13}C was detected in samples prior to ingestion of the BA, the ^{13}C isotope was confirmed in the 8–16 h urine sample from all six subjects. Its presence was determined by preliminary GC fractionation before subjecting the relevant fractions to derivatization and GC–MS. The ^{13}C isotope accounted, by selective ion monitoring, for 0.4–10.9% (median 3.4%) in the SA derivative and 6.8–43.1% (median 33.9%) in the SU derivative. In addition considerable amounts of the expected $^{13}C_6$-labelled hippuric acid were found [28].

Set against the **total** SA + SU levels the extent of the SU $^{13}C_6$ labelling found might be considered surprising but could, as well as confirming the in vivo synthesis of SA, point to possible bioregulation of the levels of endogenous serum SA.

5. Salicylic acid in the biosphere

The protean actions of aspirin in animals and man are here, in a short review by JRL an GJB, set against what is known of the role of its SA precursor in earlier life forms.

5.1 Bacteria

This complex area is here only briefly overviewed in relation to its potential for pointing to possible effects of SA preserved into animals.

Para-aminosalicylic acid (PAS), the earliest truly effective anti-tuberculous agent, was long thought an analogue for para-aminobenzoic acid and so an inhibitor of folic acid biosynthesis. That was before the discovery of the mycobacterial siderophore (iron binding molecule) mycobactin, and that SA (also formed, as an extracellular metabolite, by mycobacteria in iron deficient conditions) is its direct precursor. It appears PAS primarily inhibits the conversion of SA into myobactin. Possible secondary roles for SA are the transfer of Fe^{2+} across the cell membrane, either for direct incorporation into various porphyrins and apoproteins, or for storage of iron within the cytoplasm in bacterioferritin (both roles also potential targets for PAS) [33].

There are many kinds of bacterial siderophores but SA or one of its hydroxylated metabolites (2,3DHBA) are at the core of the aryl- capped molecules found in *E. coli* (Enterobactin); *Yersinia* sp. and *Klebsiella pneumoniae* (Yersinibactin); *Pseudomonas* sp.(Pyochelin); *Vibrio* sp. (Vibriobactin/Vulnibactin) and *Acinetobacter baumanii* (Acinetobactin) [34]. These authors described a probe for the initial aryl acid activation enzymatic step in the synthetic pathways of these "bactins" (*via a non-ribosomal peptide synthetase pathway initiated by adenylation*) and suggested lack of human homologues makes this a potential drug target—but see Section 5.3.4.

Intriguingly investigation into the bioinorganic chemistry of bacterial siderophores has revealed that many have functional capacities other than mere iron homeostasis. Examples include interactions with other metals such as zinc, copper and boron; signalling agents (referred to as "ferrimones") in the regulation of genes related to iron metabolism; protection—by those with catecholate structures—from oxidative stress and an antibiotic function in sideromycins [35].

Finally bacterial growth in the presence of salicylate can be both beneficial and detrimental. On the one hand an intrinsic multiple antibiotic resistance phenotype can be induced and on the other reduced resistance to some antibiotics might result and bacterial virulence factors may be affected [36]. While the in vivo consequences of these observations is speculative the findings highlight, the authors suggest, the ability of salicylate to alter gene expression; they claim that the only life form not yet (then) shown to be affected by salicylate is the Archaea!

5.2 Plants

While salicylic acid (initially from plant sources) has been used in therapeutics for millennia detailed knowledge of its role in plants is relatively recent. Although plant phenolics are diverse and ubiquitous they were traditionally assumed to be unimportant secondary metabolites but SA in plants is a critical hormone playing a direct role in the regulation of many aspects of growth and development as well as in thermogenesis and disease resistance [37]. The first clear evidence came, intriguingly (in relation to its antipyretic qualities in animals), from its role in voodoo lily thermogenesis; that appears to be mediated by stimulation of the mitochondrial alternative respiratory pathway [38]. Soon thereafter its role as a defence signalling hormone was documented—though the ability of plants to develop acquired immunity after pathogen infection was first proposed many years earlier. In the acquired immunity—called "systemic acquired resistance" (SAR)—of plants to biotrophic (i.e. threatening living cells) pathogens, the role of SA is pivotal. Careful study has identified two pathways for its synthesis, numerous proteins that regulate its synthesis and metabolism and some signalling components, including a large number of potential targets/receptors, which operate downstream of SA [39]. This is a perplexing field; for example while the non-specialist can readily appreciate methylation of SA to a volatile ester for transport through the phloem (before demethylation at a site where SA levels are low) subsequent steps are complex. As these authors point out it is increasingly evident that SA does not signal immune response by itself but as part of an intricate network of other plant hormones. We would highlight, from the viewpoint of the present review, their suggestion that it is important to differentiate SA "targets" from the subset (whose criteria, they concede, will be difficult to specify) that meet additional conditions to be designated "receptors" [40]. That idea is particularly relevant when later considering the propensity of aspirin to acetylate many animal protein "receptors"—see Section 5.3.4.

The wide range of basal SA levels between and within plant species, and potential for a biphasic/concentration dependent response may explain some conflicting reports on the spectrum of plant processes it influences. Despite these caveats the long list affected by exogenous SA includes resistance to biotic (pathogen-associated) stress and tolerance to many abiotic stresses (drought, chilling, heat, metal, UV radiation, and salinity/osmotic stress) as well as multiple aspects of plant growth and development. These include photosynthesis, senescence, thermogenesis, respiration, glycolysis, the Krebs cycle and the alternative respiratory pathway [40].

5.3 Salicylic acid and aspirin (ASA) in animals and man

Although the use of willow extracts had been known for centuries the report of its first well documented use—as a cheaper remedy for "the agues" than expensive cinchona bark—focused on its antipyretic properties. Then, particularly in the decades following the isolation of SA as the active principle, evidence steadily accrued for its efficacy as an analgesic and anti-inflammatory in e.g. acute rheumatic fever.

5.3.1 After the discovery of aspirin

Following Hoffman's synthesis of the apparently better tolerated ester in 1897 use of that compound prevailed. ASA was the prototype non-steroidal anti-inflammatory drug (NSAID); it seems that term arose from a need to distinguish it from the undesirable effects of synthetic steroids. As a prodrug for a long recognised active agent its mode of action was naturally linked to the effects of SA.

It was not until the 1960s that work by Vane and Piper led to the proposal of a single mode of action of ASA in the inhibition of prostaglandin synthesis. The resulting paradigm-shifting series of experiments led to the discovery that inhibition of constitutive COX-1 and of COX-2 (predominantly inducible) by serine side-chain acetylation altered levels of prostaglandins and leukotrienes. This revelation came at a time when the potency of ASA as an inhibitor of platelet aggregation in the treatment of vascular disease was coming to the fore. So Vane's work explained, in a unitary and coherent way, the multiple pharmacological actions of ASA. The ester prevailed—particularly as SA itself had no significant anti-COX-1 effect on platelets.

5.3.2 Platelet effects predominant?

This emphasis arose from the apparent efficacy, in cancer chemo-protection, of ASA at the low doses (~70–100 mg/day) used to inhibit platelet aggregation. Irreversible inhibition of COX-1 in the circulating anucleate platelets ensures that thromboxane A_2 formation is prevented throughout their lifespan without, at these doses, suppressing the production of prostacyclin (PGI_2) which mediates platelet inhibition and vasodilatation. While that is the principle effect required in vascular disease platelet activation also triggers a host of processes leading to leucocyte recruitment into various tissues and subsequent phenotypic changes in stromal cells contributing to atherosclerosis, intestinal inflammation and cancer as well as atherothrombosis [41]. That review also encompasses the non-COX effects of the widespread acetylation of other proteins by ASA—quoting one study which revealed over 12,000 ASA-mediated acetylations in over 3700 proteins!

5.3.3 Do earlier accepted effects of ASA and SA still hold?

There is a trend to describe non-COX, indeed increasingly non-platelet, effects of ASA as "non-canonical". That tag appears to include almost all actions not demonstrably due to COX acetylation with the possible exception of inhibition of COX-2 gene transcription [4].

We should, however, remind ourselves that

a. It is generally accepted that although SA is a much weaker inhibitor of COX activity in vitro their anti-inflammatory effects in vivo are comparable [3].

b. ASA has a very short serum half-life compared with SA [2]; its passage (almost certainly total salicylates were determined) through the blood/brain barrier is slow and incomplete [42]. That observation is particularly relevant to the oft forgotten central action of salicylates [43].

c. ASA's antipyretic effect was first validated centuries ago using plant extracts; it is mainly due to inhibition of COX-2 in the hypothalamus [44].

d. There is a clear dose/response relationship between the analgesic effect of ASA up to a dose of 1.2 g [45] compared with the plateau above ~100 mg/day for the effect on platelets and its efficacy in chemoprevention of colorectal adenomas [46].

5.3.4 ASA "receptors"

The eminent facility for ASA to acetylate proteins has been known for decades and proteomic studies—*see above*—have shown its very marked extent. While the functional relationship between such activity and its effects are unclear the blockade of glucose6phosphate dehydrogenase (G6PD), affecting the pentose phosphate pathway, and disruption of mitochondrial respiration may explain platelet autophagy [41]. Clearly, as for SA in plants, caution is required in the strict definition of ASA receptors [39, 40].

5.3.5 SA "receptors"

While the above caveat applies the blunderbuss masking effect of acetylation is not a consideration. At least 15 SA binding proteins are described to date [39] but some intriguing examples point to effects on proteins with plant and bacterial homologues.

Human glyceraldehyde3-phosphate dehydrogenase (HsGADPH)—has been identified as a SA binding protein—as it is in plants. In addition to its central role in glycolysis GADPH participates in pathological processes, with effects on viral replication and neuronal cell death [47]. Its suppression, by low μM levels of salicylate, in a model of cell death comparable to that induced by reactive oxygen species (ROS) was found. The authors postulate that likely due to suppression of HsGADPH nuclear translocation, mirroring the effect of the anti-Parkinsonian drug Deprenyl.

The same group have also shown [39, 48] that SA targets human high mobility group box 1 (HMGB1), an abundant chromatin associated protein, present in all animal cells; fungi and plants have related proteins. Its diverse effects modulate inflammatory processes. *HMGB1's many activities and receptors likely account for its multiple roles in human disease which include sepsis, arthritis, atherosclerotic plaque formation and cancer.* The effect of SA on HMGB1 occurs at concentrations far lower than those required to inhibit COX enzyme activity; an effect on COX2 is on synthesis rather than activity.

An example of a bacterial homologue enzyme, found in mice, is responsible for synthesis of 2,5DHBA—the iron binding moiety of a mammalian siderophore [49]; that enzyme is a homologue of bacterial EntA which catalyses 2,3DHBA production during enterobactin biosynthesis (Section 5.1). 2,5DHBA can, of course, also derive from the metabolism of SA or benzoic acid.

Other orthologs of a plant SA receptor—NAD(P)-reductase like proteins—have been characterised in the human neuroblastoma SK-N-SH cell line and mouse brain tissue [50]. Their results may point, the authors claim, to the existence of a thermoregulation system that is evolutionary conserved.

5.3.6 ASA and SA as NSAIDs

The few direct studies to validate the assertion 5.3.2a above compared salsalate (which yields only SA on absorption) with SA, generally at the higher doses used in rheumatic diseases. Given what we know about the distribution and relative inhibition of COX1 and COX2 it's not surprising that at comparable doses effects were similar with a predictable lower gastrointestinal toxicity of SA [51]. The authors suggested that, when ASA was originally marketed, commercial forces equated taste and tolerability/toxicity! These prominent rheumatologists concluded that "non-acetylated salicylates should be preferred to ASA in rheumatology". They clearly supported the German proverb:- "Bitter im Mund, gesund im Korper."

While the NSAID categorisation originally served to differentiate the side effects of SA and steroids, very early work had shown a CNS effects specific to salicylates. Later studies—stimulated by discovery of the antipyretic/anti-inflammatory actions of the neuropeptide α-melanocyte stimulating hormone (αMSH)—clearly demonstrated peripheral effects of salicylates introduced into the CNS by injection into the lateral ventricle. These experiments showed that CNS doses which had no effect systemically had a marked effect on the mouse model of inflammation used. The effect was restricted to the salicylates; central injection of an anti-inflammatory dose (when given intra-peritoneally) of indomethacin had no effect: neither did intraventricular dexamethasone or prostaglandin E_2 [43].

More recent work on peroxisome proliferator-activated receptors (PPARs) has also shown the importance of central nervous system actions. Peroxisomes are oxidative (H_2O_2 producing) organelles subserving redox regulation and metabolism of very long chain fatty acids. They are abundant in the CNS, where such fatty acids abound and their increase, when required, is receptor mediated. Studies have compared the anti-inflammatory effect of agonists of PPARα and PPARγ (themselves inactive at the site of inflammation) with the effect of dexamethasone and ASA. Only other agonists and ASA (which itself has generally no direct* PPAR agonist effect) were found to diminish inflammation when given after the inflammatory insult in contrast to the effect of dexamethasone. The conclusion was that PPARα and PPARγ regulate inflammation through a mechanism similar to salicylates and distinct from that ascribed to steroids [53]. The authors postulated that activating PPARs in the CNS could elicit **the release of a salicylate-like compound, an endosalicylate**, which may subsequently cause the release of a physiological anti-inflammatory substance such as αMSH.

These results on CNS activity point to steroid/NSAID differentiation which is at least partially dependent on how agents influence the anti-inflammatory and immunomodulatory effect of melanocortins (ACTH and MSH).

6. Conclusions

Given the ever increasing complexity of SA and ASA effects revealed by basic research it seems blinkered to increasingly restrict focus to platelet/COX effects in the biomedical field.

We reiterate our conclusion that ASA is no mere anti-platelet prototype [54]. That is the case, we aver, for most of the protean pathophysiological effects of ASA and not solely in cancer chemoprevention. The evidence summarised here, particularly our demonstration of the in-vivo synthesis of SA, points to it as a truly endogenous molecule in animals and man. Potential "preserved" receptors which have been described are there, we suggest, not simply to deal with ingested SA or other exogenous precursors.

The place of SA in the biosphere overall is, we think, as pivotal as it appears to be in plants. While a unifying hypothesis to explain its many roles is elusive we suspect they all ultimately relate to the need for evolving life to balance its requirements for oxygen and iron [55]. These authors concluded that the sequestration of iron to restrict its reaction with reactive oxygen species (ROS) is one of our major antioxidant defence mechanisms. They particularly emphasise, in that summary, how such sequestration remains critical to our ongoing resistance to bacterial infection.

The huge increase in energy production arising from enzymatic reduction of oxygen enabled evolution of multicellular animal life. While that was an evolutionary milestone ability to use the resulting reactive oxygen species (ROS) for cell signalling and regulation may have been the first true breakthrough in development of complex life [56]. By then SA was already well established and poised to interact (with ROS) as required. In animals its many effects are unlikely to be less complex than the interactions steadily becoming clarified in plants [39]. *Many may depend upon the type of intricate relationships which initiate plant systemic acquired resistance (SAR) with an initial SA induced redox change. Subsequent SA concentration sensitive*

---

* However ASA's apparently direct binding to PPARα may explain its stimulation of hippocampal plasticity [52] and potential for prevention of Alzheimers.

oligomer/monomer transformation permits nuclear translocation of a cytosolic messenger to activate immune-associated genes [40].

Re-focus on the importance of the SA moiety of ASA should also lead to further evaluation of SA derivatives which are more active than SA itself in interaction with particular "binding protein/receptors" [47, 48]. At a more basic level we have previously pointed out that, particularly to extend its use in prophylaxis, the risk/benefit profile of ASA may be improved with an SA/ASA combined formulation [54].

Given what we have learned on this investigative journey it is somewhat paradoxical that we embarked upon it driven by desire to capitalise on the hydroxylation of ASA as a biomarker of oxidative "stress" in man—see Section 2.

Acknowledgements

Dr. John Robert Paterson (1955–2004), our dear friend who initiated and steered this line of research, always—from schooldays onwards—thought of himself as a chemist first and foremost. Through his long and arduous training in pharmacy, medicinal chemistry, medicine, royal college membership and clinical biochemistry he described himself as a chemist. Most of the work summarised herein, including results published after his death, was either planned by him or arose from discussions during his life. Our prime purpose in undertaking this compilation has been to remain true to his vision. We only pray that there are no glaring chemical errors—the fault is entirely ours if there are.

We are grateful to Hannah Mortlock for the preparation of **Figure 1**.

Thanks

We wish to thank Dumfries and Galloway Health Board for their support over the many years of these studies, especially their Research and Development and Library services.

Our work has been supported financially by the Dumfries and Galloway Health Board's Salicylic Acid Research Endowment Fund.

Other declarations

We have done our utmost to accurately reflect the findings and conclusions of the many authors quoted in Section 5. Profuse apologies if our reflections on their studies appear at variance with their interpretations.

Author details

James Ronald Lawrence*, Gwendoline Joan Baxter and John Robert Paterson†
Research and Development Support Unit, Dumfries and Galloway Royal Infirmary, Cargenbridge, Dumfries, Scotland

*Address all correspondence to: jim.lawrence@nhs.net

† Deceased.

References

[1] Klessig DF, Choi HW, Dempsey DA. Systemic acquired resistance and salicylic acid. Past, present and future. Molecular Plant-Microbe Interactions. 2018;**31**(9):871-888

[2] Needs CJ, Brooks PM. Clinical pharmacokinetics of the salicylates. Clinical Pharmacokinetics. 1985;**10**: 164-177

[3] Higgs GA, Salmon JA, Henderson VJR. Pharmacokinetics of aspirin and salicylate in relation to inhibition of arachidonate cyclooxygenase and anti-inflammatory activity. Proceedings of the National Academy of Sciences of the United States of America. 1987;**84**:1417-1420

[4] Xu X-M, Sansores-Garcia L, Chen X-M, et al. Suppression of inducible cyclooxygenase 2 gene transcription by aspirin and sodium salicylate. Proceedings of the National Academy of Sciences of the United States of America. 1999;**96**:5292-5297

[5] Vree TB, Ewijk-Beneken V, EWJ K, et al. Direct gradient reversed-phase high performance liquid chromatographic determination of salicylic acid with the corresponding glycine and glucoronate conjugates in human plasma and urine. Journal of Chromatography B. 1994;**652**:161-170

[6] Coudray C, Mangournet C, Bouhadjeb S, et al. Rapid high-performance liquid chromatographic assay for salicylic acid in plasma without solvent extraction. Journal of Chromatographic Science. 1996;**34**: 166-173

[7] Ruffin MT, Krishnan K, Rock CL, et al. Suppression of human colorectal mucosal prostaglandins: Determining the lowest effective aspirin dose. Journal of the National Cancer Institute. 1997; **89**:1152-1160

[8] Paterson JR, Blacklock C, Campbell G, et al. The identification of salicylates as normal constituents of serum. A link between diet and health?Journal of Clinical Pathology. 1998;**51**: 501-505

[9] Armstrong MD, Shaw KNF, Wall PE. The phenolic acids of human urine. The Journal of Biological Chemistry. 1956; **218**:293-303

[10] Von Studnitz W, Engelman K, Sjoerdsma A. Urinary excretion of phenolic acids in human subjects on a glucose diet. Clinica Chimica Acta. 1964;**9**:224-227

[11] Young DS. Effect of a chemically defined diet on urinary excretion of minerals and aromatic compounds. Clinical Chemistry. 1970;**16**:681-686

[12] Finnie MDA, Ersser RS, Seakins JWT, Snedden W. The occurrence and identification of o-hydroxyhippuric acid (salicyluric acid) in the urine of sick children. Clinica Chimica Acta. 1976;**70**:171-178

[13] Janssen PLTMK, Hollman PCH, Reichman E, et al. Urinary salicylate excretion in subjects eating a variety of diets shows that amounts of bioavailable salicylates in food are low. The American Journal of Clinical Nutrition. 1996;**64**:743-747

[14] Baxter GJ, Lawrence JR, Graham AB, et al. Identification and determination of salicylic acid and salicyluric acid in urine of people not taking salicylate drugs. Annals of Clinical Biochemistry. 2002;**39**:50-55

[15] Anon. Salicylic acid I strawberries. Lancet. 1903;**25**:117

[16] Anon. "Natural" and synthetic salicylates. JAMA. 1913;**20**:968

[17] Acamovich T, Brooker JD. Biochemistry of plant secondary metabolites and their affects in animals. The Proceedings of the Nutrition Society. 2005;**64**:403-412

[18] Paterson JR, Lawrence JR. Salicylic acid: A link between aspirin, diet and the prevention of colorectal cancer. The Quarterly Journal of Medicine. 2001;**94**: 445-448

[19] Elwood PC, Gallagher AM, Duthie GG, et al. Aspirin, salicylates and cancer. Lancet. 2009;**373**:1301-1309

[20] Sostres C, Gargallo CJ, Lanas A. Aspirin, cyclooxygenase inhibition and colorectal cancer. World Journal of Gastrointestinal Pharmacology and Therapeutics. 2014;**5**:40-49

[21] Alfonso L, Spitali RC, Bhat GJ. Molecular targets of aspirin and cancer prevention. British Journal of Cancer. 2014;**111**:61-67

[22] Swain AR, Dutton SP. Salicylates in food. Journal of the American Dietetic Association. 1985;**85**:950-960

[23] Venema DP, Hollman PCH, Janssen PLTM, Katan MB. Determination of acetylsalicylic acid and salicylic acid in foods using HPLC with fluorescence detection. Journal of Agricultural and Food Chemistry. 1996; **44**:1762-1767

[24] Blacklock CJ, Lawrence JR, Wiles D, et al. Salicylic acid in the serum of subjects not taking aspirin. Comparison of salicylic acid concentrations in the serum of vegetarians, non-vegetarians, and in patients taking low dose aspirin. Journal of Clinical Pathology. 2001;**54**: 553-555

[25] Lawrence JR, Peter R, Baxter GJ, et al. Urinary excretion of salicyluric and salicylic acids by non-vegetarians, vegetarians and patients taking low dose aspirin. Journal of Clinical Pathology. 2003;**56**:651-653

[26] Mohandas KM. Colorectal cancer in India: Controversies, enigmas and primary prevention. Indian Journal of Gastroenterology. 2011;**30**(1):3-6

[27] Paterson JR, Srivastava R, Baxter GJ, et al. Salicylic acid content of spices and its implications. Journal of Agricultural and Food Chemistry. 2006;**54**: 2891-2896

[28] Paterson JR, Baxter GJ, Dreyer JS, et al. Salicylic acid sans aspirin in animals and man: Persistence in fasting and biosynthesis from benzoic acid. Journal of Agricultural and Food Chemistry. 2008;**56**:11648-11652

[29] Wood A, Baxter GJ, Thies F, et al. A systematic review of salicylates in foods; estimated daily intake of a Scottish population. Molecular Nutrition & Food Research. 2011;**55**:S7-S14

[30] Baxter GJ, Graham AB, Lawrence, Paterson JR. Salicylic acid in soups prepared from organically and non-organically grown vegetables. European Journal of Nutrition. 2001;**40**:289-292

[31] Spadafranca A, Bertoli S, Fiorillo G, et al. Circulating salicylic acid is related to fruit and vegetable consumption in healthy subjects. The British Journal of Nutrition. 2007;**4**:802-806

[32] Armstrong MD, Chao F-C, Parker VJ, Wall PE. Endogenous formation of hippuric acid. Proceedings of the Society for Experimental Biology and Medicine. 1955;**90**:675-679

[33] Ratledge C. Iron, mycobacteria and tuberculosis. Tuberculosis (Edinburgh, Scotland). 2004;**84**:110-130

[34] Neres J, Wilson DJ, Celia L, et al. Aryl acid adenylating enzymes involved in siderophore biosynthesis. Biochemistry. 2008;**47**(45):11735-11749

[35] Johnstone TC, Nolan EM. Beyond iron: Non-classical biological functions of bacterial siderophores. Dalton Transactions. 2015;**44**(14):6320-6339

[36] Price CTD, Lee IR, Gustafson JE. The effects of salicylate in bacteria. The International Journal of Biochemistry and Cell Biology. 2000;**32**:1029-1043

[37] Vlot AC, Dempsey DA, Klessig DF. Salicylic acid, a multifaceted hormone to combat disease. Annual Review of Phytopathology. 2009;**47**:177-206

[38] Rhoads DM, McIntosh L. Salicylic acid regulation of respiration in higher plants: Alternative oxidase expression. The Plant Cell. 1992;**4**:1131-1139

[39] Klessig DF, Choi HW, Dempsey DA. Systemic acquired Resistanc and salicylic acid; past, present, and future. Molecular Plant-Microbe Interactions. 2018;**31**:871-888

[40] Dempsey DA, Klessig DF. How does the multifaceted plant hormone salicylic acid combat disease in plants and are similar mechanisms utilized in humans. BMC Biology. 2017;**15**:23

[41] Ornelas A, Zacharias-Millward N, Menter DG, et al. Beyond COX-1: The effects of aspirin on platelet biology and potential mechanisms of chemoprevention. Cancer Metastasis Reviews. 2017;**36**:289-303

[42] Bannwarth B, Netter P, Pourel J, et al. Clinical pharmacokinetics of non-steroidal anti-inflammatory drugs in the cerebrospinal fluid. Biomedicine & Pharmacotherapy. 1989;**43**:121-126

[43] Catania A, Macaluso A, Arnold J, et al. Inhibition of acute inflammation in the periphery by the central action of salicylates. Proceedings of the National Academy of Sciences of the United States of America. 1991;**88**: 8544-8547

[44] Aronoff DM, Neilson EG. Antipyretics: Mechanisms of action and clinical use in fever suppression. The American Journal of Medicine. 2001;**111**: 304-315

[45] McQuay HJ, Moore RA. Dose-response in direct comparisons of different dose of aspirin, ibuprofen and paracetamol (acetaminophen) in analgesic studies. British Journal of Clinical Pharmacology. 2006;**63**:271-278

[46] Cole BF, Logan RF, Halabi S, et al. Aspirin for the chemoprevention of colorectal adenomas: Meta-analysis of the randomized trials. Journal of the National Cancer Institute. 2009;**101**: 256-266

[47] Choi HW, Tian M, Manohar M, et al. Human GADPH is a target of Aspirin's primary metabolite salicylic acid and its derivatives. PLoS One. 2015; **10**:e0143447. DOI: 10.1371/journal.pone.0143447

[48] Choi HW, Tian M, Song F, et al. Aspirin's active metabolite salicylic acid targets high mobility group Box1 to modulate inflammatory response. Molecular Medicine. 2015;**21**:526-535

[49] Devireddy LR, Hart DO, Goetz D, Green M. A mammalian siderophore synthesized by an enzyme with a bacterial homologue involved in Enterobactin production. Cell. 2010; **141**(6):1006-1017

[50] Skubatz H, Howald WN. Human orthology of plant salicylic acid receptor found in SK-N-SH cell line. The Protein Journal. 2013;**32**:641-648

[51] Rainsford KD, Buchanan WW. Aspirin versus the non-acetylated salicylates. Baillière's Clinical Rheumatology. 1990;**4**(2):247-268

[52] Patel D, Roy A, Kundu M, et al. Aspirin binds to PPARα to stimulate hippocampal plasticity and protect

memory. PNAS. 2018;**115**(31):E7408-E7417

[53] Youssef J, Badr M. Peroxisome proliferator activated receptors: Features, functions, and future. Nuclear Receptor Research. 2015:1-30. DOI: 10.11131/2015/101188

[54] Lawrence JR, Baxter GJ, Paterson JR. Aspirin for cancer is no mere antiplatelet prototype. There is potential in its ancient roots. Medical Hypotheses. 2016;**94**:74-76

[55] Gutteridge JMC, Halliwell B. Mini-review: Oxidative stress, redox stress or redox success. Biochemical and Biophysical Research Communications. 2018;**502**:183-186

[56] Taverne YJ, Merkus D, Bogers Ad J, et al. Reactive oxygen species: Radical factors in the evolution of animal life. BioEssays. 2018;**40**:1-9. DOI: 10.1002.bies.201700158

8

Drug Repositioning for the Treatment of Glioma: Current State and Future Perspective

Sho Tamai, Nozomi Hirai, Shabierjiang Jiapaer, Takuya Furuta and Mitsutoshi Nakada

Abstract

Gliomas are the most common primary brain tumors. Among them, glioblastoma (GBM) possesses the most malignant phenotype. Despite the current standard therapy using an alkylating anticancer agent, temozolomide, most patients with GBM die within 2 years. Novel chemotherapeutic agents are urgently needed to improve the prognosis of GBM. One of the solutions, drug repositioning, which broadens the indications of existing drugs, has gained attention. Herein, we catego-rize candidate agents, which are newly identified as therapeutic drugs for malignant glioma into 10 classifications based on these original identifications. Some drugs are in clinical trials with hope. Additionally, the obstacles, which should be overcome in order to accomplish drug repositioning as an application for GBM and the future perspectives, have been discussed.

Keywords: glioma, glioblastoma, drug repositioning, chemotherapy, temozolomide, existing drugs, pre-drugs

1. Introduction

Many diseases require the development of new drugs for effective treatment. The relevance of drug repurposing in medical science has progressively grown recently. The increasing interest in drug repurposing is realized based on the increase of related academic publications.

Annually, approximately 23 per 100,000 people suffer from tumors of the central nervous system (CNS). Gliomas, which account for 25% of all CNS tumors, are the most common primary brain tumors, and most are malignant [1]. Glioblastoma (GBM) is a malignant glioma with the worst prognosis, as it accounts for 60% of all gliomas and is classified as grade IV by the World Health Organization (WHO) [1, 2]. Despite aggressive therapies, the median overall survival (OS) of patients who suffer from GBM is only 15–18 months [1, 3].

The current treatments for GBM are maximum surgical resection and adjuvant chemoradiotherapy. The first-line agent for chemotherapy is temozolomide (TMZ), an imidazotetrazinone derivative [4]. TMZ acts as a major groove-directed deoxyribonucleic acid (DNA)-alkylating agent, and its molecular weight is only 194 Da [4]. A phase III clinical trial revealed that concomitant and adjuvant TMZ with radiotherapy is effective for the treatment of patients with primary GBM [5].

Approximately half of the cases of GBM have a methylation of the O^6-methylguanine-DNA methyltransferase (MGMT) promoter, and these cases are associated with a favorable outcome after concomitant and adjuvant TMZ with radiotherapy [6]. MGMT potentially removes methyl adducts at the O^6 position of guanine and indicates resistance to alkylating agents; however, the methylation of the MGMT promoter interferes with MGMT activity and induces glioma cell death [6].

Clinical trials have revealed the therapeutic benefit of bevacizumab (BEV), a recombinant, humanized, monoclonal antibody against vascular endothelial growth factor (VEGF), in patients with cancer [7]. Large-scale clinical studies have been performed to investigate the therapeutic effects of BEV in patients with newly diagnosed GBM [8, 9]. However, the clinical benefits of BEV in patients with glioma are still unknown.

Research into drug repositioning for GBM is now expanding, although no effective drug has yet been reported with strong and solid evidence. Herein, we focus on candidate agents with therapeutic effects in malignant glioma and that have undergone clinical trials to evaluate their efficacy in patients. We also describe the issues of drug repositioning in malignant glioma.

2. Current candidate agents for glioma

Here, we categorize candidate agents into 10 classifications (**Table 1**).

2.1 Antidiabetic drugs

2.1.1 Metformin

The intracellular metabolic pathway of cancer cells differs from that of normal cells, as represented by the Warburg effect, and is considered as a cancer therapeutic target. Metformin is a biguanide antidiabetic drug that exerts a hypoglycemic effect via the suppression of gluconeogenesis in the liver and promotion of glucose uptake in the muscle and adipose tissues. The antitumor effects of metformin are widely known and reported in various cancers, such as breast cancer [10].

Basic research with metformin in glioma cells and glioma stem-like cells (GSCs) has shown that metformin targets multiple pathways (**Figure 1**). Metformin activates AMP-activated protein kinase (AMPK) via the inhibition of oxidative phosphorylation in mitochondrial complex I, which increases the AMP/ATP ratio, thereby inhibiting the mammalian target of rapamycin (mTOR) and promoting apoptosis [11, 12]. The metformin-mediated activation of AMPK, followed by the activation of forkhead box O3 (FOXO3), induces GSC differentiation and reduces tumorigenicity [13]. The Cancer Genome Atlas has reported missense mutations in isocitrate dehydrogenase (IDH) genes 1 and 2. D-2-Hydroxyglutarate (D-2HG), a cancer metabolite produced by the mutant IDH protein, contributes to the development and progression of cancer. The conversion of glutamine to α-ketoglutarate (αKG) is catalyzed by glutamate dehydrogenase (GDH), and the inhibition of GDH by metformin reduces the production of D-2HG in glioma with the IDH 1/2 mutation [14]. Chloride intracellular channel 1 (CLIC1) is involved in the progression of various cancers, including GBM [15–17]. CLIC1 is involved in the regulation of the G1/S transition, and metformin causes G1 cell cycle arrest in GSCs by the selective inhibition of CLIC1 [18].

An epidemiological study using the Clinical Practice Research Datalink reported that the use of metformin is not associated with a reduced risk of glioma [19]. In a

	Candidate agent	Original indication disease	Mechanism of original disease	Mechanism of anti-glioma effect	CT	Refs.
2.1 Antidiabetic drugs	2.1.1 Metformin	Diabetes mellitus	Suppress gluconeogenesis in the liver	Activate AMPK Inhibit glutamate dehydrogenase	NY	[10–20]
2.2 Antihypertensive drugs	2.2.1 Angiotensin II receptor blocker	Hypertension	Block angiotensin II receptor	Inhibit vascular endothelial growth factor	III	[21–25]
	2.2.2 β-blocker	Hypertension	Block β receptor	Decrease cAMP levels	NY	[26, 27]
	2.2.3 Calcium channel blocker	Hypertension	Block calcium channel	Inhibit hippo pathway	NY	[28, 29]
2.3 Antiepileptic drugs	2.3.1 Valproic acid	Epilepsy	Block sodium channel	Inhibit GSK3β	NY	[31–39]
	2.3.2 Levetiracetam	Epilepsy	Block calcium channel	Inhibit MGMT expression	II	[40, 41]
2.4 Pesticides	2.4.1 Chloroquine	Malaria (*Plasmodium* spp.)	Inhibit heme polymerization	Inhibit TGF-β and NF-κB	II	[42–46]
	2.4.2 Pentamidine	Pneumocystis pneumonia	Inhibition of glucose metabolism, protein synthesis, amino acid transport and ribonucleic acid synthesis	Unknown	NY	[47–49]
2.5 Antipsychotic drugs	2.5.1 Fluvoxamine	Depression	Selective serotonin reuptake inhibitor	Suppress the activity of actin polymerization regulators	NY	[50–57]
	2.5.2 Fluspirilene	Schizophrenia	Dephenylbutylpiperidine	Inhibit activation of STAT3	NY	[58–62]
2.6 Antineoplastic drugs	2.6.1 Eribulin	Breast cancer	Inhibit of microtubule activity	Inhibitor of telomerase reverse transcriptase- RNA-dependent	II	[63–76]
2.7 Anti-inflammatory drugs	2.7.1 Acetylsalicylic acid drugs	Fever, inflammation disease	Inhibit cyclooxygenase	Activate connexin 43, suppress Wnt/β-catenin/T-cell factor signaling and SHH/GLI1 pathway	NY	[77–81]
	2.7.2 Sulfasalazine	Rheumatoid arthritis	Block activation of NF-κB	Block activation of NF-κB	I/II	[82–86]
2.8 Multiple drug combination therapy	2.8.1 CLOVA cocktail	–	–	Inhibit GSK3β	I/II	[87–90]
	2.8.2 CUSP9* treatment	–	–	Suppress multiple molecule pathway	NY	[91, 92]
	2.8.3 FTT cocktail	–	–	Inhibit ROCK2/moesin/β-catenin pathway, suppress TGF-β	NY	[93–96]

	Candidate agent	Original indication disease	Mechanism of original disease	Mechanism of anti-glioma effect	CT	Refs.
2.9 Other drugs	2.9.1 Disulfiram	Alcoholism	Inhibitor of ALDH	Inhibiting polo-like kinese-1	II	[97–101]
	2.9.2 Statins	Dyslipidemia	Inhibited 3-hydroxy-3-methylglutaryl-coenzyme A reductase	Activate transcription factor-2 and c-jun, suppress ERK	NY	[102–106]
2.10 Pre drugs	2.10.1 Kenpaullone	-	-	Inhibit GSK3β	NY	[107–111]
	2.10.2 2-Fluoropalmitic acid	-	-	Dephosphorylate ERK, suppress MMP-2	NY	[112–115]

ALDH, aldehyde dehydrogenase; AMPK, AMP-activated protein kinase; CT, clinical trial; ERK, extracellular signal-regulated kinase; GLI1, glioma-associated oncogene homolog 1; GSK3β, glycogen synthase kinase 3β; MGMT, O^6-methylguanine-DNA methyltransferase; MMP-2, matrix metalloproteinase-2; NF-κB, nuclear factor- kappaB; NY, not yet; ROCK2, Rho-associated protein kinase 2; SHH, sonic hedgehog; STAT3, signal transducer and activator of transcription 3; TGF-β, tumor growth factor-β.

Table 1.
The list of candidate agents.

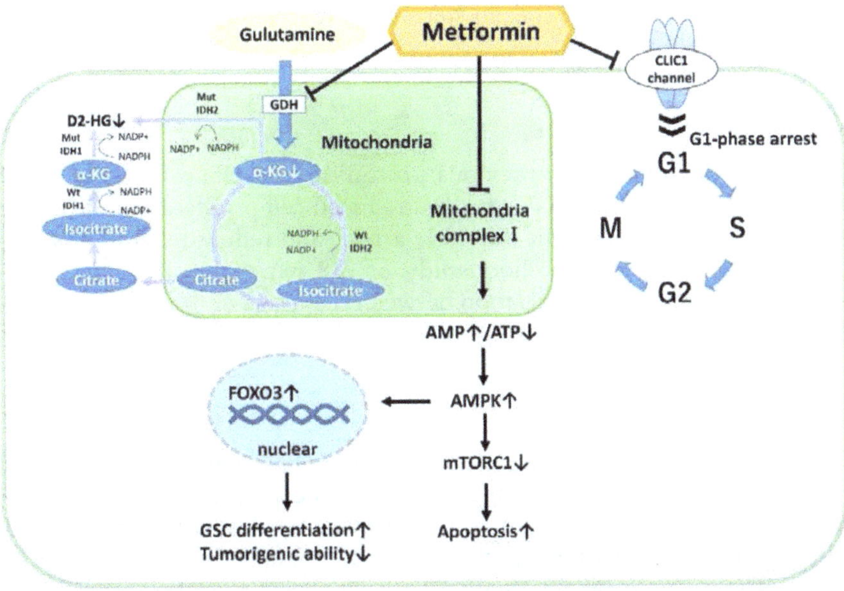

Figure 1.
Antitumor mechanisms of metformin in glioma. The inhibition of oxidative phosphorylation in mitochondrial complex I induces the inhibition of mammalian target of rapamycin complex 1 (mTORC1) and activation of FOXO3 via activating AMPK. The inhibition of GDH reduces the D-2HG production via αKG reduction in IDH 1/2 mutation glioma. Selective inhibition of CLIC1 causes G1 cell cycle arrest in GSCs.

pooled analysis that included 1731 patients from large-scale randomized controlled trials, the use of metformin was not significantly associated with OS or progression-free survival (PFS) in patients with newly diagnosed GBM [20]. Although the results of existing retrospective and epidemiological studies are somewhat discouraging, randomized clinical trials are underway, and we expect to see encouraging results in the future.

2.2 Antihypertensive drugs

2.2.1 Angiotensin II (AT2) receptor blocker

AT2 plays a major role in the renin-angiotensin-aldosterone system and regulates vascular homeostasis, mainly via the activation of angiotensin I receptor (AT1R) and AT2 receptor. Recent studies have revealed that AT2 has roles in cell proliferation, differentiation, apoptosis, and migration. Furthermore, AT2 induces angiogenesis via the stimulation of growth factors such as VEGF, which suggests that AT2 is a target for cancer therapy [21, 22]. Rivera et al. first reported the presence of AT1R in glioma cells and demonstrated that the selective blockade of AT1R with losartan in C6 glioma rats exerts antitumor effects via the inhibition of tumor growth and angiogenesis [22]. The group also showed that treatment with losartan inhibits tumor growth via the inhibition of VEGF and promotes apoptosis in vitro and in vivo [23]. A retrospective analysis of 81 patients with newly diagnosed GBM showed that the administration of an AT2R blocker or angiotensin-converting enzyme (ACE) inhibitor with the current treatment is associated with reduced brain edema and steroid requirements and improved clinical outcomes [24]. Nevertheless, the ASTER trial (NCT01805453), a randomized, placebo-controlled trial, which included losartan to the current treatment for patients with

GBM, did not show any difference in steroid requirements or a significant increase in the median OS [25].

2.2.2 β-Blocker

Tewarie et al. summarized previous preclinical and clinical studies about the effects of β-blockers on gliomas and noted reduced cell proliferation via a decrease in cAMP levels, time-dependent cell cycle arrest, and reduced cell migration [26]. However, in a retrospective cohort study of 218 patients with recurrent GBM, Johansen et al. observed no correlation between the usage of β-blockers and OS and PFS [27].

2.2.3 Calcium channel blocker

The altered expression and activity of specific Ca^{2+} channels and pumps have been reported in malignant gliomas [28]. Amlodipine, a commonly used antihypertensive drug, was shown to inhibit tumor growth by the inhibition of YAP/TAZ signaling via the hippo pathway, which is involved in tumor malignancy by the activation of store-operated Ca^{2+} entry. This allows intracellular Ca^{2+} influx [29]. Most research on calcium signaling in GBM is recent and further study is warranted.

2.3 Antiepileptic drugs

A common symptom of GBM is epilepsy, which occurs in half of all cases; thus, patients are often treated with antiepileptic drugs, such as valproic acid (VPA) and levetiracetam (LEV) (**Figure 2**). Enzymatic modifications of histone proteins that regulate gene expression have been investigated as therapeutic drug targets. Histones are modified by histone acetyltransferase (HAT) and histone deacetylase (HDAC). A HDAC inhibitor (HDACi) enhances the acetylation by HAT and causes a hyperacetylated state, which exerts multiple antitumor effects such as cell differentiation, apoptosis, cell cycle arrest, sensitivity to chemotherapy, and inhibition of migration and angiogenesis [30].

2.3.1 Valproic acid

Recently, VPA has been shown to be an effective HDACi and has been proposed as a drug for cancer treatment [31]. VPA inhibits the proliferation of glioma cells and enhances radiosensitivity by increasing hyperacetylation in vitro and in vivo [32]. Another antitumor effect of VPA is the induction of apoptosis by the inhibition of GSK3β via the activation of Akt/ERK [33]. According to several studies, the inhibition of GSK3β suppresses survival and proliferation and induces apoptosis in human GBM cells [34]. However, some meta-analyses have revealed that the clinical benefit of VPA combination treatment in patients with GBM was contraindicated [35–39], and further studies are warranted.

2.3.2 Levetiracetam

LEV has been shown to increase HDAC1 transcription, recruit the mSin3A/HDAC1 corepressor complex on the MGMT promoter, and inhibit MGMT expression through the direct binding of p53 to the MGMT promoter [40]. Thus, LEV inhibits glioma cell proliferation and significantly potentiates the cytotoxic effects of TMZ in glioma cells and GSCs [40, 41]. A phase II clinical trial (NCT02815410) is ongoing and the results are expected in the future.

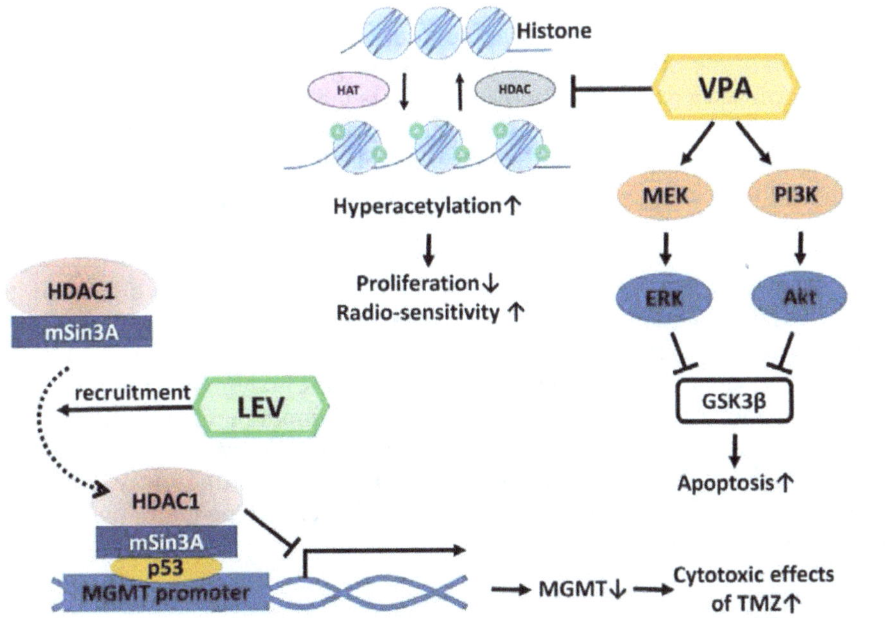

Figure 2.
Antitumor mechanisms of VPA and LEV in glioma. ***VPA:*** *hyperacetylation of histones via the inhibition of HDAC suppresses cell proliferation and increases radiosensitivity. The activation of Akt/extracellular signal-regulated kinase (ERK) inhibits glycogen synthase kinase-3β (GSK3β) and induces apoptosis.* ***LEV:*** *recruitment of the mSin3A/HDAC1 corepressor complex and direct binding to the MGMT promoter via p53. Abbreviations: HAT, histone acetyltransferase; MEK, mitogen-activated protein kinase/ERK kinase; PI3K, phosphoinositide 3-kinase; TMZ, temozolomide.*

2.4 Pesticides

2.4.1 Chloroquine (CHQ)

CHQ is a therapeutic drug for the treatment of malaria [42]. This agent has antitumor effects for some cancer cells, including glioma cells [43]. However, the mechanism of the antitumor effect of CHQ in glioma is not well known. Some studies have suggested that CHQ leads to cancer cell death by controlling autophagy [44], and recent research has revealed more effects of CHQ treatment. CHQ adjusts the metabolism of amino acids and inhibits glycogenesis [42]. CHQ administration also induces the alteration of mitochondrial membrane potential in glioma cells and causes apoptosis [45]. Some studies have investigated the molecular signaling associated with CHQ treatment. The molecular signaling changes in glioma cells caused by CHQ include the inhibition of the signaling pathway of transforming growth factor-β (TGF-β) and nuclear factor-kappaB (NF-κB), which play a role in tumorigenesis [42, 45]. CHQ treatment also suppresses glioma cell invasion by the inhibition of matrix metalloproteinase-2 (MMP-2) and improved radiosensitivity by the accumulation of glioma cells in the G2/M phase [45]. Based on the results of these in vitro studies, clinical trials that investigated the therapeutic effects of CHQ in patients with glioma have been conducted [43]. In a randomized trial (double-blind, placebo-controlled) of patients with primary GBM, there were no statistically significant differences between the CHQ treatment group and the placebo group; however, the death rate in the CHQ group was half as large as that in the placebo group [46]. Further clinical trials are in progress (NCT03243461, NCT02432417, and NCT02378532).

2.4.2 Pentamidine

Pentamidine is effective in the treatment of pneumonia caused by *Pneumocystis jirovecii*. This drug exerts its therapeutic effects via the inhibition of glucose metabolism, protein synthesis, amino acid transport, and ribonucleic acid (RNA) synthesis [47]. Previous studies have shown the therapeutic effects of pentamidine in various cancers [48]. One in vitro study revealed that pentamidine suppressed cancer activity via the inhibition of phosphatase of regenerating liver (PRL) [48] and the inhibition of PRL phosphatase suppressed the activation of Akt and ERK [49]. Based on these studies, we investigated the effect of pentamidine in glioma cells and GSCs. Pentamidine suppressed the proliferation of glioma cells and GSCs and reduced the stemness of GSCs. Additionally, there are clinical benefits to repurposing pentamidine as the therapeutic drug for malignant glioma, because the current chemoradiotherapy sometimes induces lymphopenia as a side effect and patients might suffer from pneumonia caused by *P. jirovecii*. Further research to investigate the molecular mechanism of pentamidine is in underway. In the future, clinical trials are warranted to determine the benefit of pentamidine for patients with malignant glioma.

2.5 Antipsychotic drugs

2.5.1 Fluvoxamine

Fluvoxamine has been used as an antidepressant since 1986 and is widely applied in the treatment of anxiety disorders owing to its selective serotonin reuptake inhibitor activity, which helps maintain sufficient serotonin levels in the brain to function [50, 51]. Recently, a new screening method for the quantitative determination of actin polymerization showed that fluvoxamine inhibits the formation of F-actin, which induces lamellipodial protrusions, focal adhesions, and stress fibers at the edge of GBM and is essential for the migration and invasion of GBM cells into normal brain tissues [52–54]. The molecular signal changes in fluvoxamine-treated glioma cells are achieved by the suppression of the activity of actin polymerization regulators, focal adhesion kinases, and mTOR complex 2 [55, 56]. The daily administration of fluvoxamine to an intracranial xenograft mouse model significantly prolongs survival and blocks the infiltration of tumor cells into normal brain tissues in vivo [57]. Therefore, fluvoxamine disrupts focal adhesion and actin depolymerization, blocks the migration and invasion ability of GBM cells, and prolongs patient survival. Fluvoxamine is a potentially effective anti-invasive drug for the treatment of glioma.

2.5.2 Fluspirilene

Fluspirilene, a member of the diphenylbutylpiperidine class of drugs, is an effective, traditional, long-acting antipsychotic [58, 59]. Fluspirilene displays an effective Ca^{2+} channel blocking activity [60] and inhibits synaptic transmission; thus, fluspirilene can mitigate a seizure [58]. However, recent studies have shown a new effect of fluspirilene against some incurable cancers, such as hepatocellular carcinoma [61] and GBM [62]. Fluspirilene has been identified as a potential anti-GSC drug. An in vitro investigation has shown that fluspirilene not only attenuates the cell viability, stemness, sphere-forming ability, and proliferation of GSCs but also suppresses the invasion of GBM cells via the inhibition of signal transducer and activator of transcription 3 (STAT3) activity and its nuclear reduction in GBM cells [62]. In vivo, fluspirilene significantly decreases tumor volume and prolongs survival in an intracranial xenograft mouse model [62]. These results suggest that fluspirilene is a potential novel anti-glioma candidate.

2.6 Antineoplastic drugs

2.6.1 Eribulin

Eribulin, a non-taxane inhibitor of microtubule dynamics [63, 64], was approved by the US Food and Drug Administration (FDA) in 2010 for the treatment of stage 4 breast cancer [65]. Eribulin prevents the growth of tumor cells via the inhibition of microtubule activity during cell mitosis and induces M-phase arrest, which result in cell apoptosis (**Figure 3**) [66, 67]. Eribulin also reduces the aberrance of the vascular microenvironment of a tumor [68]. Based on these effects on various cancers, recent studies have demonstrated that eribulin sensitizes a tumor to radiation via eribulin-induced M-phase arrest and causes more DNA damage than radiation alone. This induces an increase in cleaved caspase-3 and cleaved poly-ADP ribose polymerase levels and results in mitotic catastrophe (**Figure 3**) [69, 70]. An in vivo study of the concomitant administration of radiation with eribulin showed that this combination prolongs the survival of the intracranial xenograft GBM mouse model [71]. Eribulin also suppresses vascular remodeling and normalizes the radiation-induced aberrant vascular microenvironment in the xenograft mouse model [71]. A growing evidence indicates that a telomerase reverse transcriptase (TERT) promoter mutation, a common mutation in GBM [72], maintains telomerase activity to evade telomere shortening; thus, tumor cells overcome replicative senescence and proliferate infinitely [73] telomerase-independent RNA-dependent RNA polymerase (RdRP) activity [74, 75]. Eribulin has been identified as a specific inhibitor of TERT-RdRP through drug screening [76]. Thus, TERT-targeting therapies would be a novel direction to treat glioma (**Figure 3**). Both in vitro and in vivo experiments using eribulin to treat gliomas have shown that eribulin exerts an anticancer activity and suppresses glioma proliferation through its function as a TERT-RdRP inhibitor, in addition to its micro-tubule inhibitor activity. Now, eribulin is in a phase II doctor-led clinical trial in recurrent GBM (UMIN ID: 000030359).

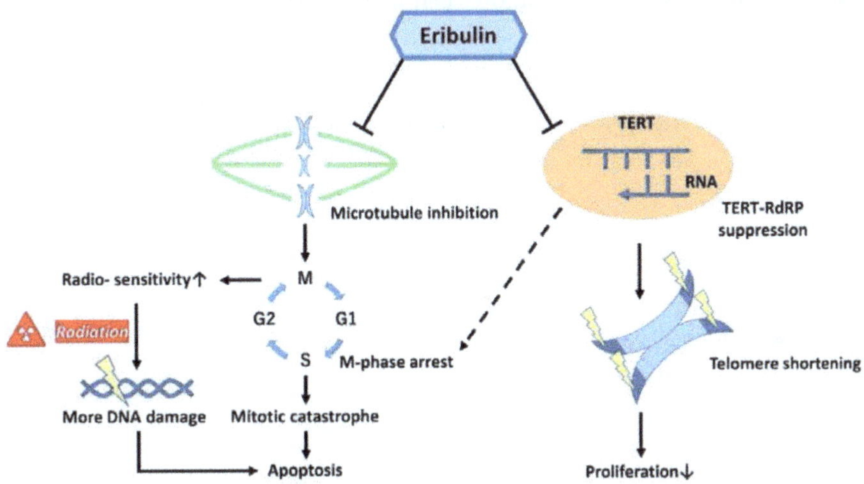

Figure 3.
Antitumor mechanisms of eribulin. The effect of eribulin against glioblastoma multiforme. Eribulin suppresses microtubule activity and induces M-phase arrest, which makes cells more radiosensitive and ends up with apoptosis. Eribulin also suppresses proliferation by inhibiting the TERT-RdRP activity.

2.7 Anti-inflammatory drugs

2.7.1 Acetylsalicylic acid (ASA)

ASA, a nonsteroidal anti-inflammatory drug, is used worldwide. Previous studies have shown the molecular signaling changes by aspirin (**Figure 4**). ASA exerts an anticancer via the inhibition of prostaglandin, including prostaglandin E2 (PGE2), synthesis through the acetylation, and inhibition of cyclooxygenase [77, 78]. ASA treatment suppresses the invasion of glioma cells via the activation of the expression of connexin 43 (Cx43), which is a major gap junction protein in astrocytes. Cx43 is normally suppressed by PGE2. Thus, ASA-treated glioma cells would overexpress Cx43 and the invasion would be inhibited [79]. Other studies have revealed that ASA suppresses the Wnt/β-catenin/T-cell factor (TCF) signaling pathway, which plays a key role in glioma progression [79]. Wnt/β-catenin/TCF pathway suppression would suppress glioma via the regulation of downstream genes, *c-myc* and *cyclin D1*. ASA inhibits the sonic hedgehog (SHH)/glioma-associated oncogene homolog 1 (GLI1) pathway and adjusts the epithelial-to-mesenchymal transition [80]. The SHH/GLI1 pathway is also associated with recovery from the damage by TMZ [80]. Based on these studies, a retrospective cohort study was performed to investigate the therapeutic effect of ASA in patients with malignant glioma. The results revealed that the use of ASA is associated with a higher OS and PFS in patients with WHO grade III glioma; however, there was no difference in OS and PFS in patients with WHO grade IV glioma [81]. In the future, prospective multicenter randomized studies are warranted to determine the effect of ASA in malignant glioma.

2.7.2 Sulfasalazine (SAS)

SAS, which is approved for the treatment of rheumatoid arthritis and inflammatory bowel diseases, may be a therapeutic drug for malignant glioma [82]. SAS exerts anti-inflammatory effects by blocking the activation of NF-κB and the X_c^- antiporter system, which usually causes the uptake of cystine, release of glutamate, and increase in the levels of reactive oxygen species (ROS) [83]. NF-κB is activated in GBM tissues and promotes cell proliferation and survival. SAS blocks

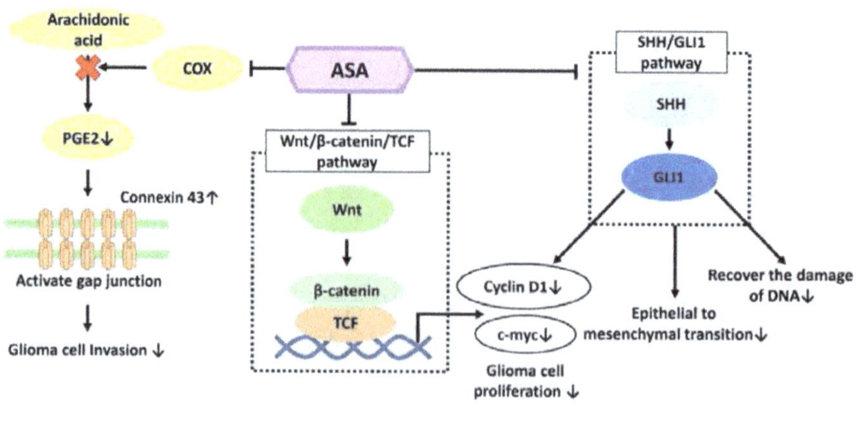

Figure 4.
Antitumor mechanisms of acetylsalicylic acid. ASA indicates multimodal effects for glioma cells. ASA suppresses the invasion of glioma cells by activating the expression of connexin 43. ASA also suppresses c-myc *and* cyclin D1 *through Wnt/β-catenin/TCF pathway and interfered the recovery of DNA damages and adjusted the epithelial-to-mesenchymal transition through SHH/GLI1 pathway. Abbreviation: PGE2, prostaglandin E2.*

the cell cycle and induces apoptosis in vitro and inhibits the growth of brain tumors in mouse xenograft models [83, 84]. However, a phase I/II study of the current therapy with SAS for patients with recurrent malignant glioma showed no clinical benefit of SAS [85]. Recently, a phase I/II study of the current therapy with SAS in patients who were newly diagnosed GBM was performed [86], which showed that there is no increase in OS and PFS in the current therapy with SAS group compared to the current therapy group. Results suggest that this new regimen would improve seizure control; however, the therapeutic effect of SAS would be limited.

2.8 Multiple-drug combination therapy

A combination therapy with different drugs targeting on multiple molecules that contribute to malignancy is rational and enhances antitumor effects, reduces side effects, and avoids resistance. This section provides an overview of the treatment of recurrent GBM with multiple existing drugs (**Figure 5**).

2.8.1 CLOVA cocktail

The CLOVA cocktail, composed of cimetidine, lithium, olanzapine, and valproate, targets dysregulated GSK3β in GBM [87–89]. The therapeutic effects of GSK3β inhibition are the suppression of tumor cell survival and proliferation, synergy with TMZ and irradiation, attenuation of invasion, and induction of GSC differentiation via various pathways [90]. Olanzapine stimulates AMPK catabolic action, followed by the induction of p53-dependent autophagy. VPA, as an HDACi, enhances the effect of radiation. A phase I/II clinical study to investigate the efficacy and safety of the CLOVA cocktail in patients with TMZ-resistant recurrent GBM revealed that this regimen is well tolerated and results in a higher OS than the control group treated with TMZ alone [87].

2.8.2 CUSP9 treatment*

The rational of the coordinated undermining of the survival paths active in GBM by nine repurposed drugs [aprepitant, artesunate, auranofin, captopril, celecoxib, disulfiram (DSF), itraconazole, ritonavir, and sertraline], termed CUSP9*, was developed to prevent therapeutic resistance in tumor cells. CUSP9* targets the diverse complementary redundant pathways to render tumor cells susceptible to the cytotoxic effects of TMZ [91] by the simultaneous administration of nine drugs with low-dose daily TMZ. Each drug exerts different inhibitory effects on the 17 molecules and pathways shown in **Figure 5**. Auranofin and DSF increase the level of intracellular reactive oxygen species [96]. Recently, the experimental CUSP9* strategy with TMZ was shown to suppress the stemness of GSCs and tumorigenesis via the blockade of the Wnt/β-catenin pathway [92].

2.8.3 FTT cocktail

A unique therapeutic approach to reprogram and reverse cancer cells to normal somatic cells has attracted attention. The combination of fasudil, tranilast, and TMZ was identified to reprogram GBM cells into neuronal like cells [93]. GBM cells treated with the FTT cocktail show normal neuronal morphology, gene expression, and electrophysiological properties and lower malignancy than untreated cells. This might be caused by the synergistic effect of the three drugs [93]. In addition, the FTT cocktail suppresses tumor growth and prolongs survival in a GBM xenograft

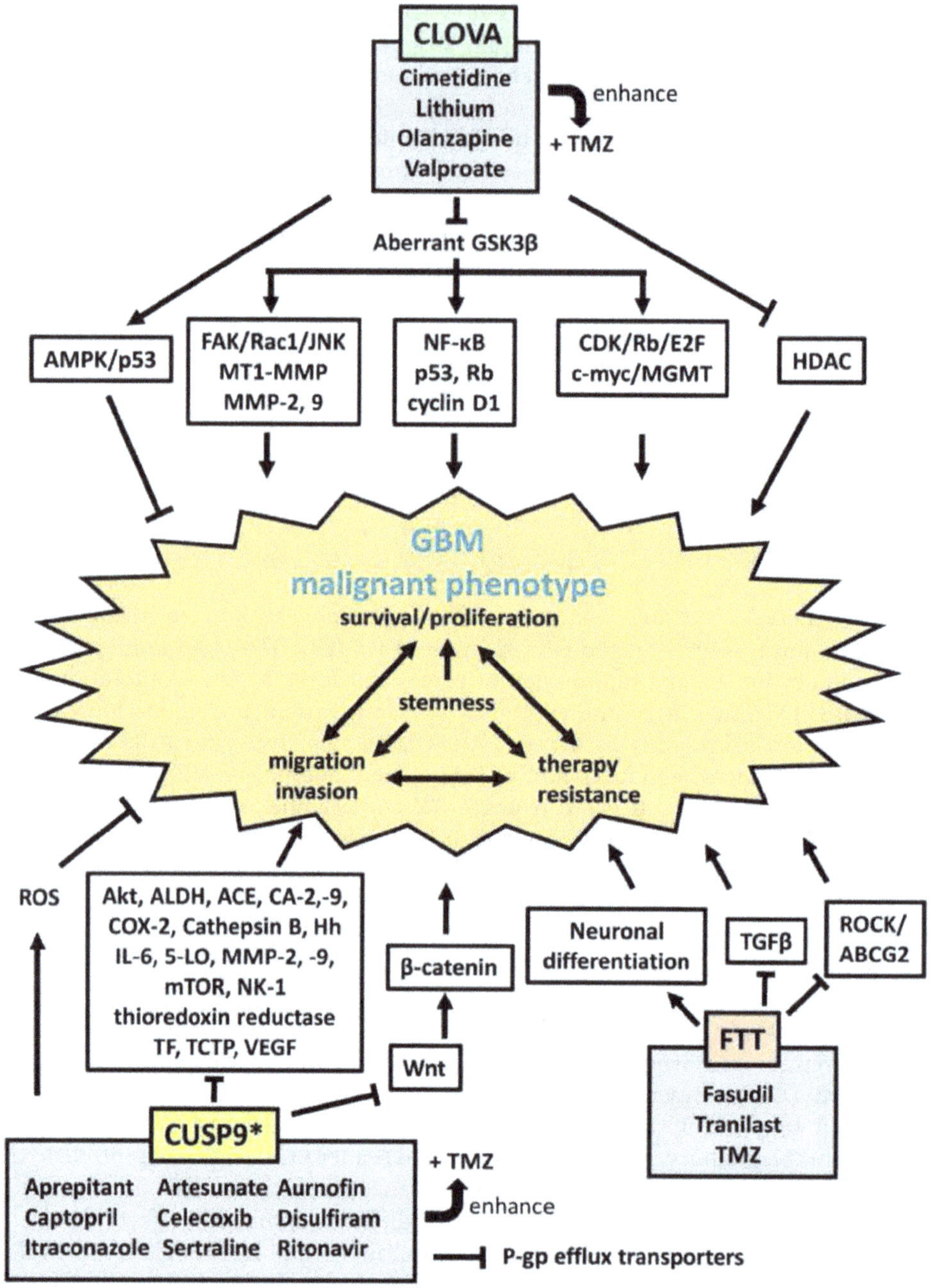

Figure 5.
Multiple molecular-targeted therapies by multiple-drug treatment with temozolomide. Multiple existing drug combination, CLOVA cocktail, CUSP9 treatment, and FTT cocktail, targets multiple signaling pathways which attribute GBM malignant phenotype. Abbreviations: 5-LO, 5-lipoxygenase; ABCG2, ATP-binding cassette super-family G member 2; ACE, angiotensin-converting enzyme; ALDH, aldehyde dehydrogenase; AMPK, adenosine monophosphate; CA, carbonic anhydrase; CDK, cyclin-dependent kinase; COX, cyclooxygenase; FAK, focal adhesion kinase; GSK3β, glycogen synthase kinase-3β; HDAC, histone deacetylase; HH, hedgehog; JNK, c-Jun N-terminal kinase; MGMT, O^6-methylguanine-DNA methyltransferase; MMP, matrix metalloproteinase; MT, membrane type; mTOR, mammalian target of rapamycin; NK-1, neurokinin-1; NF-κB, nuclear factor-kappaB; P-gp, P-glycoprotein; ROCK, rho-associated protein kinase; ROS, reactive oxygen species; TCTP, translationally controlled tumor protein; TF, tissue factor; TGF-β, transforming growth factor-β; TMZ, temozolomide; VEGF, vascular endothelial growth factor.*

model more than TMZ alone. Fasudil inhibits the ROCK2/moesin/β-catenin pathway in TMZ-resistant glioma cell lines and downregulates the ATP-binding cassette super-family G member 2 transporter to increase sensitivity to TMZ [94]. The inhibition of ROCK with mTOR inhibition exerts neuronal reprogramming more effectively in vitro and in vivo than the inhibition of ROCK alone [95], which suggests the possibility of more drug combinations. Tranilast alone inhibits glioma progression via TGF-β restriction [96]. Although the mechanism underlying the tumor-suppressive function of the FTT cocktail is not fully elucidated, this cocktail might improve the current therapy for malignant glioma.

2.9 Other drugs

2.9.1 Disulfiram

DSF, the FDA-approved drug for the treatment of alcohol abuse, may be a therapeutic drug for GBM. DSF is an irreversible inhibitor of aldehyde dehydrogenase [97], which is a functional marker of cancer stem cells [98]. An in vitro study revealed that DSF is an inhibitor of MGMT and enhances the efficacy of alkylator-induced tumor death [99]. Another study revealed that DSF suppresses the growth and self-renewal of GSCs via the inhibition of polo-like kinase-1, which controls cell progression and cytokinesis [97]. The activity of DSF is potentiated by copper and induces GSC death [100]. However, an open-label, single-arm phase II study of TMZ plus DSF for patients with recurrent TMZ-resistant GBM showed that the objective response rate is 0% and DSF combination therapy would have only limited therapeutic effects for patients with GBM [101].

2.9.2 Statins

Statins, a therapeutic drug for dyslipidemia, inhibit 3-hydroxy-3-methylglutaryl-coenzyme A reductase. Some statins have a therapeutic effect on glioma cells [102, 103]. In vitro, simvastatin induces the apoptosis of C6 glioma cells by phosphorylation of activating transcription factor-2 and c-Jun [102]. Lovastatin suppresses the proliferation and migration of glioma cell lines via the suppression of the activation of ERK [103]. A retrospective cohort study suggested that the long-term prediagnostic statin intake increases the OS in patients with GBM [104]. Another retrospective cohort study suggested that statin intake is associated with fewer seizures in patients with GBM [105]. However, other cohort studies have not indicated a survival rela-tionship between malignant glioma and statin intake. Finally, a meta-analysis of these retrospective cohort studies revealed that statins do not increase the PFS and OS in patients with GBM [106]. In the future, prospective multicenter randomized studies are warranted to determine the effect of statins in malignant glioma.

2.10 Pre-drugs

2.10.1 Kenpaullone

Kenpaullone, a potent and nonselective inhibitor of GSK3 [107], is a serine/threonine kinase that regulates numerous signaling pathways involved in cell cycle control, proliferation, differentiation, and apoptosis [108, 109]. Kenpaullone treatment inhibits glioma cell proliferation, suppresses anti-apoptotic mechanisms in the mitochondria, inhibits pro-survival factors, and attenuates the stemness and viability of GSCs via the downregulated activity of GSK3β [88, 110, 111]. The combination of low-dose kenpaullone with TMZ enhances cytotoxicity against glioma via the induction of c-Myc-mediated apoptosis [110]. These results suggest that kenpaullone is a potential compound for the treatment of glioma.

2.10.2 2-Fluoropalmitic acid (2-FPA)

Recently, 2-FPA, a new fatty acid inhibitor compound, has been identified as a potential anti-glioma agent through a drug screening system for drugs that target cancer stem cells using existing drug libraries [62]. As an active chemical compound, the safety of 2-FPA for normal brain cells has not yet been revealed. There are no reports that have mentioned the effect of 2-FPA in other cancers. An in vitro investigation using GSCs and GBM cells [112] has shown that 2-FPA suppresses the viability and sphere-forming ability of GSCs; inhibits the proliferation of GBM cells via the dephosphorylation of ERK, which is essential for the proliferation and invasion of glioma [113]; and blocks the invasion of GBM cells via the suppression of the activity of MMP-2, which plays an important role in cell invasion [114]. In addition to its mono activity against glioma, the combination of 2-FPA with TMZ synergistically enhances the efficacy of TMZ against glioma in vitro via the increase in MGMT promoter methylation and downregulation of MGMT, the main and predominant reasons for TMZ resistance [115], which suggest that combination therapy may be one strategy to improve TMZ efficacy and overcome resistance. Overall, 2-FPA is a potential therapeutic agent against GBM. To extend these results, physiological studies are required.

3. Issues of drug repositioning for glioma

Despite these studies, some problems remain in drug repositioning for the treatment of glioma because of the uniqueness of this brain tumor.

The biggest problem is the penetration of the blood-brain barrier (BBB), which restricts the passage of molecules, including candidate agents. The BBB is a multilayered barrier between the blood and brain tissues to regulate the environment of the brain. The BBB has a good permeability for nutrients that are required for nerve cells [116]. Additionally, the BBB adjusts the ionic composition and the concentration of neurotransmitters, such as neuroexcitatory amino acids, to maintain the optimal environment for synapses. If ions and neurotransmitters spread into the CNS in an uncontrolled manner, the synapse is insufficiently stimulated and brain tissue is damaged [116]. The BBB also prevents the penetration of macromolecules more than 400–500 Da to exclude neurotoxic molecules [117]. Some plasma proteins induce the apoptosis of nerve cells [116]. This multilayered barrier blocks these proteins and would block the penetration of candidate agents. To overcome this problem, techniques are being explored. Some studies have investigated a new drug delivery system that uses an ultrasound-sensitizing nanoparticle complex, as preliminary studies have revealed that an ultrasound with microbubbles could open the BBB locally [118]. Other studies have evaluated the usefulness of convention-enhanced delivery therapy, which is a local infusion therapeutic technique to directly introduce a drug to brain neoplasms [119, 120].

A malignant glioma has features that are different from those in other malignant tumors. First, a malignant glioma has heterogeneity. Some malignant cancers, such as acute leukemia, are homogeneous; thus, the appropriate candidate agent would induce remission because "the weak point" of all tumor cells is the same.

However, a malignant glioma is a complicated aggregation, once called "glioblastoma multiforme" [121]. If one candidate agent exerts therapeutic effects for some glioma cells, other resistant glioma cells would multiply. To overcome this problem, several previous studies have performed multiple-drug combination therapy. This therapy would focus on multiple therapeutic targets at once with minimal side effects [85]; however, currently, there are no combination treatments that can replace the current treatments. Second, despite its clinical aggressiveness, 60–70% of the tumor cells in malignant glioma are in the nonproliferating phase [122]. This indicates that not only heterogeneous cells but also the cell cycle must be considered because resting cells indicate resistance to chemoradiotherapy [122]. Based on this, some studies have focused on candidate agents that can change the phase of the cell cycle [18, 45].

4. Perspective

The strategy to discover the most effective drug is the key to accomplish a successful drug repositioning. One of the main methods is an in vitro or in vivo drug screening system in which target cells are treated by various existing drugs and the alteration to the malignant phenotype, such as by cytotoxicity, is analyzed. Drugs that exert cytotoxicity in GBM cells, especially GSCs, at low concentrations would be good candidates. Since the previous reports mention that GSCs were the cause of recurrence of GBM [100], GSCs can be good target. Lower drug concentration can minimize side effects. However, to achieve this strategy, appropriate experimental resources, including candidate agents, drug screening systems, and established cell lines are required. Epidemiological discovery is another option, such as the measurement of the incidence of a certain disease in the population to which specific drugs are administered. Serendipity is an important factor in this strategy. For instance, a prospective cohort study revealed a lower cancer incidence in people with schizophrenia [123]. This led us to the idea that antipsychotic drugs possess therapeutic effects against cancers including glioma [57, 62]. However, the most efficient method might be mutual molecular and structure analyses between target cells and drugs using artificial intelligence (AI). Different biochemical and mathematical techniques have been designed and optimized to accurately infer links between target cells and drugs. Drug-target interaction prediction is an important part of most rational drug repositioning pipelines. The major target molecules for malignant glioma are Akt, ERK, and STAT3, which sustain malignant phenotype [62, 103, 113].

The supply of research resources is also important. Pharmaceutical companies hold the materials for drug repositioning such as drug libraries and useful knowledge for bringing new drugs to market. Thus, a collaboration between researchers who establish efficient screening systems and pharmaceutical companies that own various drugs, including those that failed in clinical trials, can lead to a successful drug repositioning.

Although drug repositioning may be useful in the future, there are hurdles to the transition of this research into clinical practice owing to financial problems. Drug repositioning involves reinvestment in inexpensive drugs with expired patents; therefore, the benefits to pharmaceutical companies are small, which results in a reluctance to cooperate to broaden the indications of their drugs. This is especially true for rare diseases, such as glioma. Currently, the only way for researchers to raise public and private funds is by themselves, and they must conduct physician-led clinical trials without the support of pharmaceutical companies. An effective system in which the government supports drug repositioning is required to overcome the issue of budget constraints. From an economic perspective, it would be beneficial to patients and countries to treat patients with inexpensive drugs with expired patents.

After the appearance of TMZ, drug development for GBM has stagnated. A huge advance in the treatment of patients with GBM can be expected if effective drugs are identified via drug repurposing.

5. Conclusion

Drug repositioning is a useful research strategy to identify the therapeutic agents for glioma. Here, we discuss the current drug repositioning and its perspective for glioma treatment. Despite many efforts to date, no agents are widely used in the current clinical practice. For breaking down the current situation, appropriate screening system, suitable animal model, well-designed clinical trials, and tight collaboration with pharmaceutical companies are warranted. From now on, the drastic progress in this field would be occurred by new methods including AI.

Abbreviations

2-FPA	2-fluoropalmitic acid
AI	artificial intelligence
AMPK	AMP-activated protein kinase
ASA	acetylsalicylic acid
AT1R	angiotensin I receptors
AT2	angiotensin II
BBB	blood-brain barrier
BEV	bevacizumab
CHQ	chloroquine
CLIC1	chloride intracellular channel 1
CNS	central nervous system
Cx43	connexin 43
D-2HG	D-2-hydroxyglutarate
DSF	disulfiram
ERK	extracellular signal-regulated kinase
FDA	Food and Drug Administration
GBM	glioblastoma
GDH	glutamate dehydrogenase
GLI1	glioma-associated oncogene homolog 1
GSC	glioma stem-like cell
GSK3	glycogen synthase kinase 3
HAT	histone acetyltransferase
HDAC	histone deacetylase
HDACi	histone deacetylase inhibitor
IDH	isocitrate dehydrogenase
LEV	levetiracetam
MGMT	O^6-methylguanine-DNA methyltransferase

MMP-2	matrix metalloproteinase-2
mTOR	mammalian target of rapamycin
NF-κB	nuclear factor-kappaB
OS	overall survival
PFS	progression-free survival
PGE2	prostaglandin E2
PRL	phosphatase of regenerating liver
RdRP	RNA-dependent RNA polymerase
ROCK	Rho-associated protein kinase
SAS	sulfasalazine
SHH	sonic hedgehog
STAT3	signal transducer and activator of transcription 3
TCF	T-cell factor
TERT	telomerase reverse transcriptase
TGF-β	transforming growth factor-β
TMZ	temozolomide
VEGF	vascular endothelial growth factor
VPA	valproic acid
WHO	World Health Organization

Author details

Sho Tamai[1], Nozomi Hirai[1], Shabierjiang Jiapaer[1], Takuya Furuta[2] and Mitsutoshi Nakada[1*]

1 Department of Neurosurgery, Graduate School of Medical Science, Kanazawa University, Kanazawa, Japan

2 Department of Pathology, Kurume University, Kurume, Japan

*Address all correspondence to: mnakada@med.kanazawa-u.ac.jp

References

[1] Ostrom QT, Cioffi G, Gittleman H, Patil N, Waite K, Kruchko C, et al. CBTRUS statistical report: Primary brain and other central nervous system tumors diagnosed in the United States in 2012-2016. Neuro-Oncology. 2019;**21** (Suppl 5):v1-v100

[2] Louis DN, Perry A, Reifenberger G, von Deimling A, Figarella-Branger D, Cavenee WK, et al. The 2016 World Health Organization classification of tumors of the central nervous system: A summary. Acta Neuropathologica. 2016; **131**(6):803-820

[3] Dolecek TA, Propp JM, Stroup NE, Kruchko C. CBTRUS statistical report: Primary brain and central nervous system tumors diagnosed in the United States in 2005-2009. Neuro-Oncology. 2012;**14**(Suppl 5):v1-v49

[4] Stupp R, Gander M, Leyvraz S, Newlands E. Current and future developments in the use of temozolomide for the treatment of brain tumours. The Lancet Oncology. 2001; **2**(9):552-560

[5] Stupp R, Mason WP, van den Bent MJ, Weller M, Fisher B, Taphoorn MJ, et al. Radiotherapy plus concomitant and adjuvant temozolomide for glioblastoma. The New England Journal of Medicine. 2005; **352**(10):987-996

[6] Hegi ME, Diserens AC, Gorlia T, Hamou MF, de Tribolet N, Weller M, et al. MGMT gene silencing and benefit from temozolomide in glioblastoma. The New England Journal of Medicine. 2005;**352**(10):997-1003

[7] Ferrara N, Hillan KJ, Novotny W. Bevacizumab (Avastin), a humanized anti-VEGF monoclonal antibody for cancer therapy. Biochemical and Biophysical Research Communications. 2005;**333**(2):328-335

[8] Chinot OL, Wick W, Mason W, Henriksson R, Saran F, Nishikawa R, et al. Bevacizumab plus radiotherapy-temozolomide for newly diagnosed glioblastoma. The New England Journal of Medicine. 2014;**370**(8):709-722

[9] Gilbert MR, Dignam JJ, Armstrong TS, Wefel JS, Blumenthal DT, Vogelbaum MA, et al. A randomized trial of bevacizumab for newly diagnosed glioblastoma. The New England Journal of Medicine. 2014; **370**(8):699-708

[10] Jiralerspong S, Palla SL, Giordano SH, Meric-Bernstam F, Liedtke C, Barnett CM, et al. Metformin and pathologic complete responses to neoadjuvant chemotherapy in diabetic patients with breast cancer. Journal of Clinical Oncology. 2009;**27**(20): 3297-3302

[11] Wurth R, Pattarozzi A, Gatti M, Bajetto A, Corsaro A, Parodi A, et al. Metformin selectively affects human glioblastoma tumor-initiating cell viability: A role for metformin-induced inhibition of Akt. Cell Cycle. 2013;**12**(1): 145-156

[12] Aldea MD, Petrushev B, Soritau O, Tomuleasa CI, Berindan-Neagoe I, Filip AG, et al. Metformin plus sorafenib highly impacts temozolomide resistant glioblastoma stem-like cells. Journal of BUON. 2014;**19**(2):502-511

[13] Sato A, Sunayama J, Okada M, Watanabe E, Seino S, Shibuya K, et al. Glioma-initiating cell elimination by metformin activation of FOXO3 via AMPK. Stem Cells Translational Medicine. 2012;**1**(11):811-824

[14] Molenaar RJ, Coelen RJS, Khurshed M, Roos E, Caan MWA, van Linde ME, et al. Study protocol of a phase IB/II clinical trial of metformin and chloroquine in patients with

IDH1-mutated or IDH2-mutated solid tumours. BMJ Open. 2017;7(6):e014961

[15] Zhang J, Li M, Song M, Chen W, Mao J, Song L, et al. Clic1 plays a role in mouse hepatocarcinoma via modulating Annexin A7 and Gelsolin in vitro and in vivo. Biomedicine & Pharmacotherapy. 2015;**69**:416-419

[16] Tian Y, Guan Y, Jia Y, Meng Q, Yang J. Chloride intracellular channel 1 regulates prostate cancer cell proliferation and migration through the MAPK/ERK pathway. Cancer Biotherapy & Radiopharmaceuticals. 2014;**29**(8):339-344

[17] Setti M, Savalli N, Osti D, Richichi C, Angelini M, Brescia P, et al. Functional role of CLIC1 ion channel in glioblastoma-derived stem/progenitor cells. Journal of the National Cancer Institute. 2013;**105**(21):1644-1655

[18] Barbieri F, Verduci I, Carlini V, Zona G, Pagano A, Mazzanti M, et al. Repurposed Biguanide drugs in Glioblastoma exert Antiproliferative effects via the inhibition of intracellular Chloride Channel 1 activity. Frontiers in Oncology. 2019;**9**:135

[19] Seliger C, Ricci C, Meier CR, Bodmer M, Jick SS, Bogdahn U, et al. Diabetes, use of antidiabetic drugs, and the risk of glioma. Neuro-Oncology. 2016;**18**(3):340-349

[20] Seliger C, Genbrugge E, Gorlia T, Chinot O, Stupp R, Nabors B, et al. Use of metformin and outcome of patients with newly diagnosed glioblastoma: Pooled analysis. International Journal of Cancer. 2020;**146**(3):803-809

[21] Ager EI, Neo J, Christophi C. The renin-angiotensin system and malignancy. Carcinogenesis. 2008; **29**(9):1675-1684

[22] Rivera E, Arrieta O, Guevara P, Duarte-Rojo A, Sotelo J. AT1 receptor is present in glioma cells; its blockage reduces the growth of rat glioma. British Journal of Cancer. 2001;**85**(9):1396-1399

[23] Arrieta O, Guevara P, Escobar E, Garcia-Navarrete R, Pineda B, Sotelo J. Blockage of angiotensin II type I receptor decreases the synthesis of growth factors and induces apoptosis in C6 cultured cells and C6 rat glioma. British Journal of Cancer. 2005;**92**(7): 1247-1252

[24] Januel E, Ursu R, Alkhafaji A, Marantidou A, Doridam J, Belin C, et al. Impact of renin-angiotensin system blockade on clinical outcome in glioblastoma. European Journal of Neurology. 2015;**22**(9):1304-1309

[25] Ursu R, Thomas L, Psimaras D, Chinot O, Le Rhun E, Ricard D, et al. Angiotensin II receptor blockers, steroids and radiotherapy in glioblastoma-a randomised multicentre trial (ASTER trial). An ANOCEF study. European Journal of Cancer. 2019;**109**: 129-136

[26] Tewarie IA, Senders JT, Hulsbergen AFC, Kremer S, Broekman MLD. Beta-blockers and glioma: A systematic review of preclinical studies and clinical results. Neurosurgical Review. 2020

[27] Johansen MD, Urup T, Holst CB, Christensen IJ, Grunnet K, Lassen U, et al. Outcome of Bevacizumab therapy in patients with recurrent Glioblastoma treated with angiotensin system inhibitors. Cancer Investigation. 2018; **36**(9–10):512-519

[28] Maklad A, Sharma A, Azimi I. Calcium signaling in brain cancers: Roles and therapeutic targeting. Cancers (Basel). 2019;**11**(2):145

[29] Liu Z, Wei Y, Zhang L, Yee PP, Johnson M, Zhang X, et al. Induction of store-operated calcium entry (SOCE) suppresses glioblastoma growth by

inhibiting the hippo pathway transcriptional coactivators YAP/TAZ. Oncogene. 2019;**38**(1):120-139

[30] Witt O, Deubzer HE, Milde T, Oehme I. HDAC family: What are the cancer relevant targets? Cancer Letters. 2009;**277**(1):8-21

[31] Phiel CJ, Zhang F, Huang EY, Guenther MG, Lazar MA, Klein PS. Histone deacetylase is a direct target of valproic acid, a potent anticonvulsant, mood stabilizer, and teratogen. The Journal of Biological Chemistry. 2001; **276**(39):36734-36741

[32] Chinnaiyan P, Cerna D, Burgan WE, Beam K, Williams ES, Camphausen K, et al. Postradiation sensitization of the histone deacetylase inhibitor valproic acid. Clinical Cancer Research. 2008; **14**(17):5410-5415

[33] Zhang C, Liu S, Yuan X, Hu Z, Li H, Wu M, et al. Valproic acid promotes human Glioma U87 cells apoptosis and inhibits glycogen synthase kinase-3beta through ERK/Akt signaling. Cellular Physiology and Biochemistry. 2016; **39**(6):2173-2185

[34] Pyko IV, Nakada M, Sabit H, Teng L, Furuyama N, Hayashi Y, et al. Glycogen synthase kinase 3beta inhibition sensitizes human glioblastoma cells to temozolomide by affecting O6-methylguanine DNA methyltransferase promoter methylation via c-Myc signaling. Carcinogenesis. 2013;**34**(10):2206-2217

[35] Weller M, Gorlia T, Cairncross JG, van den Bent MJ, Mason W, Belanger K, et al. Prolonged survival with valproic acid use in the EORTC/NCIC temozolomide trial for glioblastoma. Neurology. 2011;**77**(12):1156-1164

[36] Yuan Y, Xiang W, Qing M, Yanhui L, Jiewen L, Yunhe M. Survival analysis for valproic acid use in adult glioblastoma multiforme: A meta-analysis of individual patient data and a systematic review. Seizure. 2014;**23**(10): 830-835

[37] Barker CA, Bishop AJ, Chang M, Beal K, Chan TA. Valproic acid use during radiation therapy for glioblastoma associated with improved survival. International Journal of Radiation Oncology, Biology, Physics. 2013;**86**(3):504-509

[38] Kerkhof M, Dielemans JC, van Breemen MS, Zwinkels H, Walchenbach R, Taphoorn MJ, et al. Effect of valproic acid on seizure control and on survival in patients with glioblastoma multiforme. Neuro-Oncology. 2013;**15**(7):961-967

[39] Happold C, Gorlia T, Chinot O, Gilbert MR, Nabors LB, Wick W, et al. Does Valproic acid or Levetiracetam improve survival in Glioblastoma? A pooled analysis of prospective clinical trials in newly diagnosed Glioblastoma. Journal of Clinical Oncology. 2016; **34**(7):731-739

[40] Bobustuc GC, Baker CH, Limaye A, Jenkins WD, Pearl G, Avgeropoulos NG, et al. Levetiracetam enhances p53-mediated MGMT inhibition and sensitizes glioblastoma cells to temozolomide. Neuro-Oncology. 2010; **12**(9):917-927

[41] Scicchitano BM, Sorrentino S, Proietti G, Lama G, Dobrowolny G, Catizone A, et al. Levetiracetam enhances the temozolomide effect on glioblastoma stem cell proliferation and apoptosis. Cancer Cell International. 2018;**18**:136

[42] Weyerhauser P, Kantelhardt SR, Kim EL. Re-purposing Chloroquine for Glioblastoma: Potential merits and confounding variables. Frontiers in Oncology. 2018;**8**:335

[43] Verbaanderd C, Maes H, Schaaf MB, Sukhatme VP, Pantziarka P,

Sukhatme V, et al. Repurposing drugs in oncology (ReDO)-chloroquine and hydroxychloroquine as anti-cancer agents. Ecancermedicalscience. 2017; **11**:781

[44] Golden EB, Cho HY, Hofman FM, Louie SG, Schonthal AH, Chen TC. Quinoline-based antimalarial drugs: A novel class of autophagy inhibitors. Neurosurgical Focus. 2015;**38**(3):E12

[45] Roy LO, Poirier MB, Fortin D. Chloroquine inhibits the malignant phenotype of glioblastoma partially by suppressing TGF-beta. Investigational New Drugs. 2015;**33**(5):1020-1031

[46] Sotelo J, Briceno E, Lopez-Gonzalez MA. Adding chloroquine to conventional treatment for glioblastoma multiforme: A randomized, double-blind, placebo-controlled trial. Annals of Internal Medicine. 2006;**144**(5):337-343

[47] Pesanti EL, Cox C. Metabolic and synthetic activities of pneumocystis carinii in vitro. Infection and Immunity. 1981;**34**(3):908-914

[48] Pathak MK, Dhawan D, Lindner DJ, Borden EC, Farver C, Yi T. Pentamidine is an inhibitor of PRL phosphatases with anticancer activity. Molecular Cancer Therapeutics. 2002;**1**(14):1255-1264

[49] Bai Y, Yu ZH, Liu S, Zhang L, Zhang RY, Zeng LF, et al. Novel anticancer agents based on targeting the Trimer Interface of the PRL phosphatase. Cancer Research. 2016;**76**(16):4805-4815

[50] Irons J. Fluvoxamine in the treatment of anxiety disorders. Neuropsychiatric Disease and Treatment. 2005;**1**(4):289-299

[51] Hartter S, Wetzel H, Hammes E, Hiemke C. Inhibition of antidepressant demethylation and hydroxylation by fluvoxamine in depressed patients. Psychopharmacology. 1993;**110**(3): 302-308

[52] Pollard TD, Borisy GG. Cellular motility driven by assembly and disassembly of actin filaments. Cell. 2003;**112**(4):453-465

[53] Nurnberg A, Kitzing T, Grosse R. Nucleating actin for invasion. Nature Reviews. Cancer. 2011;**11**(3):177-187

[54] Le Clainche C, Carlier MF. Regulation of actin assembly associated with protrusion and adhesion in cell migration. Physiological Reviews. 2008; **88**(2):489-513

[55] Serrels B, Serrels A, Brunton VG, Holt M, McLean GW, Gray CH, et al. Focal adhesion kinase controls actin assembly via a FERM-mediated interaction with the Arp2/3 complex. Nature Cell Biology. 2007;**9**(9): 1046-1056

[56] Huang W, Zhu PJ, Zhang S, Zhou H, Stoica L, Galiano M, et al. mTORC2 controls actin polymerization required for consolidation of long-term memory. Nature Neuroscience. 2013;**16**(4): 441-448

[57] Hayashi K, Michiue H, Yamada H, Takata K, Nakayama H, Wei FY, et al. Fluvoxamine, an anti-depressant, inhibits human glioblastoma invasion by disrupting actin polymerization. Scientific Reports. 2016;**6**:23372

[58] Wang SJ, Lu KT, Gean PW. Inhibition of synaptic transmission and epileptiform activity in central neurons by fluspirilene. British Journal of Pharmacology. 1997;**120**(6):1114-1118

[59] Abhijnhan A, Adams CE, David A, Ozbilen M. Depot fluspirilene for schizophrenia. Cochrane Database of Systematic Reviews. 2007;**1**:CD001718

[60] Galizzi JP, Fosset M, Romey G, Laduron P, Lazdunski M. Neuroleptics of the diphenylbutylpiperidine series are potent calcium channel inhibitors. Proceedings of the National Academy of

Sciences of the United States of America. 1986;**83**(19):7513-7517

[61] Shi XN, Li H, Yao H, Liu X, Li L, Leung KS, et al. In Silico identification and In vitro and In vivo validation of anti-psychotic drug Fluspirilene as a potential CDK2 inhibitor and a candidate anti-cancer drug. PLoS One. 2015;**10**(7):e0132072

[62] Dong Y, Furuta T, Sabit H, Kitabayashi T, Jiapaer S, Kobayashi M, et al. Identification of antipsychotic drug fluspirilene as a potential anti-glioma stem cell drug. Oncotarget. 2017; **8**(67):111728-111741

[63] Jordan MA, Kamath K, Manna T, Okouneva T, Miller HP, Davis C, et al. The primary antimitotic mechanism of action of the synthetic halichondrin E7389 is suppression of microtubule growth. Molecular Cancer Therapeutics. 2005;**4**(7):1086-1095

[64] Okouneva T, Azarenko O, Wilson L, Littlefield BA, Jordan MA. Inhibition of centromere dynamics by eribulin (E7389) during mitotic metaphase. Molecular Cancer Therapeutics. 2008;**7**(7):2003-2011

[65] Donoghue M, Lemery SJ, Yuan W, He K, Sridhara R, Shord S, et al. Eribulin mesylate for the treatment of patients with refractory metastatic breast cancer: Use of a "physician's choice" control arm in a randomized approval trial. Clinical Cancer Research. 2012;**18**(6): 1496-1505

[66] Kuznetsov G, Towle MJ, Cheng H, Kawamura T, TenDyke K, Liu D, et al. Induction of morphological and biochemical apoptosis following prolonged mitotic blockage by halichondrin B macrocyclic ketone analog E7389. Cancer Research. 2004; **64**(16):5760-5766

[67] Towle MJ, Salvato KA, Wels BF, Aalfs KK, Zheng W, Seletsky BM, et al. Eribulin induces irreversible mitotic blockade: Implications of cell-based pharmacodynamics for in vivo efficacy under intermittent dosing conditions. Cancer Research. 2011;**71**(2):496-505

[68] Funahashi Y, Okamoto K, Adachi Y, Semba T, Uesugi M, Ozawa Y, et al. Eribulin mesylate reduces tumor microenvironment abnormality by vascular remodeling in preclinical human breast cancer models. Cancer Science. 2014;**105**(10):1334-1342

[69] Pawlik TM, Keyomarsi K. Role of cell cycle in mediating sensitivity to radiotherapy. International Journal of Radiation Oncology, Biology, Physics. 2004;**59**(4):928-942

[70] Oehler C, von Bueren AO, Furmanova P, Broggini-Tenzer A, Orlowski K, Rutkowski S, et al. The microtubule stabilizer patupilone (epothilone B) is a potent radiosensitizer in medulloblastoma cells. Neuro-Oncology. 2011;**13**(9):1000-1010

[71] Miki S, Imamichi S, Fujimori H, Tomiyama A, Fujimoto K, Satomi K, et al. Concomitant administration of radiation with eribulin improves the survival of mice harboring intracerebral glioblastoma. Cancer Science. 2018; **109**(7):2275-2285

[72] Arita H, Narita Y, Fukushima S, Tateishi K, Matsushita Y, Yoshida A, et al. Upregulating mutations in the TERT promoter commonly occur in adult malignant gliomas and are strongly associated with total 1p19q loss. Acta Neuropathologica. 2013;**126**(2): 267-276

[73] Chiba K, Johnson JZ, Vogan JM, Wagner T, Boyle JM, Hockemeyer D. Cancer-associated TERT promoter mutations abrogate telomerase silencing. eLife. 2015;**4**

[74] Ozturk MB, Li Y, Tergaonkar V. Current insights to regulation and role

of telomerase in human diseases. Antioxidants (Basel). 2017;**6**(1)

[75] Maida Y, Yasukawa M, Furuuchi M, Lassmann T, Possemato R, Okamoto N, et al. An RNA-dependent RNA polymerase formed by TERT and the RMRP RNA. Nature. 2009;**461**(7261): 230-235

[76] Yamaguchi S, Maida Y, Yasukawa M, Kato T, Yoshida M, Masutomi K. Eribulin mesylate targets human telomerase reverse transcriptase in ovarian cancer cells. PLoS One. 2014; **9**(11):e112438

[77] Vane JR. Inhibition of prostaglandin synthesis as a mechanism of action for aspirin-like drugs. Nature: New Biology. 1971;**231**(25):232-235

[78] Qin LJ, Jia YS, Zhang YB, Wang YH. Cyclooxygenase inhibitor induces the upregulation of connexin-43 expression in C6 glioma cells. Biomed Reports. 2016;**4**(4):444-448

[79] Lan F, Yue X, Han L, Yuan X, Shi Z, Huang K, et al. Antitumor effect of aspirin in glioblastoma cells by modulation of beta-catenin/T-cell factor-mediated transcriptional activity. Journal of Neurosurgery. 2011;**115**(4):780-788

[80] Ming J, Sun B, Li Z, Lin L, Meng X, Han B, et al. Aspirin inhibits the SHH/GLI1 signaling pathway and sensitizes malignant glioma cells to temozolomide therapy. Aging (Albany NY). 2017;**9**(4): 1233-1247

[81] Seliger C, Schaertl J, Gerken M, Luber C, Proescholdt M, Riemenschneider MJ, et al. Use of statins or NSAIDs and survival of patients with high-grade glioma. PLoS One. 2018;**13**(12):e0207858

[82] Farr M, Tunn EJ, Symmons DP, Scott DG, Bacon PA. Sulphasalazine in rheumatoid arthritis: Haematological problems and changes in haematological indices associated with therapy. British Journal of Rheumatology. 1989;**28**(2): 134-138

[83] Sleire L, Skeie BS, Netland IA, Forde HE, Dodoo E, Selheim F, et al. Drug repurposing: Sulfasalazine sensitizes gliomas to gamma knife radiosurgery by blocking cystine uptake through system xc-, leading to glutathione depletion. Oncogene. 2015;**34**(49):5951-5959

[84] Robe PA, Bentires-Alj M, Bonif M, Rogister B, Deprez M, Haddada H, et al. In vitro and in vivo activity of the nuclear factor-kappaB inhibitor sulfasalazine in human glioblastomas. Clinical Cancer Research. 2004;**10**(16): 5595-5603

[85] Robe PA, Martin DH, Nguyen-Khac MT, Artesi M, Deprez M, Albert A, et al. Early termination of ISRCTN45828668, a phase 1/2 prospective, randomized study of sulfasalazine for the treatment of progressing malignant gliomas in adults. BMC Cancer. 2009;**9**:372

[86] Takeuchi S, Wada K, Nagatani K, Otani N, Osada H, Nawashiro H. Sulfasalazine and temozolomide with radiation therapy for newly diagnosed glioblastoma. Neurology India. 2014; **62**(1):42-47

[87] Furuta T, Sabit H, Dong Y, Miyashita K, Kinoshita M, Uchiyama N, et al. Biological basis and clinical study of glycogen synthase kinase- 3beta-targeted therapy by drug repositioning for glioblastoma. Oncotarget. 2017;**8**: 22811-22824

[88] Kotliarova S, Pastorino S, Kovell LC, Kotliarov Y, Song H, Zhang W, et al. Glycogen synthase kinase-3 inhibition induces glioma cell death through c-MYC, nuclear factor-kappaB, and glucose regulation. Cancer Research. 2008;**68**:6643-6651

[89] Miyashita K, Kawakami K, Nakada M, Mai W, Shakoori A,

Fujisawa H, et al. Potential therapeutic effect of glycogen synthase kinase 3beta inhibition against human glioblastoma. Clinical Cancer Research. 2009;**15**: 887-897

[90] Domoto T, Pyko IV, Furuta T, Miyashita K, Uehara M, Shimasaki T, et al. Glycogen synthase kinase-3beta is a pivotal mediator of cancer invasion and resistance to therapy. Cancer Science. 2016;**107**:1363-1372

[91] Kast RE, Karpel-Massler G, Halatsch ME. CUSP9* treatment protocol for recurrent glioblastoma: aprepitant, artesunate, auranofin, captopril, celecoxib, disulfiram, itraconazole, ritonavir, sertraline augmenting continuous low dose temozolomide. Oncotarget. 2014;**5**: 8052-8082

[92] Skaga E, Skaga IO, Grieg Z, Sandberg CJ, Langmoen IA, Vik-Mo EO. The efficacy of a coordinated pharmacological blockade in glioblastoma stem cells with nine repurposed drugs using the CUSP9 strategy. Journal of Cancer Research and Clinical Oncology. 2019;**145**: 1495-1507

[93] Gao L, Huang S, Zhang H, Hua W, Xin S, Cheng L, et al. Suppression of glioblastoma by a drug cocktail reprogramming tumor cells into neuronal like cells. Scientific Reports. 2019;**9**:3462

[94] Zhang X, Liu X, Zhou W, Yang M, Ding Y, Wang Q, et al. Fasudil increases temozolomide sensitivity and suppresses temozolomide-resistant glioma growth via inhibiting ROCK2/ABCG2. Cell Death & Disease. 2018;**9**: 190

[95] Yuan J, Zhang F, Hallahan D, Zhang Z, He L, Wu LG, et al. Reprogramming glioblastoma multiforme cells into neurons by protein kinase inhibitors. Journal of Experimental & Clinical Cancer Research. 2018;**37**:181

[96] Platten M, Wild-Bode C, Wick W, Leitlein J, Dichgans J, Weller M. N-[3,4-dimethoxycinnamoyl] anthranilic acid (tranilast) inhibits transforming growth factor-beta release and reduces migration and invasiveness of human malignant glioma cells. International Journal of Cancer. 2001; **93**:53-61

[97] Triscott J, Rose Pambid M, Dunn SE. Concise review: Bullseye: Targeting cancer stem cells to improve the treatment of gliomas by repurposing disulfiram. Stem Cells. 2015;**33**(4): 1042-1046

[98] Ma I, Allan AL. The role of human aldehyde dehydrogenase in normal and cancer stem cells. Stem Cell Reviews and Reports. 2011;**7**(2):292-306

[99] Paranjpe A, Zhang R, Ali-Osman F, Bobustuc GC, Srivenugopal KS. Disulfiram is a direct and potent inhibitor of human O6-methylguanine-DNA methyltransferase (MGMT) in brain tumor cells and mouse brain and markedly increases the alkylating DNA damage. Carcinogenesis. 2014;**35**(3): 692-702

[100] Hothi P, Martins TJ, Chen L, Deleyrolle L, Yoon JG, Reynolds B, et al. High-throughput chemical screens identify disulfiram as an inhibitor of human glioblastoma stem cells. Oncotarget. 2012;**3**(10):1124-1136

[101] Huang J, Chaudhary R, Cohen AL, Fink K, Goldlust S, Boockvar J, et al. A multicenter phase II study of temozolomide plus disulfiram and copper for recurrent temozolomide-resistant glioblastoma. Journal of Neuro-Oncology. 2019;**142**(3):537-544

[102] Koyuturk M, Ersoz M, Altiok N. Simvastatin induces proliferation inhibition and apoptosis in C6 glioma

cells via c-Jun N-terminal kinase. Neuroscience Letters. 2004;**370**(2–3): 212-217

[103] Afshordel S, Kern B, Clasohm J, Konig H, Priester M, Weissenberger J, et al. Lovastatin and perillyl alcohol inhibit glioma cell invasion, migration, and proliferation—Impact of Ras-/rho-prenylation. Pharmacological Research. 2015;**91**:69-77

[104] Gaist D, Hallas J, Friis S, Hansen S, Sorensen HT. Statin use and survival following glioblastoma multiforme. Cancer Epidemiology. 2014;**38**(6): 722-727

[105] Henker C, Kriesen T, Scherer M, Glass A, von Deimling A, Bendszus M, et al. Association between tumor compartment volumes, the incidence of pretreatment seizures, and statin-mediated protective effects in Glioblastoma. Neurosurgery. 2019; **85**(4):E722-E7e9

[106] Xie Y, Lu Q, Lenahan C, Yang S, Zhou D, Qi X. Whether statin use improves the survival of patients with glioblastoma?: A meta-analysis. Medicine (Baltimore). 2020;**99**(9):e18997

[107] Leost M, Schultz C, Link A, Wu YZ, Biernat J, Mandelkow EM, et al. Paullones are potent inhibitors of glycogen synthase kinase-3beta and cyclin-dependent kinase 5/p25. European Journal of Biochemistry. 2000;**267**(19):5983-5994

[108] Doble BW, Woodgett JR. GSK-3: Tricks of the trade for a multi-tasking kinase. Journal of Cell Science. 2003;**116** (Pt 7):1175-1186

[109] Cohen P, Goedert M. GSK3 inhibitors: Development and therapeutic potential. Nature Reviews. Drug Discovery. 2004;**3**(6):479-487

[110] Kitabayashi T, Dong Y, Furuta T, Sabit H, Jiapaer S, Zhang J, et al. Identification of GSK3beta inhibitor kenpaullone as a temozolomide enhancer against glioblastoma. Scientific Reports. 2019;**9**(1):10049

[111] Tran NL, McDonough WS, Savitch BA, Fortin SP, Winkles JA, Symons M, et al. Increased fibroblast growth factor-inducible 14 expression levels promote glioma cell invasion via Rac1 and nuclear factor-kappaB and correlate with poor patient outcome. Cancer Research. 2006;**66**(19): 9535-9542

[112] Jiapaer S, Furuta T, Dong Y, Kitabayashi T, Sabit H, Zhang J, et al. Identification of 2-fluoropalmitic acid as a potential therapeutic agent against glioblastoma. Current Pharmaceutical Design. DOI: 10.2174/ 1381612826666200429092742

[113] Wu H, Li X, Feng M, Yao L, Deng Z, Zao G, et al. Downregulation of RNF138 inhibits cellular proliferation, migration, invasion and EMT in glioma cells via suppression of the Erk signaling pathway. Oncology Reports. 2018; **40**(6):3285-3296

[114] Aroui S, Aouey B, Chtourou Y, Meunier AC, Fetoui H, Kenani A. Naringin suppresses cell metastasis and the expression of matrix metalloproteinases (MMP-2 and MMP-9) via the inhibition of ERK-P38-JNK signaling pathway in human glioblastoma. Chemico-Biological Interactions. 2016;**244**:195-203

[115] Chen X, Zhang M, Gan H, Wang H, Lee JH, Fang D, et al. A novel enhancer regulates MGMT expression and promotes temozolomide resistance in glioblastoma. Nature Communications. 2018;**9**(1):2949

[116] Abbott NJ, Patabendige AA, Dolman DE, Yusof SR, Begley DJ. Structure and function of the blood-brain barrier. Neurobiology of Disease. 2010;**37**(1):13-25

[117] Pardridge WM. The blood-brain barrier: Bottleneck in brain drug development. NeuroRx. 2005;**2**(1):3-14

[118] Ha SW, Hwang K, Jin J, Cho AS, Kim TY, Hwang SI, et al. Ultrasound-sensitizing nanoparticle complex for overcoming the blood-brain barrier: An effective drug delivery system. International Journal of Nanomedicine. 2019;**14**:3743-3752

[119] Sugiyama S, Yamashita Y, Kikuchi T, Sonoda Y, Kumabe T, Tominaga T. Enhanced antitumor effect of combined-modality treatment using convection-enhanced delivery of hydrophilic nitrosourea with irradiation or systemic administration of temozolomide in intracranial brain tumor xenografts. Neurological Research. 2008;**30**(9):960-967

[120] Tosi U, Souweidane MM. Longitudinal monitoring of Gd-DTPA following convection enhanced delivery in the brainstem. World Neurosurgery. 2020;**137**:38-42

[121] Patel AP, Tirosh I, Trombetta JJ, Shalek AK, Gillespie SM, Wakimoto H, et al. Single-cell RNA-seq highlights intratumoral heterogeneity in primary glioblastoma. Science. 2014;**344**(6190): 1396-1401

[122] Hoshino T, Wilson CB, Rosenblum ML, Barker M. Chemotherapeutic implications of growth fraction and cell cycle time in glioblastomas. Journal of Neurosurgery. 1975;**43**(2):127-135

[123] Chou FH, Tsai KY, Su CY, Lee CC. The incidence and relative risk factors for developing cancer among patients with schizophrenia: A nine-year follow-up study. Schizophrenia Research. 2011; **129**(2–3):97-103

9

Drugs Repurposing for Multi-Drug Resistant Bacterial Infections

Andrea Vila Domínguez, Manuel Enrique Jiménez Mejías and Younes Smani

Abstract

Different institutions recognized that antimicrobial resistance is a global health threat that has compounded by the reduction in the discovery and development of new antimicrobial agents. Therefore, the development of new antimicrobial therapeutic strategies requires immediate attention to avoid the 10 million deaths predicted to occur by 2050 as a result of multidrug-resistant (MDR) bacteria. Despite the great interest in the development of repurposing drugs, only few repurposing drugs are under clinical development against Gram-negative critical-priority pathogens. In this chapter, we aim: (i) to discuss the therapeutic potential of the repurposing drugs for treating MDR bacterial infections, (ii) to summarize their mechanism of action, and (iii) to provide an overview for their preclinical and clinical development against these critical-priority pathogens.

Keywords: repurposing drug, infection, bacteria, nosocomial, clinical

1. Introduction

Antimicrobial resistance poses a well-recognized global health threat due to the global dissemination of bacteria resistants to multiple antibiotic classes. This situation is deemed a global priority by the World Health Organization and the European Centre for Disease Prevention and Control [1, 2]. Currently, global deaths due to antimicrobial resistance are more than 70,000 in USA and in Europe together [3, 4]. Therefore, the development of new antimicrobial therapeutic strategies requires immediate attention to avoid the high number of deaths predicted to occur in the future as a result of multidrug-resistant (MDR) bacteria [5]. It is clear that effective solutions such as the establishment of antimicrobial stewardship programs to optimize the use of existing antibiotics, the promotion of novel rapid diagnostics to curtail the unnecessary use of antimicrobial agents; the promotion, development, and use of vaccines and novel antibiotic classes are urgently needed [5]. However, the increased prevalence of infections by MDR bacteria and the scarcity of novel antibiotic families that are under clinical development could warrant the development of new antimicrobial therapeutic strategies for use alone or together with one of the scarce but clinically relevant antibiotics.

Repurposing drugs have been gained renewed interest in the last decade as reflected by several recent studies [6–9]. Since then, 4% of the 407 preclinical antibiotic projects from 314 institutions are related with repurposing drugs evaluated against bacterial infections [10]. Further evidence of the increased interest in these drugs class is that the development process for repurposed drugs benefits from a large body of available knowledge and reduces the time and cost of develop-ment [9]. The majority of repurposed drugs developed to treat bacterial infections are approved or in advanced clinical stages as anticancer drugs, anti-inflammatory/ immunomodulatory drugs, antipsychotic and antidepressant drugs, statins and iron-storage drugs [9]. The large difference between the numerous drugs approved or in development for oncologic indications and the small number of new anti-biotics is surprising given that over the past decades antimicrobial resistance has emerged as an important public health with high associated mortality, and in 2050 antimicrobial resistance would result in 10 million more deaths than those caused by cancers [5]. Although multiple factors contribute to the scarcity of new antibiotics for bacterial infections, the success of repurposing drugs-based antibi-otic therapy as an alternative approach can be reached. Repurposing drugs-based approaches could provide a viable alternative for the treatment of certain MDR bacterial infections. This could be especially important for certain infections caused by MDR Gram-negative infections such as *Acinetobacter baumannii, Pseudomonas aeruginosa* and *Enterobacterales* carbapenems-resistants, for which current antimi-crobial treatments are not active. The WHO has classified as critical priority these pathogens for research and development of new antibiotics [1].

In this chapter, we focus on the current state of knowledge regarding the potential benefits and disadvantages of repurposing drugs treatments for MDR Gram-negative infections. We outline the advances to-date in their preclinical and clinical development as antimicrobial agents. To this end, we introduce in Pubmed database different key words such as repurposing drug, repositioning, antimicrobial and/or antibacterial in order to find published literature about the repurposing drugs for treatment of bacterial infections.

2. Therapeutic potential of repurposing drugs

There is a widely acknowledged that repurposing drugs could address the global increase in antimicrobial resistance and especially the treatment of MDR Gram-negative bacteria. This could be due by the fact that repurposing drugs might exhibit some advantageous characteristics. Repurposing drugs target some genes and surface proteins that are not targets of currently used antimicrobials [9]. Of note, it is unlikely that their antibacterial activities can be disturbed by existing antimicrobial resistance mechanisms. The most of repurposing drugs increased the permeability and damaged the bacterial membrane without killing the bacteria. They enhanced the activity of the current antibiotics [9]. Furthermore, repurposing drugs are drugs approved by the Federal Drug Administration (FDA), information about their pharmacological characteristics (both safety and pharmacokinetic) in preclinical and clinical trials is widely available. Therefore, the time and economic costs associated with the repurposing of these drugs for other therapeutic applica-tions such as the treatment of bacterial infections will be minimized [11]. Finally, to our knowledge, it was not reported that repurposing drugs produce selective pressure on the human microbiome.

Substantial progress has been made in the development of repurposed drugs against bacterial infections. Although some current compounds in the pipeline have exhibited promising results, existing pharmacokinetic characteristics limits the activity of many of them. It should be taken into account in the preclinical development of repurposing drugs the possible need for new formulations to increase their bioavailability and absorption. This aspect is relevant for the development of anthelmintics. Extensive binding to plasma proteins has been reported for oxyclozanide and other salicylanilides, which currently limits their systemic and intravenous applications [12]. Of note, positive results have been seen with niclosamide derivative O-alkylamino-tethered, which has a potent antibacterial effect against carbapenemase producing and colistin resistant *Enterobacterales* isolates [13]. Inhalable nanosuspension and salt form of niclosamide, niclosamide ethanolamine, have presented better solubility profile and inhibited the *P. aeruginosa* quorum sensing (QS) [14, 15]. An additional relevant issue should be taken into account is that their administration route can be changed. ADMET tests should be performed before the development of these repurposing drugs in clinical trials. The choice of the route is a relevant aspect in serious infections in hospitalized patients such as ventilated-associated pneumonia who patients are intubated and other circumstances in which the oral route is not available.

3. Mechanisms of action of repurposing drugs against Gram-negative bacilli

Different agents are promising both in vitro and in vivo candidates to be repositioned as antimicrobial agents to treat infections caused by MDR Gram-negative bacilli. A variety of drugs with different mechanisms of action and targets have been selected including: DNA, RNA and proteins inhibitors [16–20], QS regulators [15, 17, 21–25], biofilm formation inhibitors and disruptors [26, 27], drugs that interact with cell membrane [28–30], drugs that interact with iron metabolism [31–35], and host immune system modulators [36–39]. These drugs and their mechanisms of action against critical-priority pathogens (*A. baumannii*, *P. aeruginosa* and *Enterobacterales*) are summarized in **Figure 1** and **Table 1**.

3.1 DNA, RNA and proteins inhibitors

Anticancer and anti-inflammatory drugs that interact with DNA, RNA and proteins have been reported. Mitomycin C, used in several types of carcinomas such

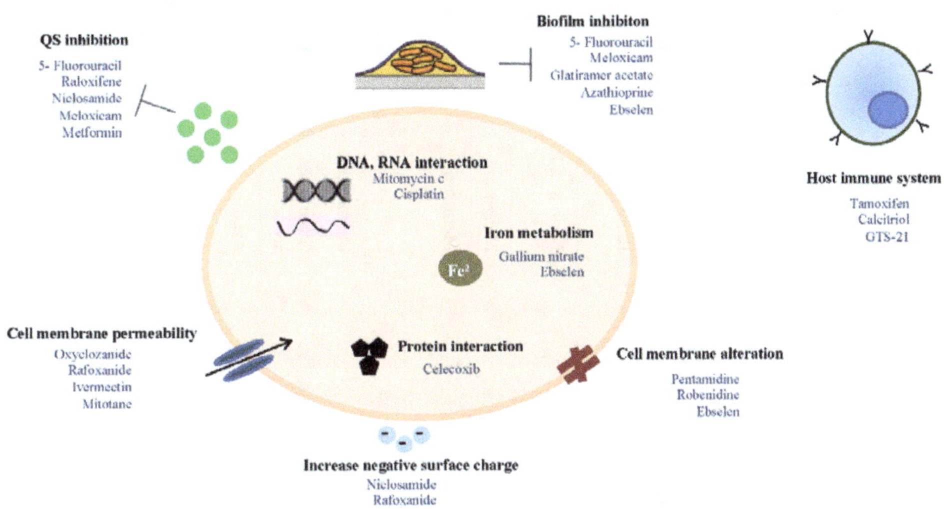

Figure 1.
Mechanisms of action of repurposed drugs against Gram-negative critical-priority pathogens.

Bacterial target	Repurposed drug	Clinical indications	Mechanism of action	Reference
DNA, RNA & proteins	Mitomycin c	Superficial vesical carcinoma	Binding to DNA during DNA synthesis and causes inhibition of its synthesis and function in *P. aeruginosa* and *E. coli*	[18]
	Cisplatin	Cancer	Upregulation of the *recA* gene of *P. aeruginosa*, which is known to be important for DNA repair	[20]
	Celecoxib	Inflammation	Inhibition of RNA, DNA, and protein synthesis in *S. aureus*	[19]
Quorum sensing	5-fluorouracil	Solid tumors	Inhibition of QS formation in *P. aeruginosa*	[23, 41]
	Raloxifene	Breast cancer	Binding to PhzB2 which is involved in the production of pyocyanin, a pigment related with virulence factor and QS signalling molecule in *P. aeruginosa*	[24]
	Niclosamide	Helminthiasis	Production of the QS signaling molecules N-3-oxododecanoyl-homeserine lactone and N-butanoyl-homoserine lactone in *P. aeruginosa*	[15, 25]
	Meloxicam	Inflammation	Interaction with active sites of the QS of *P. aeruginosa*	[26]
	Metformin	Diabetes	Inhibition of QS system by bind to LasR by hydrogen bonding and electrostatic interaction and to rhlR by hydrogen bonding in *P. aeruginosa*	[21]
Biofilm formation	5-Fluorouracil	Solid tumors	Regulation of different genes involved in the biofilm formation by *P. aeruginosa*	[41]
	Meloxicam	Inflammation	Decrease in the extracellular Psl, Pel, and alginate production by *P. aeruginosa*	[26, 27]
	Glatiramer acetate	Inflammation	Disruption of the biofilm formation by GNB	[42]
	Azathioprine	Crohn's disease	Inhibition of WspR, involved in the regulation of c-di-GMP known as a regulator of the bacterial biofilm formation by *P. aeruginosa* and *E. coli*	[43]
	Ebselen	Bipolar disorder and ischemic stroke	Inhibition of c-di-GMP in *P. aeruginosa*	[44, 45]

Bacterial target	Repurposed drug	Clinical indications	Mechanism of action	Reference
Cell membrane	Niclosamide	Helminthiasis	Increase of the negative surface charge of *A. baumannii* and *K. pneumoniae*	[30]
	Oxyclozanide	Helminthiasis	Reduction of the membrane potential and increase of aminoglucosides accumulation in *P. aeruginosa*. Increase of the membrane permeability of *A. baumannii*, *P. aeruginosa* and *K. pneumoniae*	[28, 46]
	Rafoxanide	Helminthiasis	Increase of the negative surface charge of *A. baumannii* and *K. pneumoniae* Increase of the membrane permeability of *A. baumannii, P. aeruginosa* and *K. pneumoniae*	[47]
	Ivermectin	Helminthiasis	Increase of the membrane permeability of *A. baumannii, P. aeruginosa* and *K. pneumoniae*	[48]
	Mitotane	Cancer	Permeabilization of the outer membrane of *A. baumannii, P. aeruginosa* and *K. pneumoniae*	[49]
	Pentamidine	Protozoal infection	Alteration of the outer membrane of GNB, due to the interaction with membrane lipopolysaccharides	[29]
	Robenidine	Protozoal infection	Alteration of the cell membrane of GNB	[50]
	Ebselen	Bipolar disorder and ischemic stroke	Inhibition of the TonB-mediated physiology of *A. baumannii* and *E. coli*	[51]
Iron metabolism	Gallium Nitrate	Lymphoma and bladder cancer	Interferance with iron-dependent metabolic pathways in GNB	[31–33]
	Ebselen	Bipolar disorder and ischemic stroke	Iinhibition of TonB involved in iron acquisition by *A. baumannii* and *E. coli*	[51]
Host immune system	Tamoxifen	Breast cancer	Reduction in the migration of immune cells from bone marrow to blood through the reduction of MCP-1 and IL-18 in presence of *A. baumannii, P. aeruginosa* and *E. coli*	[36]
	Calcitriol		Enhancement of the killing activity of monocytes and macrophages towards *P. aeruginosa.*	[37]
	GTS-21	Inflammation	Enhancement of the macrophage function towards *P. aeruginosa* via inhibiting the release of nuclear protein high mobility group box-1 Reduction of pro-inflammatory cytokines (TNF-α, IL-1β, and IL-6) release	[38, 39]

Table 1.
Repurposing drugs and their mechanisms of action.

as the superficial vesical carcinoma [40], has shown activity against *A. baumannii*, *P. aeruginosa* and *E. coli in vitro* and *in vivo* [16–18]. Mitomycin C binds to DNA during DNA synthesis and causes inhibition of its synthesis and function in *P. aeruginosa* and *E. coli* [18]. Cisplatin, approved for treatment of a number of cancers, was found to inhibit microbial cells growth [17, 20]. The mechanism of action of this drug has been attributed to the upregulation of the recA gene in *P. aeruginosa*, which is important for DNA repair, implicating that cisplatin could interfere with DNA replication [20]. Moreover, celecoxib, a non-steroidal anti-inflammatory drug (NSAID), has been tested in a *Caenorhabditis elegans* and in whole-animal *A. baumannii* and *P. aeruginosa* infection models. It was suggested that inhibit dose-dependently the DNA, RNA and protein synthesis as in *Staphylococcus aureus* [19].

3.2 Quorum sensing regulators

QS inhibition and regulation have been reported as antibacterial properties of anticancer, anthelminthic, anti-inflammatory and hypoglycemic drugs such as 5-fluorouracil, raloxifene, niclosamide, meloxicam and metformin. 5-fluorouracil is a potent drug indicated for the treatment of different types of solid tumors, that has shown antibacterial activity *in vitro* [17, 22, 23]. The antibacterial mechanism of this drug has been proposed as QS inhibitor [23, 41]. Also, 5-fluorouracil has dual inhibition mechanisms including functioning as an alternative substrate resulting in miscoding DNA and RNA, and inhibiting thymidylate synthase [22]. Moreover, the selective estrogen receptor modulator (SERM) raloxifene, used in the preven-tion of osteoporosis and invasive breast cancer in post-menopausal women, has presented activity against Gram-negative bacilli (GNB). Raloxifene binds to PhzB2 which is involved in the production of pyocyanin, a pigment related with both the virulence factor and the QS signaling molecule in *P. aeruginosa* [24]. Regarding the anthelmintic drugs, niclosamide, used for the treatment of helminthiasis, has been reported to inhibit QS in *P. aeruginosa* in *Galleria mellonella* model by hindering the cell's response and production of the QS signaling molecules as N-3-oxododecanoyl-homeserine lactone and N-butanoyl-homoserine lactone [15, 25]. Finally, meloxi-cam, a NSAID used to manage moderate-to-severe pain, and metformin, one of the most commonly prescribed oral hypoglycemic for treatment of type 2 diabetes, have been reported to interact with active sites and to inhibit the QS of *P. aeruginosa*, respectively [21, 26, 27]. Molecular docking study has shown that metformin could bind to LasR by hydrogen bonding and electrostatic interaction and to rhlR by hydrogen bonding only [21].

3.3 Biofilm formation inhibitors and disruptors

Compared with QS, much less drugs have been act on the biofilm formation. 5-fluorouracil has been revealed to regulate different genes involved in the biofilm formation by *P. aeruginosa* [41]. More specifically, meloxicam has been reported to inhibit biofilm formation of *P. aeruginosa* by decreasing the extracellular Psl, Pel and alginate production, three vital biofilm exopolysaccharides in this pathogen [26, 27]. Moreover, glatiramer acetate, a drug used in the treatment of multiple sclerosis, has also been shown to disrupt biofilm formation by GNB [42]. Finally, azathioprine, an immunosuppressive drug used for the treatment of Crohn's disease and other autoimmune diseases, has exhibited anti-biofilm activity against *P. aeruginosa* and *E. coli* through the inhibition of WspR [43]. WspR is a diguanylate cyclase involved in the regulation of a signal molecule called cyclic-di-GMP (c-di-GMP) known as a regulator of the bacterial biofilm formation [43]. The same mechanism of action has been used by ebselen to exhibit anti-biofilm activity against *P. aeruginosa* [44, 45]. Ebselen, despite the fact that it is not an FDA-approved drug, it is being investigated in clinical trials for the treatment of bipolar disorder, hearing loss and tinnitus and ischemic stroke.

3.4 Interaction with cell membrane

Various anthelmintic, anticancer and antiprotozoal drugs such as niclosamide, oxyclozanide, rafoxanide, ivermectin, mitotane, pentamidine and robenidine have been reported to interact with the bacterial cell membrane. Three anthelmintic drugs in combination with colistin have shown activity against GNB by the regulation of electric charges. Niclosamide and rafoxanide were discovered to increase the negative surface charge of bacterial membrane in *A. baumannii* and *K. pneumoniae* clinical strains *in vitro* [30, 47]. In turn, oxyclozanide has enhanced the activity of additional tobramycin against *P. aeruginosa* by reducing the membrane potential and increasing tobramycin accumulation [28]. This increase in the negative surface charges allow to restore the activity of colistin in colistin-resistant (Col-R) *A. baumannii* and *K. pneumoniae*, and the activity tobramycin in tobramycin-resistant *P. aeruginosa* [30, 47]. Not only the regulation of electric charges has been reported as mechanism of action of anthelmintic drugs, but the increase of bacterial membrane permeabilization has also been reported. Oxyclozanide, rafoxanide and ivermectin have been shown to increase the membrane permeability of *A. baumannii*, *P. aeruginosa* and *K. pneumoniae*, especially in Col-R strains [46–48]. Moreover, Tran et al. have demonstrated that mitotane, a FDA-approved antineoplastic drug, in combination of polymyxin B lead mitotane to enter inside *A. baumannii*, *P. aeruginosa* and *K. pneumoniae* through the permeabilization of the outer membrane by polymyxin B [49]. Additionally, antiprotozoal drugs, pentamidine and robenidine, possess a mechanism of action that disturbs the outer membrane of GNB, due to the interaction with membrane lipopolysaccharides (LPS) [29, 50]. Finally, ebselen has also presented antibacterial effect against *A. baumannii* and *E. coli* by inhibiting the TonB-mediated physiology, which is involved in iron acquisition from host sources [51].

3.5 Interaction with iron metabolism

Antunes et al. have demonstrated that virulent bacteria are able to acquire iron in the blood and tissues [33]. Given the essential role of iron in bacterial physiology and pathogenicity, iron uptake and metabolism have become attractive targets for the development of new antibacterial agents [52, 53]. The ion gallium [Ga(III)], a ferric iron [Fe(III)] mimetic, has been shown to inhibit the growth of many bacterial species by interfering with iron-dependent metabolic pathways. Therefore, gallium drugs have gained special interest in the fight of MDR-GNB infections [31]. Gallium nitrate is an anticancer drug that was approved by the FDA for the treatment of cancer-associated hypercalcemia. Antibacterial properties of gallium nitrate have been previously reported against GNB infections, both *in vitro* and *in vivo* [31–35]. In addition, Ebselen as mentioned before has the characteristic to inhibit TonB in *A. baumannii* and *E. coli* [51].

3.6 Host immune system modulators

Also, some drugs that modulate host immune system have reported antibacterial activity against GNB. Tamoxifen, a SERM used for breast cancer treatment, can reduced the migration of immune cells from bone marrow to blood through the reduction of monocytes chemoattractant protein 1 (MCP-1) and IL-18 in a murine model of sepsis by *A. baumannii*, *P. aeruginosa* and *E. coli* [36]. Moreover, tamoxifen has been shown to enhance the killing activity of macrophages and neutrophils against *A. baumannii* and *E. coli in vitro* [36]. Calcitriol, a bioactive form of vitamin D3 used to treat hypocalcemic conditions and renal osteodystrophy, has a similar mechanism of action which it has been described to enhance the killing activity of monocytes and macrophages towards *P. aeruginosa* [37]. Moreover, GTS-21, an anti-inflammatory drug, has presented therapeutic efficacy against *P. aeruginosa in vivo* by enhancing macrophage function via inhibiting the release of nuclear protein high mobility group box-1 (HMGB1) [39]. When GTS-21 is combined with M1 muscarinic acetylcholine receptor agonist and α7n-acetylcholine receptor agonist against *E. coli in vivo*, the blood concentrations of pro-inflammatory cytokines TNF-α, IL-1β, and IL-6 were reduced significantly [38].

4. Repurposing drugs against MDR Gram-negative bacilli

There are currently multiple repurposing drugs in preclinical development for the treatment of infections by Gram-negative critical-priority pathogens. Few of them have been evaluated in early and late stage clinical trials. A summary of recent developments in repurposing drugs *in vitro*, in animal models and in clinical trials is presented below. The different clinical trials with repurposing drugs against these pathogens are listed in **Table 2**.

4.1 *Acinetobacter baumannii*

MDR *A. baumannii* is a well-recognized current global health threat that needs urgent effective solutions [1, 2]. Last-resort treatments such as colistin are no longer effective in an increasing number of cases, leading to a mortality rate of around 35–60% in hospitalized patients with ventilator-associated pneumonia [54, 55]. The number of antibiotics approved by the FDA cannot keep up with the pace at which resistance is acquired by *A. baumannii*. The therapeutic potential of different repurposing drugs against *A. baumannii* has been tested in preclinical models, most of them in combination with polymyxins (colistin and polymyxin B) or its prodrug colistimethate sodium (CMS).

Repurposing drug	Clinical indication	Target bacteria	New clinical indication	Clinical trial phase	Clinical trial identifier
GTS-21	Inflammation	*E. coli*	Endotoxemia	Interventional (Clinical trial)	NCT00783068
Sodium nitrite	Acute cyanide poisoning	*P. aeruginosa*	Cystic fibrosis (antimicrobial agent)	Phase I/II	NCT02694393
Sodium nitrite	Acute cyanide poisoning	*P. aeruginosa*	Cystic fibrosis (biofilm disruptor)	Phase II	NCT02295566
Gallium nitrate	Cancer-associated hypercalcemia	*P. aeruginosa*	Cystic fibrosis	Phase II	NCT02354859
Amitriptyline	Depression	*P. aeruginosa*	Cystic fibrosis	Phase II	NCT00515229
Atorvastatin	Hyper cholestremia	*P. aeruginosa*	bronchiectasis and infection	Phase IV	NCT01299194

Table 2.
List of repurposing drugs under clinical trial development against Gram-negative critical-priority pathogens.

4.1.1 Anticancer drugs

The antibacterial activity of anticancer drugs has been reported *in vitro* and *in vivo* non-vertebrate and vertebrate models by *A. baumannii*. Gallium nitrate has demonstrated an inhibitory effect on bacterial growth in a collection of 58 MDR clinical isolates of *A. baumannii in vitro* [33]. This antibacterial activity is maintained in *G. mellonella* model. The administration of this drug alone and in combination with colistin, at concentrations mimicking the human therapeutic dose of gallium nitrate used for cancer patients (28 μM), significantly increased the survival of larvae after infection by A. baumannii [33]. When a vertebrate model was used such as murine models of acute and chronic lung infections by *A. baumannii*, gallium nitrate has reduced lung injury and bacterial loads in tissues [32]. Moreover, the combination of mitomycin C with tobramycin and ciprofloxacin together has increased *in vitro* the activity of this anticancer drug against MDR clinical isolates of *A. baumannii* [17]. Whereas, mitotane combined with polymyxin B against polymyxin B-resistant *A. baumannii* has presented synergy with polymyxin B, increasing the activity of polymyxin B *in vitro* and in murine model of burn wound infection by reducing the bacterial load in wounds [49]. Another group of anticancer drugs developed to combat breast cancer is the SERMs. Tamoxifen has been reported to exhibit activity in the immunocompetent and neutropenic murine model of peritoneal sepsis by ATCC 17978 strain by decreasing the bacterial loads in spleen, lungs and blood and increasing the mice survival [36]. Tamoxifen metabolites (N-desmethyltamoxifen, 4-hydroxytamoxifen and endoxifen), produced after tamoxifen metabolizing by cytochrome P450 [56], have presented antibacterial activity in vitro with MIC50 and MIC90 of 8 and 16 mg/L, respectively, against a collection 100 MDR and pan-drug resistant (PDR) clinical isolates of *A. baumannii* [36].

4.1.2 Anthelmintic drugs

The potential activity of the anthelmintic drug has been also tested *in vitro* and in animal models by *A. baumannii*. Niclosamide, oxyclozanide, rafoxanide and ivermectin have been shown to potentiate the activity of colistin against clinical isolates of Col-R *A. baumannii in vitro* [30, 46–48, 57]. In the murine model of peritoneal sepsis by Col-R *A. baumannii* clinical isolate, rafoxanide plus CMS, a prodrug of colistin, compared with CMS alone increased mice survival to 53.8% and reduced bacterial loads in tissues and blood between 3 and 4 log10 cfu/g or mL, respectively [47]. Only, rafoxanide has exhibited antibacterial activity in monotherapy in this model of infection, but not *in vitro* [47].

4.1.3 Anti-inflammatory drugs

As is the case with anthelmintic drugs, anti-inflammatory drugs have demonstrated antibacterial activity against *A. baumannii* in monotherapy and in combination with polmyxins *in vitro*. Glatiramer acetate has presented activity against reference strains and clinical bacteremic isolates of A. baumannii by disrupting the biofilm formation [42]. In addition, ebselen has presented antibacterial effect against *A. baumannii* by reducing their bacterial growth at MICs of 32 μM due to the inhibition of the siderephore TonB [51]. In combination with polymyxins, auranofin, a drug used for the treatment of rheumatoid arthritis, and celecoxib have exhibited synergy with polymyxin B and colistin against reference strains of *A. baumannii* respectively [19, 58].

4.1.4 Other drugs

Other drugs with different modes of action and clinical indications have been evaluated as antibacterial agents against *A. baumannii* in monotherapy and in combination with antibiotics. Simvastatin, used in the treatment of atherosclerotic cardiovascular disease and hypercholesterolemia, has exhibited antibacterial activity in combination with sub-inhibitory concentrations of colistin against a collection of clinical isolates of *A. baumannii*, reducing the MIC of simvastatin from >256 mg/L to a range between 8 and 32 mg/L [59]. Two antiprotozoal drugs have been also evaluated in monotherapy and in combination with antibiotics. Robenidine has presented bactericidal activity alone and in combination with polymyxin B nanopeptide against reference strains of *A. baumannii in vitro* [60]. Pentamidine, in turn, has present synergy with novobiocin, a drug used for Gram-positive cocci infections, in vitro and in murine sepsis model by a reference strain of *A. baumannii* [29].

4.2 *Pseudomonas aeruginosa*

Pseudomonas aeruginosa is one of the most relevant pathogens causing human opportunistic infections in immunocompromised patients and severe nosocomial infections [61–63]. Indeed, *P. aeruginosa* is the top pathogen causing ventilator-associated pneumonia and burn wound infections and is a major cause of nosocomial bacteremia [62–64]. An MDR pattern is commonly observed in *P. aeruginosa* clinical isolates, raising the threat of difficult-to-treat infections [65–67]. These MDR isolates are generally susceptible to polymyxins and resistant to imipenem and ceftazidime [68]. New beta-lactamases inhibitors, combined with existing antibiotic families, such as ceftazidime/avibactam, ceftolozane/tazobactam, and imipenem/relebactam, against specific carbapenemases, have recently been developed [69]. Compared with *A. baumannii*, much more work has been done regarding the development of repurposing drugs for *P. aeruginosa* in preclinical and clinical stages.

4.2.1 Anticancer drugs

Different studies have been performed on *P. aeruginosa* to evaluate the antibacterial effect of anticancer drugs. Regarding SERM drugs, raloxifene attenuated *in vitro* and in *C. elegans* model the virulence of *P. aeruginosa* by binding to PhzB2 which is involved in the production of pyocyanin [24]. Whereas, tamoxifen exhibit therapeutic efficacy in murine model of peritoneal sepsis by PAO1 strain by decreasing the bacterial loads in spleen, lungs and blood and increasing the mice survival [36]. In addition, cisplatin was found to inhibit microbial cells growth [17, 20] by the upregulation of the recA gene in *P. aeruginosa* [20]. 5-fluorouracil, in turn, has been used against a collection of 5850 mutants of the PA14 strain, revealing positive activity via the regulation of a large number of genes involved in QS and biofilm formation [41, 70]. In combination with antibiotics, two anticancer drugs have been tested. Mitomycin C and mitotante in combination with tobramycin-ciprofloxacin [17] and polymyxin B [49], respectively, have shown synergy against MDR clinical and polymyxin-resistant isolates of *P. aeruginosa*, respectively. Finally, gallium nitrate is one the most studied and advanced cancer drug in clinical development against *P. aeruginosa* infection with promising data. Gallium nitrate has demonstrated an inhibitory effect on bacterial growth in *P. aeruginosa* at concentrations >3.13 μM *in vitro* [71, 72]; although the presence of pyoverdine and proteases in human serum reduce the efficacy of gallium nitrate against *P. aeruginosa* [73]. At non-bactericidal concentrations, gallium nitrate can affect the production of virulence factors of *P. aeruginosa* [71, 74]. In murine mod-els of acute and chronic lung infections by *P. aeruginosa* gallium nitrate has reduced the lung injury and bacterial loads in tissues of animals [71]. At clinical stage, a phase II clinical trial has been started in 2016 evaluating the capacity of gallium nitrate to improve the pulmonary function in 60 patients with cystic fibrosis by *P. aeruginosa*. The results of this trial showed that treatment with gallium nitrate increase the forced expiratory volume in these patients [75].

4.2.2 Anthelmintic drugs

The anthelmintic drugs niclosamide, oxyclozanide, rafoxanide and ivermectin have been shown to restore the activity of colistin against a collection of Col-R *P. aeruginosa in vitro* [46–48, 57]. Not only in combination with colistin, oxyclozanide has presented synergy with tobramycin to destruct the biofilm formation, permeabilizing the cells membrane and depolarizing the membrane potential of *P. aeruginosa* strains resistant to tobramycin *in vitro* [28]. In the murine model of peritoneal sepsis by Col-R *P. aeruginosa* clinical isolate, rafoxanide plus CMS compared with CMS alone, increased mice survival to 73.3%, and reduced bacterial loads in tissues and blood between 3 and 5 log10 cfu/g or mL, respectively [47]. In monotherapy, niclosamide and rafoxanide have exhibited antibacterial activity against *P. aeruginosa*. One *in vitro* study has indicated that niclosamide presented an anti-virulent effect against *P. aeruginosa* via the inhibition of QS and virulence genes, reducing elastase and pyocyanin levels [15]. Two additional *in vivo* studies have reported that niclosamide and rafoxanide showed therapeutic efficacy in *G. mellonella* larvae and in murine peritoneal sepsis models by a reference strain and Col-R clinical isolate of *P. aeruginosa*, respectively [15, 47]. Nevertheless, the absorption of niclosamide is lower. To increase this absorption, formulation of niclosamide under nanosuspension has been performed and showed lower toxicity in a rat lung infection model involving *P. aeruginosa* [14].

4.2.3 Anti-inflammatory and immunosuppressive drugs

Similar with *A. baumannii*, anti-inflammatory and immunosuppressive drugs have presented antibacterial activities in monotherapy and in combination with antibiotics against *P. aeruginosa*. The activity of glatiramer acetate against reference and clinical isolates of *P. aeruginosa* from chronic respiratory infections in cystic fibrosis patients has been observed by disruption of the biofilm formation [42]. With the same mechanism of action, ebselen and azathioprine has exhibited activity against *P. aeruginosa* [43, 45]. In turns, celecoxib and betamethasone have presented synergy with colistin, and with ceftazidime, erythromycin and ofloxacin against *P. aeruginosa* in vitro, respectively [19, 76]. Similarly, meloxicam has been reported to be in vitro active alone and in combination with the sub-MIC of tetracycline, gentamicin, tobramycin, ciprofloxacin, ceftriaxone, ofloxacin, norfloxacin, ceftazidime against PAO1 strain, by inhibiting the biofilm formation [27]. Finally, GTS-21 has improved *P. aeruginosa* clearance in a murine model of ventilator-associated pneumonia and reduced acute lung injury by enhancing macrophage function [39].

4.2.4 Antidepressive drugs

Regarding the antidepressive drugs, amitriptyline has reduced the inflammation in the lung of cystic fibrosis mice and prevented infection by *P. aeruginosa* [77]. At clinical stage, a phase II clinical trial evaluating the effect of amitriptyline on the improvement of lung function in 18 patients with cystic fibrosis patients showed that amitriptyline improves the lung function by increasing the forced expiratory volume and weight of these patients [78, 79].

4.2.5 Other drugs

Other drugs with different modes of action and clinical indications have been evaluated as antibacterial agents against *P. aeruginosa*. Metformin has been reported to inhibit QS, biofilm formation, and swimming and twitching motilities of PAO1 strain [21]. Calcitriol has enhanced the bactericidal activity against *P. aeruginosa*, modulating the activity of monocytes and macrophages to increase their bacterial killing [37]. Compared with *A. baumannii*, robenidine has been recently showed to present only synergy with polymyxin B nanpeptide against reference strains of *P. aeruginosa in vitro* [60]. Polymyxin B and colistin have been also combined with auronafin and simvastatin, respectively. Both drugs exhibited synergy with sub-inhibitory concentrations of polymyxin B and colistin against a collection of reference strains of *P. aeruginosa*, reducing the MIC of auronafin from >256 mg/L to 0.125–0.5 mg/L and the MIC of simvastatin from >256 mg/L to 16–32 mg/L [58, 59]. At clinical stage, a phase IV trial determining the role of atorvastatin, another statin, in patients with bronchiectasis and infection with *P. aeruginosa* showed that atorvastatin reduced systemic inflammation and improved quality of life of these patients [80, 81]. In addition, sodium nitrite, used for treatment of acute cyanide poisoning, has been shown in vitro to kill mucoid *P. aeruginosa* strains isolated from patients with cystic fibrosis, under anaerobic planktonic and biofilm conditions [82, 83]. Two early stage (I/II and II) clinical trials have been conducted to evaluate sodium nitrite as antimicrobial agent and as disrupter of biofilm formation in patients with cystic fibrosis by *P. aeruginosa* [84, 85]. The results from both studies have not yet published.

4.3 *Enterobacterales*

Escherichia coli and *Klebsiella pneumoniae* are of the most important pathogens in humans involved in different community and nosocomial infections, including bloodstream infections, urinary tract infections, intraabdominal infections and pneumonia [86–89]. The success of *E. coli* and *K. pneumoniae* as a community and nosocomial pathogens is attributed to their resistance to several antibiotic categories [86, 90]. Similar to *P. aeruginosa* the repurposing drugs developed today for *E. coli* and *K. pneumoniae* are in the preclinical and clinical stages of development.

4.3.1 Anticancer drugs

Anticancer drugs were developed against *E. coli* and *K. pneumoniae in vitro* and in animal models. Tamoxifen has been reported to exhibit activity in the immunocompetent and neutropenic murine model of peritoneal sepsis by *E. coli* ATCC 25922 strain by decreasing the bacterial loads in spleen, lungs and blood and increasing the mice survival [36]. Tamoxifen metabolites N-desmethyltamoxifen, 4-hydroxytamoxifen and endoxifen have presented antibacterial activity *in vitro* with MIC50 and MIC90 of 16 mg/L, against a 47 MDR clinical isolates of *E. coli* [36]. The activity of mitomycin C in monotherapy and in combination with tobramycin and ciprofloxacin together was increased against MDR clinical isolates of *E. coli* and *K. pneumoniae in vitro* [17, 18]. While, mitotane in combination with polymyxin B against polymyxin-resistant *K. pneumoniae* increased the activity of polymyxin B *in vitro* [49].

4.3.2 Anthelmintic drugs

Four anthelmintic drugs, niclosamide, oxyclozanide, rafoxanide and ivermectin were shown to present synergy with colistin against Col-R *K. pneumoniae* [30, 46–48, 57]. Compared to Col-R isolates of *A. baumannii* and *P. aeruginosa* much lesser effect has been observed regarding the effect of these drugs in combination with colistin against Col-R isolates of *K. pneumoniae*. Additionally, in the murine model of peritoneal sepsis model by Col-R clinical isolate of *K. pneumoniae*, rafoxanide in monotherapy and in combination with CMS compared with control animals and with CMS alone, increased mouse survival to 50 and 67%, and reduced bacterial loads in tissues and blood between 2.5 and 3 log10 cfu/g or mL, and 2 and 3 log10 cfu/g or mL, respectively [47].

4.3.3 Anti-inflammatory drugs

In the case of anti-inflammatory drugs, two drugs have presented synergistic effect with antibiotics against *E. coli* and *K. pneumoniae*. The first one is celecoxib which has potentiated the activity of colistin against *E. coli* and *K. pneumoniae* [19]. In turn, betamethasone has presented synergy with ceftazidime and ofloxacin against some isolates of *E. coli* [76]. Similar to *A. baumannii* and *P. aeruginosa*, glatiramer acetate has presented antibacterial effect against reference strains of *E. coli* by disrupting the biofilm formation [42]. Moreover, ebselen has been shown to present antibacterial effect against *E. coli* by reducing their bacterial growth at MICs <128 μM due to the inhibition of TonB [51], and azathioprine has exhibited anti-biofilm activity against *E. coli* through the inhibition of WspR *in vitro* [43]. Finally, GTS-21 in combination with M1 muscarinic acetylcholine receptor agonist have been shown to reduce the mortality of mice in sepsis model by *E. coli* in 4 and 24 h [38]. At clinical stage, an interventional clinical trial on anti-inflammatory effects of oral administration of GTS-21 on the inflammatory response in 7 patients with endotoxemia by LPS of *E. coli* showed that GTS-21 reduced the levels of proinflammatory cytokines in the plasma of these patients [91, 92].

4.3.4 Other drugs

Other drugs with different modes of action and clinical indications have been evaluated as antibacterial agents in monotherapy and in combined therapy with a large list of antibiotics against *E. coli* and *K. pneumoniae in vitro* and in animal models. Amoxapine has been reported to present therapeutic efficacy in an experimental murine model of respiratory infection by *K. pneumoniae* [93]. In addition, pentamidine in combination with different antibiotics ([novobiocin, erythromycin and rifampin] and [amikacin, tobramycin, tigecycline and rifampin]) has presented synergistic activity *in vitro* against different clinical isolates of *E. coli* harboring *mcr-1* and *K. pneumoniae* producing carbapenemases, respectively [94]. In turn, robenidine has been recently showed to present only synergy with polymyxin B nanopeptide against reference strains of *K. pneumoniae in vitro* [60]. Finally, auronafin and simvastatin exhibited synergy with sub-inhibitory concentrations of polymyxin B and colistin against a collection of reference strains of *E. coli* and *K. pneumoniae in vitro*, reducing the MIC of auronafin from >256 mg/L to 0.25–1 mg/L and the MIC of simvastatin from >256 mg/L to 8–32 mg/L, respectively [58, 59].

5. Conclusions

The retreat of the pharmaceutical sector from new antibiotic development has exacerbated the challenge of widespread resistance and signals a critical need for innovation. Repurposing drugs are an increasingly common practice in the pharmaceutical industry where an already existing drug is applied in a new, previously unknown, way. This is advantageous mainly because these drugs are already cleared for human use and thus may skip straight to phase II clinical trials which presents considerably less risk and costs compared to developing new drugs. They could represent a promising approach to enrich the therapeutic arsenal against Gram-negative critical-priority pathogens.

Some drugs indicated for human and veterinary use have been developed in combination with antibiotics; almost of them with polymyxins. They have yielded promising data in preclinical studies, specifically those with activity against biofilm formation and quorum sensing. However, additional relevant issues are required such as new formulations to increase their bioavailability and ADMET tests if the administration route is changed. Other drugs indicated for human use who have showed good activity against these pathogens in preclinical studies can be tested in advanced clinical trials. Early and late stages clinical trials with four repurposing drugs to treat cystic fibrosis and bronchiectasis by *P. aeruginosa*, and endotexemia by *E. coli* have provided promising results. Nevertheless, further clinical studies with extended clinical indications are needed to address the urgent demand for new treatments targeting infections caused by Gram-negative critical-priority pathogens.

Acknowledgements

This study was supported by the Instituto de Salud Carlos III, Proyectos de Investigación en Salud (Grant No. PI19/01435). YS is supported by the Subprograma Miguel Servet Tipo I from the Ministerio de Economía y Competitividad of Spain (CP15/00132).

Author details

Andrea Vila Domínguez, Manuel Enrique Jiménez Mejías and Younes Smani*
Institute of Biomedicine of Seville (IBiS), University Hospital Virgen del Rocío/CSIC/University of Seville, Seville, Spain

*Address all correspondence to: ysmani-ibis@us.es

References

[1] Tacconelli E, Carrara E, Savoldi A, Harbarth S, Mendelson M, Monnet DL, et al. WHO pathogens priority list working group: Discovery, research, and development of new antibiotics: The WHO priority list of antibiotic-resistant bacteria and tuberculosis. Lancet Infectious Diseases. 2018;**18**:318-327. DOI: 10.1016/S1473-3099(17)30753-3

[2] European Centre for Disease Prevention and Control. Surveillance of Antimicrobial Resistance in Europe 2018. Stockholm: ECDC; 2019

[3] Centers for Disease Control and Prevention (CDC). Antibiotic Resistance Threats in the United States, 2019. Atlanta, GA: U.S: Department of Health and Human Services, CDC; 2019

[4] Cassini A, Diaz Högberg L, Plachouras D, Quattrocchi A, Hoxha A, Skov Simonsen G, et al. Attributable deaths and disability-adjusted life-years caused by infections with antibiotic-resistant bacteria in the EU and the European economic area in 2015: A population-level modelling analysis. Lancet Infectious Diseases. 2019;**19**:56-66. DOI: 10.1016/S1473-3099(18)30605-4

[5] O'Neill J. Tackling Drug-Resistant Infections Globally: Final Report, and Recommendations The Review on Antimicrobial Resistance. 2016. Available from: https://amr-review.org/sites/default/files/160525_Final%20 paper_with%20cover.pdf [Accessed: 15 April 2020]

[6] Fischbach MA, Walsh CT. Antibiotics for emerging pathogens. Science. 2009;**325**:1089-1093. DOI: 10.1126/science.1176667

[7] Brown D. Antibiotic resistance breakers: Can repurposed drugs fill the antibiotic discovery void? Nature Reviews Drug Discovery. 2015;**4**: 821-832. DOI: 10.1038/nrd4675

[8] Rampioni G, Visca P, Leoni L, Imperi F. Drug repurposing for antivirulence therapy against opportunistic bacterial pathogens. Emerging Topics in Life Sciences. 2017;**1**:13-23. DOI: 10.1042/ETLS20160018

[9] Miró-Canturri A, Ayerbe-Algaba R, Smani Y. Drug repurposing for the treatment of bacterial and fungal infections. Frontiers in Microbiology. 2019;**10**:41. DOI: 10.3389/fmicb.2019.00041

[10] Theuretzbacher U, Outterson K, Engel A, Karlén A. The global preclinical antibacterial pipeline. Nature Reviews Microbiology. 2020;**18**(5):275- 285. DOI: 10.1038/s41579-019-0288-0

[11] Farha MA, Brown ED. Drug repurposing for antimicrobial discovery. Nature Microbiology. 2019;**4**:565-577

[12] Swan GE. The pharmacology of halogenated salicylanilides and their anthelmintic use in animals. Journal of the South African Veterinary Association. 1999;**70**:61-70. DOI: 10.4102/jsava.v70i2.756

[13] Xu J, Pachón-Ibáñez ME, Cebrero-Cangueiro T, Chen H, Sánchez-Céspedes J, Zhou J. Discovery of niclosamide and its O-alkylamino-tethered derivatives as potent antibacterial agents against carbapenemase-producing and/or colistin resistant Enterobacteriaceae isolates. Bioorganic and Medicinal Chemistry Letters. 2019;**29**:1399-1402. DOI: 10.1016/j.bmcl.2019.03.032

[14] Costabile G, d'Angel I, Rampion G, Bondi R, Pompili B, Ascenzioni F, et al. Toward repositioning niclosamide for antivirulence therapy of Pseudomonas aeruginosa lung infections: Development of inhalable formulations through nanosuspension

technology. Molecular Pharmaceutics. 2015;**12**:2604-2617. DOI: 10.1021/acs.molpharmaceut.5b00098

[15] Imperi F, Massai F, Ramachandran Pillai C, Longo F, Zennaro E, Rampioni G, et al. New life for an old drug: The anthelmintic drug niclosamide inhibits *Pseudomonas aeruginosa* quorum sensing. Antimicrobial Agents and Chemotherapy. 2013;**57**:996-1005. DOI: 10.1128/AAC.01952-12

[16] Cruz-Muñiz MY, López-Jacome LE, Hernández-Durán M, Franco-Cendejas R, Licona-Limón P, Ramos-Balderas JL, et al. Repurposing the anticancer drug mitomycin C for the treatment of persistent Acinetobacter baumannii infections. International Journal of Antimicrobial Agents. 2017;**49**(1):88-92. DOI: 10.1016/j. ijantimicag.2018.10.001

[17] Domalaon R, Ammeter D, Brizuela M, Gorityala BK, Zhanel GG, Schweizer F. Repurposed antimicrobial combination therapy: Tobramycin-ciprofloxacin hybrid augments activity of the anticancer drug mitomycin C against multidrug-resistant Gram-negative bacteria. Frontiers in Microbiology. 2019;**10**:1556. DOI: 10.3389/fmicb.2019.01556

[18] Kwan BW, Chowdhury N, Wood TK. Combatting bacterial infections by killing persister cells with mitomycin C. Environmental Microbiology. 2015;**17**(11):4406-4414. DOI: 10.1111/1462-2920.12873

[19] Thangamani S, Younis W, Seleem MN. Repurposing celecoxib as a topical antimicrobial agent. Frontiers in Microbiology. 2015;**6**(7):50. DOI: 10.3389/fmicb.2015.00750

[20] Yuan M, Chua SL, Liu Y, Drautz-moses DI, Kuok J, Yam H, et al. Repurposing the anticancer drug cisplatin with the aim of developing novel Pseudomonas aeruginosa infection control agents. Beilstein Journal of Organic Chemistry. 2018;**14**:3059-3069. DOI: 10.3762/bjoc.14.284

[21] Abbas HA, Elsherbini AM, Shaldam MA. Repurposing metformin as a quorum sensing inhibitor in Pseudomonas aeruginosa. African Health Sciences. 2017;**17**(3):808-819. DOI: 10.4314/ahs.v17i3.24

[22] Cheng YS, Sun W, Xu M, Shen M, Khraiwesh M, Sciotti RJ, et al. Repurposing screen identifies unconventional drugs with activity against multidrug resistant Acinetobacter baumannii. Frontiers in Cellular and Infection Microbiology. 2019;**8**:438. DOI: 10.3389/fcimb.2018.00438

[23] Imperi F, Fiscarelli EV, Visaggio D, Leoni L, Visca P, Juan C. Activity and impact on resistance development of two antivirulence fluoropyrimidine drugs in Pseudomonas aeruginosa. Frontiers in Cellular and Infection Microbiology. 2019;**9**:49. DOI: 10.3389/fcimb.2019.00049

[24] Ho Sui SJ, Lo R, Fernandes AR, Caulfield MD, Lerman JA, Xie L, et al. Raloxifene attenuates Pseudomonas aeruginosa pyocyanin production and virulence. International Journal of Antimicrobial Agents. 2012;**40**:246-251. DOI: 10.1016/j.ijantimicag.2012.05.009

[25] D'Angelo F, Baldelli V, Halliday N, Pantalone P, Polticelli F, Fiscarelli E, et al. Identification of FDA-approved drugs as antivirulence agents targeting the pqs quorum sensing system of Pseudomonas aeruginosa. Antimicrobial Agents and Chemotherapy. 2018;**62**:e1296-e1218. DOI: 10.1128/AAC.01296-18

[26] Soheili V, Bazzaz BS, Abdollahpour N, Hadizadeh F. Investigation of Pseudomonas aeruginosa quorum-sensing signaling system for

identifying multiple inhibitors using molecular docking and structural analysis methodology. Microbial Pathogenesis. 2015;**89**:73-78. DOI: 10.1016/j.micpath.2015.08.017

[27] She P, Wang Y, Luo Z, Chen L, Tan R, Wang Y, et al. Meloxicam inhibits biofilm formation and enhances antimicrobial agents efficacy by Pseudomonas aeruginosa. Microbiology. 2018;**7**(1):e00545. DOI: 10.1002/mbo3.545

[28] Maiden MM, Zachos MP, Waters CM. The ionophore oxyclozanide enhances tobramycin killing of Pseudomonas aeruginosa biofilms by permeabilizing cells and depolarizing the membrane potential. Journal of Antimicrobial Chemotherapy. 2019;**74**(4):894-906. DOI: 10.1093/jac/dky545

[29] Stokes JM, MacNair CR, Ilyas B, French S, Cote JP, Bouwman C, et al. Pentamidine sensitizes Gram-negative pathogens to antibiotics and overcomes acquired colistin resistance. Nature Microbiology. 2017;**2**:17028. DOI: 10.1038/nmicrobiol.2017.28

[30] Ayerbe-Algaba R, Gil-Marqués ML, Jiménez-Mejías ME, Sánchez-Encinales V, Parra-Millán R, Pachón-Ibáñez ME, et al. Synergistic activity of niclosamide in combination with colistin against colistin-susceptible and colistin-resistant Acinetobacter baumannii and Klebsiella pneumoniae. Frontiers in Cellular and Infection Microbiology. 2018;**8**:348. DOI: 10.3389/fcimb.2018.00348

[31] Runci F, Bonchi C, Frangipani E, Visaggio D, Visca P. Acinetobacter baumannii biofilm formation in human serum and disruption by gallium. Antimicrobial Agents and Chemotherapy. 2017;**61**(1):e01563-e01516. DOI: 10.1128/AAC.01563-16

[32] De Léséleuc L, Harris G, KuoLee R, Chen W. In vitro and in vivo biological activities of iron chelators and gallium nitrate against Acinetobacter baumannii. Antimicrobial Agents and Chemotherapy. 2012;**56**:5397-5400. DOI: 10.1128/AAC.00778-12

[33] Antunes LCS, Imperi F, Minandri F, Visca P. In vitro and in vivo antimicrobial activities of gallium nitrate against multidrug-resistant Acinetobacter baumannii. Antimicrobial Agents and Chemotherapy. 2012;**56**(11):5961-5970. DOI: 10.1128/AAC.01519-12

[34] Hijazi S, Visaggio D, Pirolo M, Frangipani E, Bernstein L, Visca P. Antimicrobial activity of gallium compounds on ESKAPE pathogens. Frontiers in Cellular and Infection Microbiology. 2018;**8**:316. DOI: 10.3389/fcimb.2018.00316

[35] Rezzoagli C, Wilson D, Weigert M, Wyder S, Ku R. Probing the evolutionary robustness of two repurposed drugs targeting iron uptake in Pseudomonas aeruginosa. Evolution, Medicine, and Public Health. 2018;**2018**(1):246-259. DOI: 10.1093/emph/eoy026

[36] Miró Canturri A, Ayerbe Algaba R, del Toro R, Pachón J, Smani Y. Tamoxifen repurposing to combat infections by multidrug-resistant Gram-negative bacilli. bioRxiv 2020. 2020.03.30.017475. doi: 10.1101/2020.03.30.017475

[37] Nouari W, Ysmail-Dahlouk L, Aribi M. Vitamin D3 enhances bactericidal activity of macrophage against Pseudomonas aeruginosa. International Immunopharmacology. 2015;**30**:94-101. DOI: 10.1016/j.intimp.2015.11.033

[38] Zabrodskii PF, Gromov MS, Maslyakov VV. Combined effects of M1 muscarinic acetylcholine receptor

agonist TBPB and α7n-acetylcholine receptor activator GTS-21 on mouse mortality and blood concentration of proinflammatory cytokines in sepsis. Bulletin of Experimental Biology and Medicine. 2017;**162**(6):750-753. DOI: 10.1007/s10517-017-3704-3

[39] Sitapara RA, Antoine DJ, Sharma L, Patel VS, Ashby CR Jr, Gorasiya S, et al. The α7 nicotinic acetylcholine receptor agonist GTS-21 improves bacterial clearance in mice by restoring hyperoxia-compromised macrophage function. Molecular Medicine. 2014;**20**:238-247. DOI: 10.2119/molmed.2013.00086

[40] Janeiro -Pais JM, Pastor-Casas-Agudo V, López-Garcia D, González-Dacal J, Lamas-Meilán C, González-Martín M. Mitomicina C endovesical y fibrosis pulmonar. Actas Urologicas Españolas. 2009;**33**(7):822-825. DOI: 10.1016/s0210-4806(09)74237-8

[41] Ueda A, Attila C, Whiteley M, Wood TK. Uracil influences quorum sensing and biofilm formation in Pseudomonas aeruginosa and fluorouracil is an antagonist. Microbial Biotechnology. 2009;**2**:62-74. DOI: 10.1111/j.1751-7915.2008.00060.x

[42] Christiansen SH, Murphy RA, Juul-Madsen K, Fredborg M, Hvam ML, Axelgaard E, et al. The immunomodulatory drug glatiramer acetate is also an effective antimicrobial agent that kills Gram-negative bacteria. Scientific Reports. 2017;**7**:15653. DOI: 10.1038/s41598-017-15969-3

[43] Antoniani D, Rossi E, Rinaldo S, Bocci P, Lolicato M, Paiardini A, et al. The immunosuppressive drug azathioprine inhibits biosynthesis of the bacterial signal molecule cyclic-di-GMP by interfering with intracellular nucleotide pool availability. Applied Microbiology and Biotechnology. 2013;**97**:7325-7336. DOI: 10.1007/s00253-013-4875-0

[44] Gi M, Jeong J, Lee K, Lee KM, Toyofuku M, Yong DE, et al. A drug-repositioning screening identifies pentetic acid as a potential therapeutic agent for suppressing the elastase-mediated virulence of Pseudomonas aeruginosa. Antimicrobial Agents and Chemotherapy. 2014;**58**:7205-7214. DOI: 10.1128/AAC.03063-14

[45] Lieberman OJ, Orr MW, Wang Y, Lee VT. High-throughput screening using the differential radial capillary action of ligand assay identifies ebselen as an inhibitor of diguanylate cyclases. ACS Chemical Biology. 2014;**9**:183-192. DOI: 10.1021/cb400485k

[46] Ayerbe-Algaba R, Gil-Marqués ML, Miró-Canturri A, Parra-Millán R, Pachón-Ibáñez ME, Jiménez-Mejías ME, et al. The anthelmintic oxyclozanide restores the activity of colistin against colistin-resistant Gram-negative bacilli. International Journal of Antimicrobial Agents. 2019;**54**(4):507-512. DOI: 10.1016/j.ijantimicag.2019.07.006

[47] Miró-Canturri A, Ayerbe-Algaba R, Villodres ÁR, Pachón J, Smani Y. Repositioning rafoxanide to treat Gram-negative bacilli infections. The Journal of Antimicrobial Chemotherapy. 2020;**75**(7):1895-1905. DOI: 10.1093/jac/dkaa103

[48] Miró Canturri A, Algaba RA, Pachón-Ibáñez M, Pachon-Diaz J, Smani Y. In vitro activity of ivermectin in combination with colistin against Gram-negative bacilli. In: 29th European Congress of Clinical Microbiology and Infectious Diseases; 16-19 April 2019. Amsterdam, Netherlands; 2019

[49] Tran TB, Wang J, Doi Y, Velkov T, Bergen PJ, Pereira MO. Novel polymyxin combination with antineoplastic mitotane improved the bacterial killing

against polymyxin-resistant multidrug-resistant Gram-negative pathogens. Frontiers in Microbiology. 2018;**9**:721. DOI: 10.3389/fmicb.2018.00721

[50] Ogunniyi AD, Khazandi M, Stevens AJ, Sims SK, Page SW, Garg S, et al. Evaluation of robenidine analog NCL195 as a novel broad-spectrum antibacterial agent. PLoS One. 2017;**12**(9):e0183457. DOI: 10.1371/journal.pone.0183457

[51] Nairn BL, Eliasson OS, Hyder DR, Long NJ, Majumdar A, Chakravorty S, et al. Fluorescence high-throughput screening for inhibitors of TonB action. Journal of Bacteriology. 2017;**199**:e889-e816. DOI: 10.1128/JB.00889-16

[52] Ballouche M, Cornelis P, Baysse C. Iron metabolism: A promising target for antibacterial strategies. Recent Patents on Anti-Infective Drug Discovery. 2009;**4**:190-205. DOI: 10.2174/157489109789318514

[53] Foley TL, Simeonov A. Targeting iron assimilation to develop new antibacterials. Expert Opinion on Drug Discovery. 2012;**7**:831-847. DOI: 10.1517/17460441.2012.708335

[54] Garnacho-Montero J, Ortiz- Leyba C, Jiménez Jiménez FJ, Barrero-Almodóvar AE, García- Garmendia JL, Bernabeu-Wittell M, et al. Treatment of multidrug-resistant Acinetobacter baumannii ventilator-associated pneumonia (VAP) with intravenous colistin: A comparison with imipenem-susceptible VAP. Clinical Infectious Diseases. 2003;**36**:1111-1118. DOI: 10.1086/374337

[55] Markou N, Markantonis SL, Dimitrakis E, Panidis D, Boutzouka E, Karatzas S, et al. Colistin serum concentrations after intravenous administration in critically ill patients with serious multidrug-resistant, Gram negative bacilli infections: A prospective, open-label, uncontrolled study. Clinical Therapy. 2008;**30**:143-511. DOI: 10.1016/j.clinthera.2008.01.015

[56] Hoskins JM, Carey LA, McLeod HL. CYP2D6 and tamoxifen: DNA matters in breast cancer. Nature Reviews. Cancer. 2009;**9**:576-586. DOI: 10.1038/nrc2683

[57] Domalaon R, Malaka P, Silva D, Kumar A, Zhanel GG, Schweizer F. The anthelmintic drug niclosamide synergizes with colistin and reverses colistin resistance in Gram-negative bacilli. Antimicrobial Agents and Chemotherapy. 2019;**63**(4):e02574-e02518. DOI: 10.1128/AAC.02574-18

[58] Thangamani S, Mohammad H, Abushahba MF, Sobreira TJ, Hedrick VE, Paul LN, et al. Antibacterial activity and mechanism of action of auranofin against multi-drug resistant bacterial pathogens. Scientific Reports. 2016;**6**:22571. DOI: 10.1038/srep22571

[59] Thangamani S, Mohammad H, Abushahba MFN, Hamed MI, Sobreira TJP, Hedrick VE, et al. Exploring simvastatin, an antihyperlipidemic drug, as a potential topical antibacterial agent. Scientific Reports. 2015;**5**:16407. DOI: 10.1038/srep16407

[60] Khazandi M, Pi H, Chan WY, Ogunniyi AD, Sim JXF, Venter H, et al. In vitro antimicrobial activity of robenidine, ethylenediaminetetraacetic acid and polymyxin B nonapeptide against important human and veterinary pathogens. Frontiers in Microbiology. 2019;**10**:837. DOI: 10.3389/fmicb.2019.00837

[61] Gellatly SL, Hancock REW. Pseudomonas aeruginosa: New insights into pathogenesis and host defenses. Pathogens and Disease. 2013;**67**:159-173. DOI: 10.1111/2049-632X.12033

[62] Kang CI, Kim SH, Kim HB, Park SW, Choe YJ, Oh MD, et al. Pseudomonas aeruginosa bacteremia: Risk factors for mortality and influence of delayed receipt of effective antimicrobial therapy on clinical outcome. Clinical Infectious Diseases. 2003;**37**:745-751. DOI: 10.1086/377200

[63] Vidal F, Mensa J, Almela M, Martínez JA, Marco F, Casals C, et al. Epidemiology and outcome of Pseudomonas aeruginosa bacteremia, with special emphasis on the influence of antibiotic treatment: Analysis of 189 episodes. Archives of Internal Medicine. 1996;**156**:2121-2126

[64] Vincent JL. Nosocomial infections in adult intensive-care units. Lancet. 2003;**361**:2068-2077. DOI: 10.1016/S0140-6736(03)13644-6

[65] Ali Z, Mumtaz N, Naz SA, Jabeen N, Shafique M. Multi-drug resistant Pseudomonas aeruginosa: A threat of nosocomial infections in tertiary care hospitals. Journal of the Pakistan Medical Association. 2015;**65**(1):12-16

[66] Micek ST, Wunderink RG, Kollef MH, Chen C, Rello J, Chastre J, et al. An international multicenter retrospective study of Pseudomonas aeruginosa nosocomial pneumonia: Impact of multidrug resistance. Critical Care. 2015;**19**:219. DOI: 10.1186/s13054-015-0926-5

[67] Kaye KS, Pogue JM. Infections caused by resistant Gram-negative bacteria: Epidemiology and management. Pharmacotherapy. 2015;**35**:949-962. DOI: 10.1002/phar.1636

[68] El Solh AA, Alhajhusain A. Update on the treatment of Pseudomonas aeruginosa pneumonia. The Journal of Antimicrobial Chemotherapy. 2009;**64**:229-238. DOI: 10.1093/jac/dkp201

[69] Wright H, Bonomo RA, Paterson DL. New agents for the treatment of infections with Gram-negative bacteria: Restoring the miracle or false dawn? Clinical Microbiology and Infection. 2017;**23**:704-712. DOI: 10.1016/j.cmi.2017.09.001

[70] Rangel-Vega A, Bernstein LR, Mandujano-Tinoco EA, García-Contreras SJ, García-Contreras R. Drug repurposing as an alternative for the treatment of recalcitrant bacterial infections. Frontiers in Microbiology. 2015;**6**:282. DOI: 10.3389/fmicb.2015.00282

[71] Kaneko Y, Thoendel M, Olakanmi O, Britigan BE, Singh PK. The transition metal gallium disrupts Pseudomonas aeruginosa iron metabolism and has antimicrobial and antibiofilm activity. Journal of Clinical Investigation. 2007;**117**:877-888. DOI: 10.1172/JCI30783

[72] Frangipani E, Bonchi C, Minandri F, Imperi F, Visca P. Pyochelin potentiates the inhibitory activity of gallium on Pseudomonas aeruginosa. Antimicrobial Agents and Chemotherapy. 2014;**58**:5572-5575. DOI: 10.1128/AAC.03154-14

[73] Bonchi C, Frangipani E, Imperi F, Visca P. Pyoverdine and proteases affect the response of Pseudomonas aeruginosa to gallium in human serum. Antimicrobial Agents and Chemotherapy. 2015;**59**:5641-5646. DOI: 10.1128/AAC.01097-15

[74] García-Contreras R, Pérez- Eretza B, Lira-Silva E, Jasso-Chávez R, Coria-Jiménez R, Rangel-Vega A, et al. Gallium induces the production of virulence factors in Pseudomonas aeruginosa. Pathogens and Disease. 2014;**1**:95-98. DOI: 10.1111/2049-632X.12105

[75] ClinicalTrials.gov [Internet]. Bethesda (MD): National Library

of Medicine (US). Identifier NCT02354859, A Phase 2 IV gallium study for patients with cystic fibrosis (IGNITE Study). 2015. Available from: https://clinicaltrials.gov/ct2/show/NCT02354859

[76] Artini M, Cellini R, Tilota A, Barbato M, Koverech A, Selan L. Effect of betamethasone in combination with antibiotics on gram positive and gram negative bacteria. International Journal of Immunopathology and Pharmacology. 2014;**27**:675-682. DOI: 10.1177/039463201402700426

[77] Becker KA, Riethmüller J, Lüth A, Döring G, Kleuser B, Gulbins E. Acid sphingomyelinase inhibitors normalize pulmonary ceramide and inflammation in cystic fibrosis. American Journal of Respiratory Cell and Molecular Biology. 2010;**42**(6):716-724. DOI: 10.1165/rcmb.2009-0174OC

[78] ClinicalTrials.gov [Internet]. Bethesda (MD): National Library of Medicine (US). Identifier NCT00515229, Anti-Inflammatory pulmonal therapy of CF-patients with amitriptyline and placebo. 2007. Available from: https://clinicaltrials.gov/ct2/show/NCT00515229 [Accessed: 11 July 2016]

[79] Adams C, Icheva V, Deppisch C, Lauer J, Herrmann G, Graepler-Mainka U, et al. Long-term pulmonal therapy of cystic fibrosis-patients with amitriptyline. Cellular Physiology and Biochemistry. 2016;**39**(2):565-572. DOI: 10.1159/000445648

[80] ClinicalTrials.gov [Internet]. Bethesda (MD): National Library of Medicine (US). Identifier NCT01299194, Atorvastatin in bronchiectasis in patients with *Pseudomonas aeruginosa*. 2011. Available from: https://clinicaltrials.gov/ct2/show/NCT01299194 [Accessed: 27 May 2017]

[81] Bedi P, Chalmers JD, Graham C, Clarke A, Donaldson S, Doherty C, et al. A randomized controlled trial of atorvastatin in patients with bronchiectasis infected with Pseudomonas aeruginosa: A proof of concept study. Chest. 2017;**152**(2):368-378. DOI: 10.1016/j.chest.2017.05.017

[82] Yoon SS, Coakley R, Lau GW, Lymar SV, Gaston B, Karabulut AC, et al. Anaerobic killing of mucoid Pseudomonas aeruginosa by acidified nitrite derivatives under cystic fibrosis airway conditions. Journal of Clinical Investigation. 2006;**116**:436-446. DOI: 10.1172/JCI24684

[83] Major TA, Panmanee W, Mortensen JE, Gray LD, Hoglen N, Hassett DJ. Sodium nitrite-mediated killing of the major cystic fibrosis pathogens Pseudomonas aeruginosa, Staphylococcus aureus, and Burkholderia cepacia under anaerobic planktonic and biofilm conditions. Antimicrobial Agents and Chemotherapy. 2010;**54**(11):4671-4677. DOI: 10.1128/AAC.00379-10

[84] ClinicalTrials.gov [Internet]. Bethesda (MD): National Library of Medicine (US). Identifier NCT02694393, Inhaled sodium nitrite as an antimicrobial for cystic fibrosis. 2016. Available from: https://www.clinicaltrials.gov/ct2/show/NCT02694393

[85] ClinicalTrials.gov [Internet]. Bethesda (MD): National Library of Medicine (US). Identifier NCT02295566, RATNO, Reducing Antibiotic Tolerance Using Nitric Oxide in CF - a Phase 2 pilot study (RATNO). 2014. Available from: https://clinicaltrials.gov/ct2/show/NCT02295566

[86] Vila J, Sáez-López E, Johnson JR, Römling U, Dobrindt U, Cantón R, et al. Escherichia coli: An old friend with new tidings. FEMS Microbiology Reviews.

2016;**40**:437-463. DOI: 10.1093/femsre/fuw005

[87] Manges AR, Geum HM, Guo A, Edens TJ, Fibke CD, Pitout JDD. Global extraintestinal pathogenic Escherichia coli (ExPEC) lineages. Clinical Microbiology Reviews. 2019;**32**:e00135-e00118. DOI: 10.1128/CMR.00135-18

[88] Solomkin JS, Mazuski JE, Bradkey JS, Rodvold KA, Goldstein EJC, Baron EJ, et al. Diagnosis and management of complicated intra-abdominal infection in adults and children: Guidelines by the surgical infection society and the Infectious Diseases Society of America. Clinical Infectious Diseases. 2010;**50**:133-164. DOI: 10.1089/sur.2009.9930

[89] Paczosa MK, Mecsas J. Klebsiella pneumoniae: Going on the offense with astrong defense. Microbiology and Molecular Biology Reviews. 2016;**80**:629-661. DOI: 10.1128/MMBR.00078-15

[90] Poirel L, Jayol A, Nordmann P. Polymyxins: Antibacterial activity, susceptibility testing, and resistance mechanisms encoded by plasmids or chromosomes. Clinical Microbiology Reviews. 2017;**30**(2):557-596. DOI: 10.1128/CMR.00064-16

[91] ClinicalTrials.gov [Internet]. Bethesda (MD): National Library of Medicine (US). Identifier NCT00783068, Anti-inflammatory effects of GTS-21 after LPS. 2008. Available from: https://clinicaltrials.gov/ct2/show/NCT00783068

[92] Kox M, Pompe JC, Gordinou de Gouberville MC, van der Hoeven JG, Hoedemaekers CW, Pickkers P. Effects of the α7 nicotinic acetylcholine receptor agonist GTS-21 on the innate immune response in humans. Shock. 2011;**36**(1):5-11. DOI: 10.1097/SHK.0b013e3182168d56

[93] Andersson JA, Sha J, Kirtley ML, Reyes E, Fitts EC, Dann SM, et al. Combating multidrug-resistant pathogens with host-directed nonantibiotic therapeutics. Antimicrobial Agents and Chemotherapy. 2017;**62**(1):e1943-e1917. DOI: 10.1128/AAC.01943-17

[94] Cebrero-Cangueiro T, Álvarez-Marín R, Labrador-Herrera G, Smani Y, Cordero-Matía E, Pachón J, et al. In vitro activity of pentamidine alone and in combination with aminoglycosides, tigecycline, rifampicin, and doripenem against clinical strains of carbapenemase-producing and/or colistin-resistant Enterobacteriaceae. Frontiers in Cellular and Infection Microbiology. 2018;**8**:363. DOI: 10.3389/fcimb.2018.00363

10

Risk-Benefit Events Associated with the Use of Aspirin for Primary Prevention of Cardiovascular Disorders

Deepak Kumar Dash, Vishal Jain, Anil Kumar Sahu, Rajnikant Panik and Vaibhav Tripathi

Abstract

Aspirin had been introduced as a nonsteroidal anti-inflammatory molecule. As further research on aspirin started, other therapeutic effects have been revealed. Now, this molecule has become the polychrest in medical science. Aspirin has served as a drug of choice for the primary prevention of cardiovascular disease (CVD) for the last few decades. However, recent trials have raised questions on the use of aspirin for CVD prevention due to some life-threatening adverse drug events. In spite of that, outcomes of trials will surely assist to frame a guideline for anoxic administration regimen of aspirin in order to prevent CVD.
Keywords: aspirin, CVD, clinical trial, adverse drug events

1. Introduction

In 1859, Hermann Kolbe was paved the foundation for the development of Aspirin moiety for clinical practice. Whilst, there were no scientific resemblance established for aspirin as medicine [1]. After a long laboratory modification Felix Hoffman had succeeded to evolve the finest, clinical molecule by means of acetylation. Clinical investigation had passed the salicylate compound with intended therapeutic effects with no or minimum side effect. Clinicians had accepted this molecule open handedly. On February 1, 1899 Aspirin is registered as an authentic molecule (**Figure 1**) [2]. Currently, aspirin has become renowned and huge blockbuster molecule as NSAIDs followed by primary prevention of CVD [3].

2. Chemistry of aspirin

Production of aspirin is completed as single chain reaction. Acidic and alkaline both medium are suitable for synthesis. In chemistry language, aspirin is produced by the mixing of salicylic acid and acetic anhydride with the aid of phosphoric acid. Acetylsalicylic acid possesses three functional groups, namely hydroxyl, acetyl and ester. It is due to the presence of hydroxyl group polarity index of salicylic acid is high than that of aspirin. The reaction equation is displayed (**Figure 2**) [4].

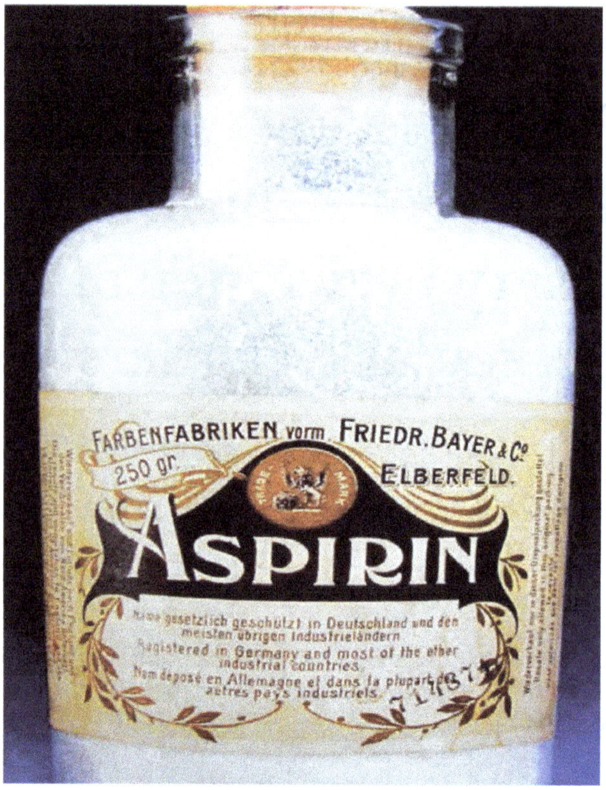

Figure 1.
First container of aspirin.

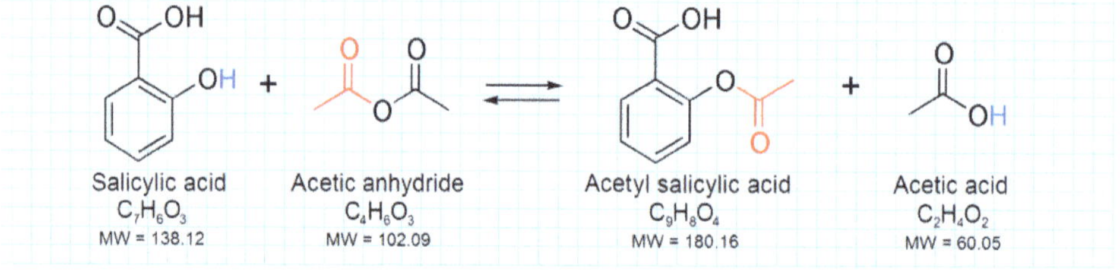

Figure 2.
Production reaction.

Aspirin is an O-acetyl derivative of salicylic acid (ASA—acetylsalicylic acid) and its dominant mechanism of action is believed to be through the transfer of this acetyl group to (–OH) and amino (–NH_2) functionalities present in biological macromolecules as depicted in **Figure 3**. The acyl ester group is also unstable under basic conditions, and its hydrolysis to acetate is believed to proceed by a general base-assisted mechanism as described previously [5, 6]. More recent computational studies have suggested an $n \rightarrow \pi^*$ interaction between the aromatic carboxylic acid and the carbonyl carbon of the acetate group [7]. This is consistent with a nuclear magnetic resonance spectroscopy (NMR) study [8], which posits the formation of a cyclic hemi-orthoester under basic conditions which can rearrange to give either the parent aspirin anion or a mixed anhydride.

Although the prevalence and role of the mixed anhydride in the biochemistry of aspirin has yet to be determined, the broad scope of anhydride reactivity may help to explain promiscuous acetylation activity of aspirin in biological systems [9, 10].

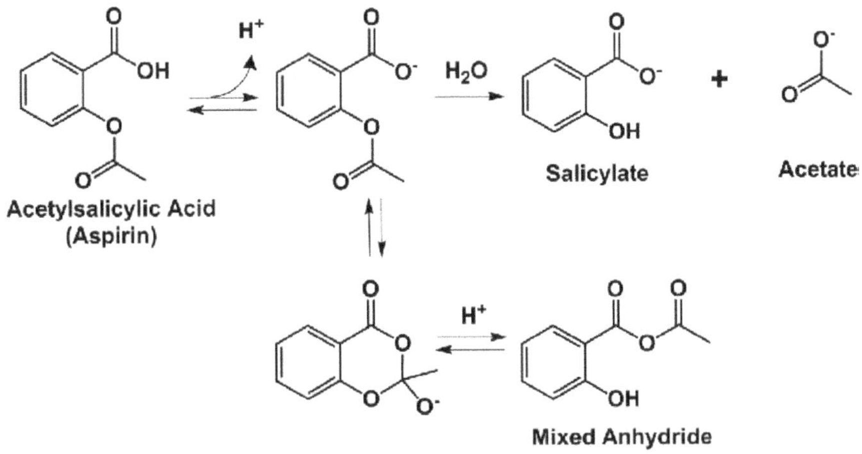

Figure 3.
Chemical reaction at molecular level.

Interestingly, it has also been shown that the mixed anhydride can react with the primary amino group of glycine in organic solvents to form N-salicyloylglycine, suggesting a second class of aspirin-mediated protein modifications [11]. The nonselectivity of aspirin-mediated acetylation was demonstrated by Richard Farr and co-workers in 1968 [12]. In these experiments, aspirin labeled with 14C at the acetyl carbonyl carbon was incubated with a series of blood proteins as well as common enzymes and nucleic acids. Following dialysis, substantial radiolabeling of albumin, immunoglobulins, α-macroglobulin, and other enzymes was observed. More recent mass spectrometry-based studies have validated this initial finding and the list of proteins acetylated by aspirin has grown to include histones, IKKβ (I-kappa-β-kinase beta), and many others [13]. At high concentrations (micromolar to millimolar), aspirin has been shown to react with nucleophilic groups on proteins resulting in irreversible acetylation. These include the functional groups of the residues lysine (–NH_2), arginine (–NH_2), serine (–OH), threonine (–OH), tyrosine (–OH), and cysteine (–SH) [31, 32]. Synthesis of ^{13}C- or ^{14}C-labeled aspirin has also facilitated the real-time analysis of acetylation of ubiquitin, hemoglobin, and human serum albumin [14].

3. Pharmacokinetics of aspirin

After absorption, as acetylsalicylic acid is rapidly converted to salicylic acid by hydrolysis and first-pass metabolism, peak plasma concentrations of acetylsalicylic acid are extremely sensitive to minor variations in solid dosage form dissolution and disintegration. In contrast, plasma concentrations of salicylic acid are predictable and relatively stable [15].

3.1 Absorption

Absorption of salicylate occurs rapidly by passive diffusion of un-ionized lipophilic molecules from the stomach at the low pH of the milieu. Aspirin (pKa 3.5) and salicylic acid (pKa 3.0) are weak acids, being 99% un-ionized at pH 1 and able to diffuse through lipid membranes. Less rapid absorption is observed with other formulations due to the rate limiting step of tablet disintegration; this latter factor being maximal in alkaline pH. Although aspirin can spontaneously hydrolyze, this is slow so that there is little or no free salicylate in the intestine and it is absorbed as aspirin rather than salicylic acid. A complete picture of absorption track of aspirin is represented in **Figure 4** [16]. Approximately 70% of aspirin reaches the peripheral circulation intact with maximum serum concentrations observed at 25 min after administration. After entering the bloodstream, aspirin undergoes enzymatic hydrolysis to yield acetate and salicylic acid. The major enzymes hydrolyzing aspirin in plasma are believed to be cholinesterases [17]. Acetylhydrolase-I, an intracellular erythrocyte platelet-activating factor, has been characterized as the major aspirin hydrolase of human blood [18].

Intravenous aspirin has a distribution half-life of about 3 min and inhibits prostaglandin biosynthesis within 5 min of administration, reflecting the rapid onset of inhibition compared to oral dosing [19].

Recent studies by Lichtenberger et al. demonstrated that aspirin could enter the lymph fluid directly when administered intragastrically or intraduodenally, potentially increasing its pharmacologic activity as a chemopreventive agent for colorectal cancer [20].

Rectal absorption of salicylate is also possible and cutaneous absorption may occur from salicylate containing rubefacients. Following oral administration of an aqueous solution, the absorption kinetics of aspirin is found to follow a first-order process [21].

The factors affecting absorption of salicylate are Rate of gastric emptying volume of food, pH of stomach contents, nervous state, concurrent drugs, exercise, posture, formulation and Disease states associated with altered gastrointestinal transit time.

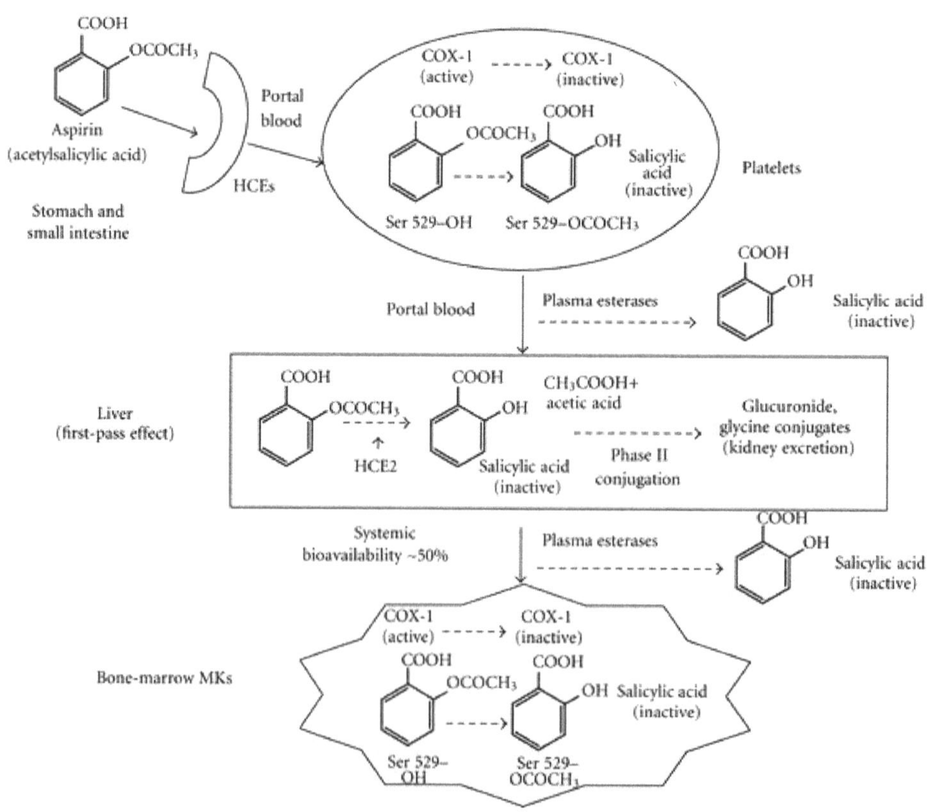

Figure 4.
In vivo reaction of aspirin.

3.2 Distribution

Once absorbed, salicylates are distributed extensively through body fluids. Reported values for the apparent volume of distribution (Vd) of salicylate range from 9.6 to 12.7 L in adults with similar values (0.12–0.14 L/kg) in children [22].

Both aspirin and salicylic acid are partially bound to serum proteins. The distribution of aspirin is further enhanced by binding to human serum albumin [23, 24]. Human serum albumin is the most abundant protein found in blood and is often used as a plasma shuttle for steroids, hormones, and other small molecules. Binding studies suggest a conformational change in albumin upon acetylation that can influence transport and metabolism of other critical metabolites and drugs. For example, aspirin-induced acetylation of albumin can inhibit glucose binding [25], while increasing the binding of other molecules, as observed with the increased affinity of acetylated albumin for the marker anion acetrizoate [26]. Aspirin's pharmacodynamic is also influenced by the interaction of other metabolites and serum albumin [24]. However, aspirin acetylation of serum albumin likely inhibits the binding of other metabolites commonly transported by albumin. In vitro studies have shown serum albumin binding and acetylation is dependent upon fatty acid binding, pH and temperature [27].

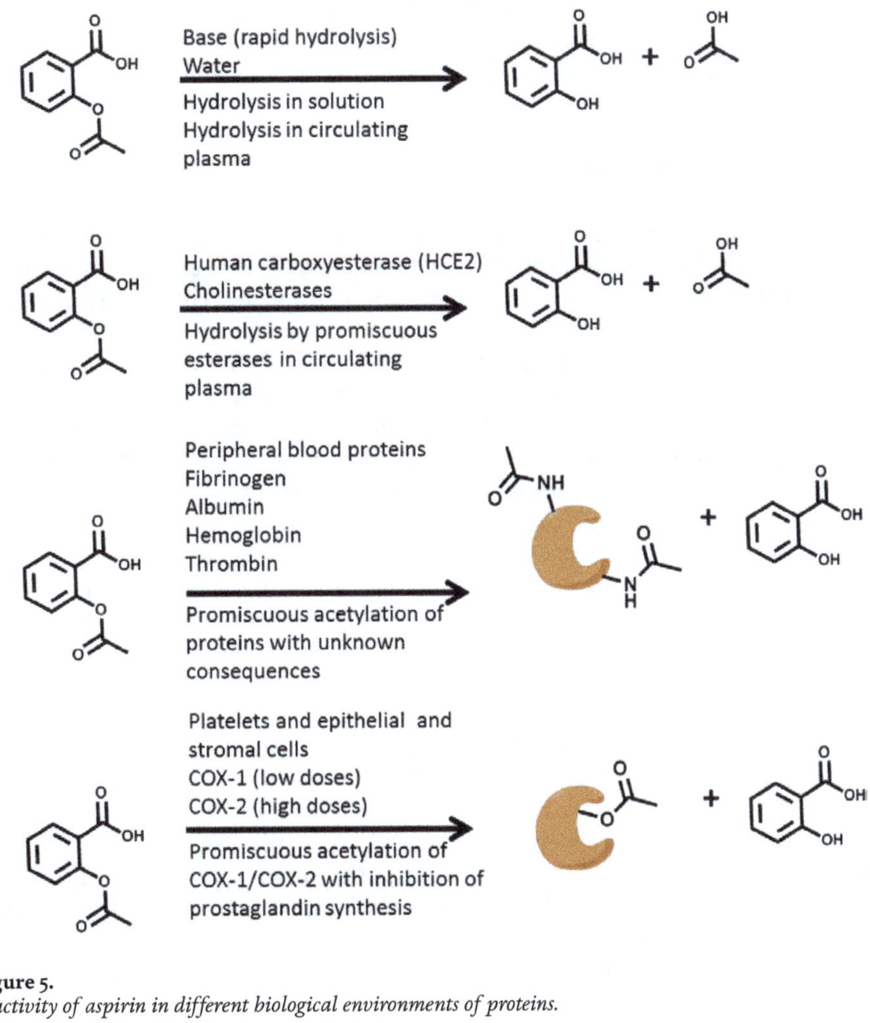

Figure 5.
Reactivity of aspirin in different biological environments of proteins.

Both salicylic acid and aspirin have been found to diffuse slowly into the cerebrospinal fluid (CSF) due to the high degree of ionization of salicylic acid at the pH (7.4) of plasma. Salicylic acid readily crosses the placenta, fetal plasma concentrations being higher at birth than concurrent maternal concentrations [28].

3.3 Metabolism and excretion

Aspirin is rapidly converted to salicylic acid with a half-life of only 15–20 minutes [19]. This hydrolysis is due to nonspecific esterases found in many body. The acetyl component of aspirin after oral and intravenous dosing is found in gastric mucosal cells or is excreted as carbon dioxide after passing through the Krebs cycle [29]. During absorption, aspirin esterase activity in the gastrointestinal mucosal membranes contributes 28–35% of the hydrolysis of aspirin; though the activity of esterase enzyme may vary in relation to age and gender. Aspirin esterase activity is reduced in patients with alcoholic liver disease [17].

The major route of elimination of aspirin is through its hydrolyzed product salicylic acid. Salicylic acid is cleared from circulation via the kidneys with a serum half-life of approximately 2 h. A summary of the most common reactions of aspirin in biological systems are summarized in **Figure 5**.

Salicylic acid is partly excreted unchanged and partly metabolized. Free salicylic acid diffuses readily across the glomerulus and is also actively secreted by the proximal tubule. The conjugates of salicylic acid are also excreted via kidney, being dependent on glomerular filtration and tubular secretion. The hydroxylated metabolite gentisic acid is excreted in the same way as free salicylic acid [30].

4. Pharmacodynamics of aspirin

The most recognized mechanism of action of aspirin is to inhibit the synthesis of prostaglandins but this by itself does not explain the repertoire of anti-inflammatory effects of aspirin. Later, another mechanism was described: the induction of the production of aspirin-triggered lipoxins (ATLs) from arachidonic acid by acetylation of the enzyme cyclooxygenase-2. The availability of a stable analog of ATL has stimulated investigations on the use of this analog and it has been found that, similar to endogenously produced lipoxins, ATL resolves inflammation and acts as antioxidant and immunomodulator. If we consider that in PE and in the obstetric APS, there is an underlying inflammatory process; aspirin might be used based on the induction of ATL [31].

The COX-inhibitory activity of aspirin is contingent on the administered dose. Low doses, those ranging from 75 to 300 mg, result in selective inhibition in platelet TXA2 production without suppressing prostacyclin (PGI2), a common platelet antagonist and vasodilator. PGI2 is expected to be derived mainly from vascular COX-2 suggesting that COX- 2 inhibition is minimal in the low-dose regime. Increased doses (>1200 mg) have analgesic and anti-inflammatory properties, properties associated with the pathophysiological inhibition of COX-1 and COX-2. It is important to note that COX- 2 can also utilize arachidonic acid for synthesis of lipoxins, particularly 15-hydroxyeicosatetraenoic acid [32, 33]. It is unlikely that the COX-2 is more than 5% acetylated while platelet-derived COX-1 is likely to be >70% acetylated. This suggests that regular low-dose aspirin will invariably maintain COX-1 inhibition in circulating platelets, with minimal effect in the inhibition of peripheral COX-2 [34].

A summary of the pharmacodynamic action of aspirin is summarized in **Figure 6** [35, 36].

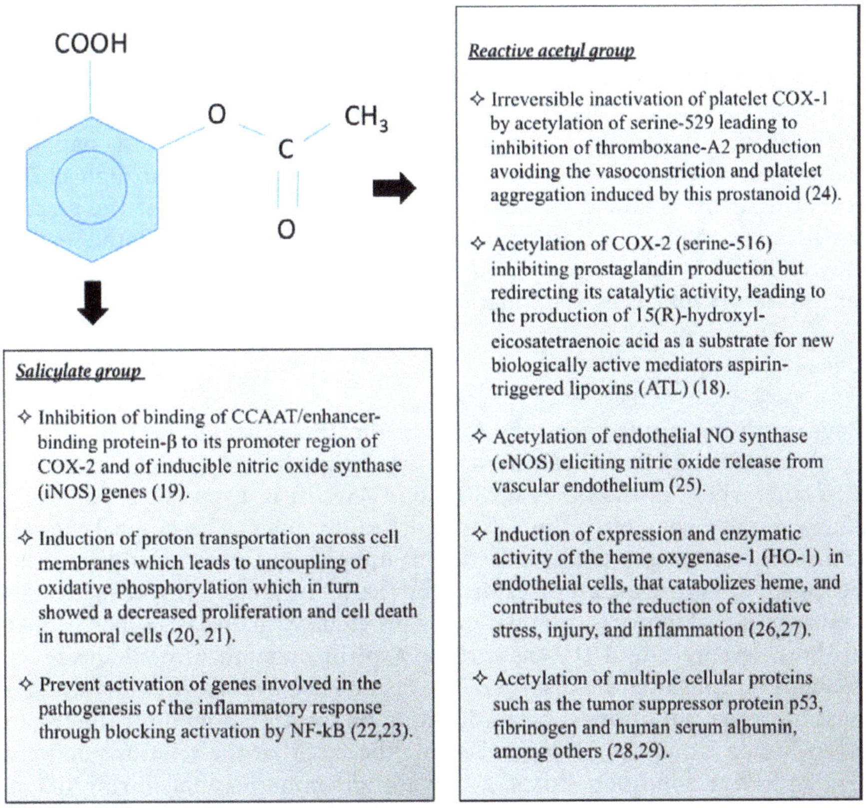

Figure 6.
Pharmacodynamics of aspirin.

5. Pharmacological action of aspirin

5.1 Therapeutic effects

Beneficial clinical impaction of aspirin is mainly anti-inflammatory and anti-pyretic action. Evidence suggests that aspirin is a better analgesic than salicylic acid [37, 38]. The analgesia produced by aspirin is dose-dependent, although the response does not parallel serum aspirin concentrations [39]. The dose of aspirin required for its antipyretic action is less than that required for analgesia [40].

The generally accepted therapeutic plasma concentration range of salicylate for the treatment of chronic inflammatory disease is 15–30 mg/100 ml (150–300 mg/L or 1–2 mmol/L), requiring daily doses in excess of 3 g [41].

Other indications for aspirin use are angina pectoris, angina pectoris prophylaxis, ankylosing spondylitis, cardiovascular risk reduction, colorectal cancer, ischemic stroke, ischemic stroke (prophylaxis), myocardial infarction, myocardial infarction (prophylaxis), osteoarthritis, revascularization procedures (prophylaxis), rheumatoid arthritis and systemic lupus erythematosus [42].

5.2 Adverse effects

The most common side effect of aspirin is gastrointestinal upset ranging from gastritis to gastrointestinal bleed. Other adverse effects are as followed:

5.2.1 Hypersensitivity

Excessive sensitivity to NSAIDs is normal among everyone. The rate is about 1–2%. Unwanted effects could be as gentle as a simple rash to angioedema and hypersensitivity. In case of asthmatic or interminable rhino-sinusitis patients, the predominance of these allergic susceptible indications could be as high as 26%. In the event that this is joined by nasal polyps and inflammation of the respiratory tract with eosinophils, it is known as aspirin triad. NSAID-exacerbated respiratory malady (NERD) is new term related with this disorder because of upper just as lower respiratory mucosal inflammation [43].

5.2.2 Reye syndrome

Reye condition, named after the Australian pathologist, Dr. R.D. Reye was first portrayed in 1963. It is an uncommon yet deadly condition with an expected death pace of somewhere in the range of 30% and 45%. It is a type of encephalopathy auxiliary to fatty changes in an otherwise healthy liver. The clinical vignette of Reye disorder comprises a viral infection of upper respiratory tract disease in kids and corresponding ingestion of aspirin for the treatment of fever. It is imagined that mitochondrial injury is optional to the previous viral disease which is the main hit to both the liver and the cerebrum. Aspirin or similar medicine gives the subsequent hit finishing the disorder. The occurrence has significantly diminished because of better mindfulness and utilization of acetaminophen for the treatment of fever in kids rather than aspirin. Despite the fact that the relationship between aspirin and Reye condition exists, a few authors contend that during diagnosis, salicylate levels were not routinely checked, biopsies were not acquired, and hereditary/intrinsic blunders of metabolism were not precluded [44, 45].

5.2.3 Intracerebral hemorrhage

Aspirin increases the risk of intracranial bleeding versus placebo [46].

5.2.4 Nephrotoxicity

Previous studies have shown conflicting results about the use of aspirin and the risk of chronic kidney diseases. Some earlier studies have shown that the use of aspirin is associated with chronic kidney disease [47].

5.2.5 Bleeding

Aspirin makes 2 3-crease increment in the danger of dose related peptic ulcer bleeding, a hazard that does not appear to be diminished by the utilization of enteric-covered aspirin. Sung et al. demonstrated that among people who had peptic ulcer blood loss, constant low-dose aspirin utilize expanded the danger of repetitive bleeding yet brought about lower overall cardiovascular and cerebrovascular mortality rates [48].

5.3 Contraindication

Aspirin is contraindicated in patients who salicylate sensitive, hemophilic, in peptic/bleeding ulcers, in children suffering from chicken pox or influenza. Cautious use is desirable in patients with anemia, impaired hepatic or renal functions, and asthma and in pregnant or nursing mothers. It should be avoided in diabetics with low cardiac reserve or frank CHF and in juvenile rheumatoid arthritis [49].

5.4 Drug interactions

Aspirin displaces warfarin, naproxen, sulfonylurea, phenytoin and methotrexate from binding sites. It antagonizes uricosuric action of probenacid. It blunts diuretic action of furosemide and thiazides and reduces the action of spironolactone. Aspirin reduces protein bound iodine levels by displacement of thyroxine; but hypothyroidism does not occur [50].

6. Role of aspirin in CVD

Efforts were being done for decades to prevent and treat cardiovascular disease (CVD). By the twentieth century, CVD had become a major cause of mortality and morbidity, and many efforts were being made to prevent it worldwide [51–53].Given the prevalence of CVD, several strategies are being considered for its prevention, including lifestyle changes as well as strict management of cardiovascular risk factors such as hypertension, diabetes, hyperlipidemia, and metabolic syndrome. In addition to traditional methods, other alternative methods have also been studied for its prevention. Along with this, some exploiters have used aspirin for the prevention of CVD, and with some controversy, it is believed that aspirin is beneficial in the primary prevention of CVD [54, 55].

Today aspirin is widely used for the primary prevention of CVD. In the United States alone, 40% of adults over the age of 50 are using aspirin for the prevention of CVD [56]. Aspirin is an irreversible and nonselective cyclo-oxygenase (COX) inhibitor class of drug, whose work is to reduce thromboxane A2 production and inhibit platelet aggregation and vasoconstriction. The ability to prevent platelet aggregation provides the potential to reduce arterial thrombosis, and when used at low doses, it is beneficial in preventing myocardial infarction (MI) and stroke. On the other hand, aspirin also inhibits the production of prostaglandin as well as reducing the side effects of GI bleeding by inhibiting COX 1 and protecting the gastrointestinal (GI) mucosa [57]. It has been assessed through successive clinical trials that aspirin is effective in the prevention of CVD. A number of tests have been performed to demonstrate its efficacy and it has been found that it is beneficial in secondary prevention of CVD even in patients with previous MI or ischemic stroke and at high risk [58].

7. Risk factors

Recently, the publication of a number of studies has raised doubts about the benefits of using aspirin as a primary prevention for patients with moderate cardiovascular risk. Three of the trials were published in 2018, A Study of Cardiovascular Events in Diabetes (ASCEND), Aspirin in Reducing Events in the Elderly (ASPREE), and ARRIVE.

The ASCEND study assessed the effectiveness and safety of aspirin use by arbitrarily assigning 14,480 diabetic patients into 100 mg aspirin or placebo teams and observing them for a median of 7.4 years. Internal hemorrhage has emerged as a haul within the safety assessment. All major bleeding during this study was 29% higher with the aspirin administration cluster and a high risk of bleeding was seen in patients with a high risk of vascular events. This study has concluded that aspirin use prevented serious vascular events in patients who had diabetes and no previous CVD, however this absolute profit was for the most part balanced by the same rate of bleeding hazard [59].

In the ASPREE trial, old patients aged 70 or above who did not have CVD, dementia or disability were randomized and given 100 mg aspirin or placebo at a median of 4.7 years of follow-up. Contrary to other studies that established the incidence of CVD as the primary endpoint, ASPREE evaluated all causes of death, dementia, and chronic physical incapacity as primary endpoints. Moreover, apart from other studies, the ASPREE study evaluated the cause of mortality. Death from any cause was 12.7 per 1000 person within the aspirin group and 11.1 per 1000 people within the placebo group with a considerably accrued risk in the aspirin cluster. However, the incidence of CVD was 10.7 within the aspirin and 11.3 within the placebo teams per 1000 person-years, which indicated there was no distinction between trial groups. They completed that once aspirin was taken for the first purpose of preventing CVD in healthy old subjects without CVD, there was no profit, but the risk of bleeding was larger and also the death rate was higher. Thus, the study has proposed that aspirin is not a significant prescribing agent as a practice in order to prevent CVD for healthy old individuals. The fascinating purpose of this study is that they enclosed insanity as a primary and secondary outcome as a result of there have been some previous suggestions that aspirin will scale back vascular insanity or physical inactivity by decreasing cerebral events [60, 61].

The ARRIVE was a randomized sort of trial, conducted with 12,545 patients of 55 years (men) or 60 years (women) and older people (mean age 63.9); who had a median cardiac risk to receive 100 mg aspirin or placebo for 60 months of follow-up. They restricted the patients who were at high risk of bleeding and diabetes. The first terminus (MI, stroke, cardiovascular death, unstable angina or TIA) occurred in 4.29% of patients within the aspirin cluster versus 4.48% of patients within the placebo teams. One of the significant the protocols to note within the ARRIVE trial is that the genuine cardiovascular event rate was less than the anticipated cardiovascular rate. This implies that the cluster concerned within the ARRIVE trials man-aged the CVD risk issue higher than within the former trials [62].

Thirteen randomized controlled trials comprising 164,225 patients were observed. The danger of all-cause and cardiovascular mortality was similar for both aspirin and control teams. Aspirin reduced the relative risk (RRR) of major adverse cardiovascular events (MACE) by 9%, myocardial infraction by 14%, and cerebrovascular accident by 10 percent, however was related to a 46% relative risk increase of major bleeding events as compared with controls. Aspirin use did not transform into a net clinical profit adjusted for event connected with mortality risk. There was associate degree interaction for aspirin impact in 3 patient subgroups: (i) in patients with statin drug treatment, aspirin was related to a 12% RRR of MACE and this impact was lacking within the no-statin group; (ii) in nonsmokers, aspirin was related to a 10% RRR of MACE and this impact was not observed in smokers; and (iii) in males, aspirin resulted in a 11% RRR of MACE with a nonsignificant impact in females. Aspirin use does not scale back all-cause of cardio vascular mortality associated with insufficient profit risk quantitative relation for CVD prevention. Nonsmokers, patients treated with statins, and males had the best risk reduction of MACE across subgroups. Systematic review registration: PROSPERO CRD42019118474 [63].

A systematic search of PubMed and Embase was conducted with the assis-tance of Antithrombotic Trialists' (ATT). A set of thirteen trials randomizing 164,225 participants with 1,050,511 participant-years of follow-up were enclosed. The median age of trial participants was 62 years, 19 had diabetes along with the median baseline risk of the primary cardiovascular outcome was 9.2%. Aspirin use was related to important reductions within the composite cardiac outcome compared with no aspirin (57.1 per 10,000 participant-years with aspirin and 61.4 per 10,000 participant-years with no aspirin). Aspirin use was related to elevated degree accrued risk of major bleeding events compared with no aspirin (23.1 per 10,000 participant-years with aspirin and 16.4 per 10,000 participant-years with no aspirin). The administration of aspirin in without cardiovascular disease was related to a lower risk of cardiovascular events associated with an accrued risk of major bleeding. This data may be helpful to aware the patients concerning aspirin use for primary prevention of cardiovascular events and bleeding [64].

Another meta-analysis was performed in concurrence with the well-liked coverage things for Systematic Reviews and Meta-Analyses (PRISMA) tips. Electronic databases were explored for randomized trials that compared aspirin vs. placebo (or control) in subjects while not established atherosclerotic disease. The first efficaciousness outcome was all-cause mortality, whereas the first safety outcome was major bleeding. Outline estimates were reported employing a Der Simonian and Laird random effects model. A set of 11 trials with 157,248 volunteers were enclosed. At a mean follow-up of 6.6 years, aspirin was not related to a lower incidence of all-cause mortality. However, aspirin was related to high degree accrued incidence of major bleeding and intracranial bleeding. The same impact on all-cause mortality and major hemorrhage was incontestable in diabetic and high cardiovascular risk patients (i.e. 10-year risk >7.5%). Aspirin was related to a lower incidence of cardiac muscle infarction; but, this outcome was characterized by extensive heterogeneousness, and this impact was not evident upon limiting the analysis to the more modern trials. Trial ordered analysis confirmed the shortage of good thing about aspirin for all-cause mortality up to a relative risk reduction of 5%. Aspirin use among healthy people while known arterial sclerosis seems to be related to accrued damage and lack of mortality benefit. During this setting, aspirin is probably related to a considerable reduction in MI risk; but, this comes at a value of accrued major bleeding and together with intracranial hemorrhage. The routine use of aspirin for primary prevention has to be reconsidered [65].

8. Guideline for prevention of CVD

The most significant approach to forestall atherosclerotic vascular malady, cardiovascular breakdown, and atrial fibrillation is to advance healthy routine all through life. A group based consideration approach is a compelling technique for the avoidance of cardiovascular malady. Clinicians ought to assess the social determinants of wellbeing that influence people to advise treatment choices. Grown-ups who are 40–75 years old and are being assessed for cardiovascular illness prevention ought to experience 10-year atherosclerotic cardiovascular disease (ASCVD) hazard estimation and have a clinician–patient risk conversation before beginning on pharmacological treatment, for example, antihypertensive treatment, a statin, or aspirin [66].

To adjust the advantages and dangers, earlier US guidelines have suggested prophylactic aspirin medicine just in the setting of raised ASCVD risk (eg, as determined estimators like the PCE (Personal Care Evaluation) or dependent on the nearness of explicit ASCVD risk elements). Meta-relapse investigations of recorded trials show that watched ASCVD chance tracks sensibly well with standard assessed ASCVD hazard. Interestingly, noticed bleeding risk on aspirin medicine is less very much related with baseline evaluated ASCVD risk. (A nonthorough rundown of situations related with expanded danger of bleeding incorporates: a history with past gastrointestinal bleeding or peptic ulcer malady or seeping from different parts of body, age > 70 years, thrombocytopenia, coagulopathy, and simultaneous utilization of different prescriptions that provoke bleeding danger, for example, nonsteroidal anti-inflammatory drugs, steroids, direct oral anticoagulants, and warfarin.) In this unique circumstance, post hoc investigation of more established trials recommends that the benefit–risk proportion for prophylactic; aspirin medicine commonly turns out to be progressively great at >10% evaluated 10-year ASCVD risk [67].

Notwithstanding, the overall advantages of aspirin, explicitly in preventing nonmorbid MI and maybe stroke (with a pattern to bring down mortality) have been less apparent in later trials. Thus, in these ongoing preliminaries, the assessed ASCVD chance has for the most part surpassed the real hazard saw during development. This ongoing information are the justification for the lower COR for prophylactic aspirin in the current protocol (Class IIb) and the evacuation of a particular PCE risk threshold as an incorporation basis for aspirin. These progressions mirror the need to rather consider the totality of accessible proof for ASCVD chance [inclusive, where proper, of hazard improving components, for example, solid family ancestry of untimely MI, failure to accomplish lipid or BP or glucose targets, or huge rise in coronary artery calcium score [68]].

Recent, US guideline has recommended the use of prophylactic aspirin only in the clinically assessed parameters of elevated ASCVD risk as shown in **Figure 7**.

Recommendations for Aspirin Use Referenced studies that support recommendations

COR(Class of Recommendation)	LOE (Level of Evidence) for CVD	Recommendations
IIb (Weak) Benefit ≥ Risk	**A** (High Quality Evidence)	Low-dose aspirin (75-100 mg orally every day) may be considered for the essential avoidance of ASCVD among select grown-ups 40 to 70 years old who are at higher ASCVD risk however not at expanded bleeding danger.
III (Moderate) Benefit = Risk	**B-R** (Randomized Moderate Quality Evidence)	Low-portion aspirin medicine (75-100 mg orally day by day) ought not to be regulated on a normal reason for the essential avoidance of ASCVD among adults >70 years old.
III (Harm) Risk > Benefit	**C-LD** (Limited Evidence)	Low-portion aspirin (75-100 mg orally day by day) ought not be regulated for the essential counteraction of ASCVD among grown-ups of all ages who are at expanded danger of bleeding.

Figure 7.
Recommendations as per guideline [69].

9. Future prospects

The totality of randomized proof since 2008, and 3 trials specifically revealed in 2018, no longer exhibits a decrease in cardiovascular mortality or all-cause death among primary prevention grown-ups with low-dose aspirin. The entirety of the examinations for aspirin medicine in primary avoidance, regardless of whether pre-viously or after 2008, likewise exhibit overabundance draining risk. In this specific situation, it seems to be very conspicuous that daily dose of aspirin is not warranted for primary prevention of CVD [70].

This is with regards to current European guidelines recommendations but negates current US rules, where aspirin is still suggested if 10-year CVD chance is assessed to be >10%. Refreshed American Heart Association/American College of Cardiology guidelines for the primary avoidance of CVD, announced in March 2019, have brought down the help for primary prevention with aspirin medicine from a Class 1 sign among those at raised CVD hazard to a class 2b proposal among high risk grown-ups matured 40–70 years (aspirin is no longer suggested for primary prevention among those >70 years). The rule additionally underscores the need to initially treat other CVD hazard variables to target and afterward just that aspirin may be considered with regards to bring down nondeadly MI risk [71].

On the other hand, the consequences of ASPREE, ASCEND, and ARRIVE all repudiate the proposal that weight-based dosing parameter may have utility in primary prevention, since none of these trials discovered advantage for low-dose aspirin among people at low weight. Regardless of whether high-dose aspirin may have a role in some primary prevention grown-ups (eg, overweight) stays theoretical and difficult to legitimize dependent on current proof. A progressing trial utilizing a novel plan is the aspirin dosing: A Patient-Centric Trial Assessing Benefits and Long-term (ADAPTABLE) trial, which will analyze high against low dose aspirin in 15,000 secondary prevention patients. In the event that ADAPTABLE finds no advantage for high-dose aspirin medicine in auxiliary prevention, at that point the weight-based dosing of aspirin for primary prevention (regardless of whether it is low-or high-dose) will turn out to be significantly tougher to legitimize [72].

10. Conclusion

The advantage of aspirin for auxiliary avoidance of CVD is entrenched, with meta-examination results preferring low-dose (75–150 mg/d) over high-dose (>150 mg/d) aspirin administered comparative viability yet lower bleeding danger. Conversely, the role of aspirin medicine in primary CVD counteraction is progressively questionable; though chronicled clinical evaluation discovered aspirin as a best alternative for PCVD (Primary Cardio Vascular Disease) anticipation [73].

The need to alter aspirin dose as indicated by weight has physiological credibility. For instance, aspirin requires de-acetylation to get dynamic, and pharmacokinetic contemplates have discovered that pudginess is related with improper treatment regimen response to aspirin medicine, as surveyed by thromboxane hindrance.

A 2018 meta-examination by Rothwell et all, which incorporated 9 clinical examination of aspirin for primary prevention (counting 103,000 volunteers) and 4 trials of secondary prevention of stroke (17,000 volunteers), detailed that the viability of aspirin at a dose of ≤100 mg in lessening cardiovascular occasions diminished with expanding weight, with advantage found in patients weighing 50–69 kg yet not in those weighing 70 kg or more. Reliable with this, low-dose of aspirin medicine possibly expanded danger of bleeding when bodyweight was <90 kg. On the other hand, aspirin (≥325 mg) had the contrary interaction with body weight, diminishing cardiovascular occasions exclusively among those >70 kg [62, 74].

In spite of the debate over the security and efficacity of aspirin, low-dose of the medicine has been broadly utilized for the primary prevention of CVD. As indicated by the investigation of National Health and Nutrition Examination study information, 22.5% of patients without a mitigated CVD were delegated as high risk, and 40.9% of them were advised to take aspirin by their health care professional. Likewise, 26.0% of individuals at low risk were advised to take the medicine paying little mind to their risk category [75].

Recently, questions have been raised about the administration of aspirin medicine for primary avoidance of CVD. Specifically, there are worries that GI bloodletting and hemorrhagic stroke, side-effects that can appear in adults utilizing aspirin, are expanded [76]. Whether the advantages of aspirin in the avoidance of CVD exceed the dangers related with side-effects is at the core of the discussion. One of the significant explanations behind the change in perspective about aspirin use is a decrease in the overall frequency of CVD.

As per European CVD measurements in 2017 distributed by the European Heart Network, CVD mortality and the age-standardized pervasiveness pace of CVD are currently falling in most European nations. Besides, from 1975 through to 2019, mortality rate from CVD have fallen in US men and women [77]. Globally, the age-standardized disability adjusted life-years (DALY) rates (per 100,000) in 2005–2015 for CVD diminished from 6231.9 to 5179.7 [78].

The considerable decrease of CVD death and frequency is because of improved prevention treatments, which deal with the principle risk components of CVD, for example, smoking, physical idleness, dyslipidemia, and hypertension. Moreover, the adjustment of overall routine of life, for example, weight reduction or regular physical exercise, has become popular [79].

Moreover, current prescription use, for example, statins, new anticoagulation agents, and hypertensive medications, has added to lessening the CVD chance for the whole populace [80]. The extent of the risk decrease by aspirin in CVD primary prevention relies upon the level of profound risk in the people [81].

A few examinations have demonstrated that if a patient's danger of CVD increments (above 1% every year), the advantage of administering aspirin medicine as primary prevention is additionally expanded. Hence, the overall CVD risk decrease brought about by another preventive methodology appears to lessen the primary prevention of aspirin for CVD contrasted with previously. The way that the cardiovascular occasion rates for all patients who took an interest in the recent published Aspirin to Reduce Risk of Initial Vascular Events (ARRIVE) clinical investigation was lower than anticipated additionally underpins this hypothesis [62]. Rather than the ongoing diminishing in the effectiveness of aspirin for the primary counteraction of CVD, the bleeding danger related with aspirin medicine still exists [82].

In numerous investigations, it is notable that the application of low-dose aspirin was related with an essentially expanded risk of significant bleeding occasions. It is flawed whether the utilization of aspirin medicine for CVD primary prevention will have a critical impact when contrasted with the danger of aspirin in the current time. Ongoing patterns have seen that the utilization of aspirin for primary prevention of CVD is reducing in the United States. In this way, it is important to consider whether it is suitable to proceed with aspirin for the primary avoidance of CVD in every patient [83].

Numerous hypotheses have been taken into account regarding why low-dose aspirin no longer seems effective in primary prevention. These encompass a reducing return for efficacy with regards to contemporary consideration (e.g., smoking suspension, statins) and the likelihood that one aspirin medicine dose may not "fit for all" patients.

In this chapter, we sum up proof for and against aspirin dosing in primary prevention, place this proof with regards to current published aspirin clinical trials, and provide refreshed clinical guidance for aspirin use in the primary prevention of CVD in the year 2020 and beyond.

Author details

Deepak Kumar Dash[1], Vishal Jain[2], Anil Kumar Sahu[1], Rajnikant Panik[1] and Vaibhav Tripathi[1*]

1 Royal College of Pharmacy, Raipur, Chhattisgarh, India

2 University Institute of Pharmacy, Pt. Ravishankar Shukla University, Raipur, Chhattisgarh, India

*Address all correspondence to: vaibhu.07@gmail.com

References

[1] Jeffreys D. Aspirin: The Remarkable Story of a Wonder Drug. 1st ed. New York, NY: Bloomsbury; 2004

[2] Zundorf U. Aspirin 100 Years: The Future Has Just Begun. Leverkusen: Bayer AG, Consumer Care Business Group; 1997

[3] Campbell CL, Smyth S, Montalescot G, Steinhubl SR. Aspirin dose for the prevention of cardiovascular disease: A systematic review. Journal of the American Medical Association. 2007;**297**:2018-2024

[4] El-Magbri M. The Synthesis and Analysis of Aspirin. Washington, D.C. 20016: Department of Chemistry, American University; February 26, 2014

[5] Fersht AR, Kirby AJ. Hydrolysis of aspirin. Intramolecular general base catalysis of ester hydrolysis. Journal of the American Chemical Society. 1967;**89**(19):4857-4863. DOI: 10.1021/ja00995a007

[6] St. Pierre T, Jencks WP. Intramolecular catalysis in the reactions of nucleophilic reagents with aspirin. Journal of the American Chemical Society. 1968;**90**(14):3817-3827. DOI: 10.1021/ja01016a040

[7] Choudhary A, Kamer KJ, Raines RT. An $n \rightarrow \pi^*$ interaction in aspirin: Implications for structure and reactivity. The Journal of Organic Chemistry. 2011;**76**(19):7933-7937

[8] Chandrasekhar S, Kumar HV. The reaction of aspirin with base. Tetrahedron Letters. 2011;**52**:3561-3564

[9] Dakin HD, West RJ. A general reaction of amino acids. The Journal of Biological Chemistry. 1928;**78**:91-104

[10] Hendrix BM, Paquin F. The effect of alkali treatment upon acetyl proteins. The Journal of Biological Chemistry. 1938;**124**:135-145

[11] Bundgaard H, Larsen C. Intramolecular and intermolecular transformations of aspirin in nonhydroxylic solvents. Journal of Pharmaceutical Sciences. 1976;**65**(5):776-778

[12] Pinckard RN, Hawkins D, Farr RS. In vitro acetylation of plasma proteins, enzyme and DNA by aspirin. Nature. 1968;**219**:68-69

[13] Shamsuddin M, Mason RG, Ritchey JY, Honig GR, Klotz I. Sites of acetylation of sickle cell hemoglobin by aspirin. Proceedings of the National Academy of Sciences. 1974;**71**(12):4693-4697

[14] Xu ASL, Macdonald JM, Labotka RJ, London RE. NMR study of the sites of human hemoglobin acetylated by aspirin. Biochemica et Biophysica Acta. 1999;**1432**:333-349

[15] Angiolillo DJ, Bhatt DL, Lanza F, et al. Pharmacokinetic/pharmacodynamic assessment of a novel, pharmaceutical lipid–aspirin complex: Results of a randomized, crossover, bioequivalence study. Journal of Thrombosis and Thrombolysis. 2019;**48**:554-562

[16] Leonards JR. Presence of acetylsalicylic acid in plasma following oral ingestion of aspirin. Proceedings of the Society for Experimental Biology and Medicine. 1962;**110**(2):304-308

[17] Rowland M, Riegelman S, Harris PA, Sholkoff SD. Absorption kinetics of aspirin in man following oral administration of an aqueous solution. Journal of Pharmaceutical Sciences. 1972;**61**(3):379-385

[18] Zhou G, Marathe GK, Willard B, McIntyre TM. Intracellular

erythrocyte platelet-activating factor acetylhydrolase I inactivates aspirin in blood. The Journal of Biological Chemistry. 2011;**286**(40):34820-34829

[19] Fu CJ, Melethil S, Mason WD. The pharmacokinetics of aspirin in rats and the effect of buffer. Journal of Pharmacokinetics and Biopharmaceutics. 01 April 1991;**19**(2):157-173

[20] Lichtenberger LM, Phan T, Fang D, Edler S, Philip J, Li-Geng T, et al. Bioavailability of aspirin in rats comparing the drug uptake into gastrointestinal tissue and vascular and lymphatic systems: Implications on aspirin's chempreventive action. Journal of Physics and Pharmacology. 2016;**67**(5):635-642

[21] Poźniak B, Switała M, Jaworski K, Okoniewski P, Niewiński P. Comparative pharmacokinetics of acetylsalicylic acid and sodium salicylate in chickens and turkeys. British Poultry Science. 2013;**54**:538-544. DOI: 10.1080/00071668.2013.809403

[22] Graham GG, Champion GD, Day RO, Paull PD. Patterns of plasma concentrations and urinary excretion of salicylate in rheumatoid arthritis. Clinical Pharmacology & Therapeutics. 1977;**22**(4):410-420

[23] Verbeeck RK, Cardinal JA. Plasma protein binding of salicylic acid, phenytoin, chlorpromazine, and pethidine using equilibrium dialysis and ultracentrifugation. Arzneimittel-Forschung. 1985;**35**:903-906

[24] Aarons L, Clifton P, Fleming G, Rowland M. Aspirin binding and the effect of albumin on spontaneous and enzyme catalyzed hydrolysis. The Journal of Pharmacy and Pharmacology. 1980;**32**:537-543

[25] Rendell M, Nierenberg J, Brannan C, Valentine JL, Stephen PM, Dodds S, et al. Inhibition of glycation of albumin and hemoglobin by acetylation in vitro and in vivo. Journal of Laboratory and Clinical Medicines. 1968;**108**:286-293

[26] Hawkins D, Pinckard RN, Crawford IP, Farr RS. Structural changes in human serum albumin induced by ingestion of acetylsalicylic acid. The Journal of Clinical Investigation. 1969;**48**(3):536-542

[27] Ashton JM, Bolme P, Zerihun B. Protein binding of salicylic acid and salicyluric acid in serum from malnourished children: The influence of albumin competitive binding and non esterified fatty acids. Journal Pharmacy and Pharmacology. 1989;**41**:474-480

[28] Levy G, Procknal JA, Garrettson LK. Distribution of salicylate between neonatal and maternal serum at diffusion equilibrium. Clinical Pharmacology & Therapeutics. 1975;**18**(2):210-214

[29] Rainsford KD, Ford NLV, Brooks PM, Watson HM. Plasma aspirin esterases in normal individuals. Patients with alcoholic liver disease and rheumatoid arthritis. Characterisation and the importance of en~ymatic components. European Journal of Clinical Investigation. 1980;**10**:413-420

[30] Ornelas A, Zacharias-Millward N, Menter DG, Davis JS, Lichtenberger L, Hawke D, et al. Beyond COX-1: The effects of aspirin on platelet biology and potential mechanisms of chemoprevention. Cancer Metastasis Reviews. 2017;**362**:289-303

[31] Cadavid AP. Aspirin: The mechanism of action revisited in the context of pregnancy complications. Frontiers in Immunology. 2017;**8**:261. DOI: 10.3389/fimmu.2017.00261

[32] Rowlinson SW, Crews BC, Goodwin DC, Schneider C, Gierse JK, Marnett LJ. Spatial requirements for

15-(R)-hydroxy-5Z,8Z,11Z, 13E-eicosatetraenoic acid synthesis within the cyclooxygenase active site of murine COX-2. Why acetylated COX-1 does not synthesize 15-(R)-HETE. (15-HETE). The Journal of Biological Chemistry. 2000;**275**(9):6586-6591

[33] Blanco FJ, Guitian R, Moreno J, De Toro FJ, Galdo F. Effect of anti-inflammator drugs on COX-1 and COX-2 activity in human articular chondrocytes. The Journal of Rheumatology. 1999;**26**(6):1366-1373

[34] Dovizio M, Bruno A, Tacconelli S, Patrignani P. Mode of action of aspirin as a chemopreventive agent. Prospects for Chemoprevention and Colorectal Neopolasia. 2013:31-65

[35] Claria J, Serhan CN. Aspirin triggers previously undescribed bioactive eicosanoids by human endothelial cell-leukocyte interactions. Proceedings of the National Academy of Sciences of the United States of America. 1995;**92**(21):9475-9479. DOI: 10.1073/pnas.92.21.9475

[36] Alfonso LF, Srivenugopal KS, Bhat GJ. Does aspirin acetylate multiple cellular proteins? (Review). Molecular Medicine Reports. 2009;**2**(4):533-537. DOI: 10.3892/mmr_00000132

[37] Lasagna L. Analgesic drugs. American Journal of Medical Sciences. 1961;**242**:620-627

[38] Lim RK. Salicylate analgesia. In: Smith, Smith, editors. The Salicylates. New York: Inter Science Publishers; 1966. p. 155

[39] Levy G. Clinical pharmacokinetics of salicylates: An assessment. British Journal of Clinical Pharmacology. 1981;**10**:285S-290S

[40] Wilson JT, Brown RD, Bocchini JA, Kearns GL. Efficacy, disposition and pharmacodynamics of aspirin, acetaminophen and choline salicylate in young febrile children. Therapeutic Drug Monitoring. 1982;**4**:147-180

[41] Rumack BH. Aspirin versus acetaminophen: A comparative view. Pediatrics. 1978;**62**(5):943-946

[42] Rooney SM, Campbell JN. Aspirin's space. In: How Aspirin Entered Our Medicine Cabinet. Cham: Springer; 2017. pp. 1-3

[43] Laidlaw TM, Cahill KN. Current knowledge and management of hypersensitivity to aspirin and NSAIDs. The Journal of Allergy and Clinical Immunology: In Practice. 2017;**5**(3):537-545

[44] Schrör K. Aspirin and Reye Syndrome. Pediatric Drugs. 2007;**9**(3):195-204

[45] Belay ED, Bresee JS, Holman RC, Khan AS, Shahriari A, Schonberger LB. Reye's syndrome in the United States from 1981 through 1997. New England Journal of Medicine. 1999;**340**(18):1377-1382

[46] Huhtakangas J, Tetri S, Juvela S, Saloheimo P, Bode MK, Hillbom M. Effect of increased warfarin use on warfarin-related cerebral hemorrhage: A longitudinal population-based study. Stroke. 2011 Sep;**42**(9):2431-2435

[47] Arif H, Aggarwal S. Salicylic acid (Aspirin). In: StatPearls [Internet]. Treasure Island (FL): StatPearls Publishing; January 2020 [updated 2019 Oct 17]

[48] Sung JJ, Lau JY, Ching JY, Wu JC, Lee YT, Chiu PW, et al. Continuation of low-dose aspirin therapy in peptic ulcer bleeding: A randomized trial. Annals of Internal Medicine. 2010;**152**:1-9

[49] Barar FS. Textbook of Pharmacology. New Delhi: S. Chand Publishing; 2012

[50] Tripathi KD. Essentials of Medical Pharmacology. New Delhi: Jaypee Brothers, Medical Publishers Pvt. Limited; 2013

[51] Yusuf S, Reddy S, Ounpuu S, A nand S. Global burden of cardiovascular diseases: Part I: General considerations, the epidemiologic transition, risk factors, and impact of urbanization. Circulation. 2001;**104**:2746-2753

[52] Geldsetzer P, Manne-Goehler J, Theilmann M, Davies JI, Awasthi A, Danaei G, et al. Geographic and sociodemographic variation of cardiovascular disease risk in India: A cross-sectional study of 797,540 adults. PLoS medicine. 2018 Jun 19;**15**(6):e1002581

[53] Dalen JE, Alpert JS, Goldberg RJ, Weinstein RS. The epidemic of the 20th century: Coronary heart disease. The American Journal of Medicine. 2014;**127**:807-812

[54] Hennekens CH, Dyken ML, Fuster V. Aspirin as a therapeutic agent in cardiovascular disease: A statement for healthcare professionals from the American Heart Association. Circulation. 1997;**96**:2751-2753

[55] Antithrombotic Trialists' (ATT) Collaboration, Baigent C, Blackwell L, Collins R, Emberson J, Godwin J, et al. Aspirin in the primary and secondary prevention of vascular disease: collaborative meta-analysis of individual participant data from randomised trials. Lancet. 2009;**373**:1849-1860

[56] Williams CD, Chan AT, Elman MR, Kristensen AH, Miser WF, Pignone MP, et al. Aspirin use among adults in the U.S.: Results of a national survey. American Journal of Preventive Medicine. 2015;**48**:501-508

[57] Nemerovski CW, Salinitri FD, Morbitzer KA, Moser LR. Aspirin for primary prevention of cardiovasculardisease events. Pharmacotherapy. 2012;**32**:1020-1035

[58] Antithrombotic Trialists' Collaboration. Collaborative meta-analysis of randomised trials of antiplatelet therapy for prevention of death, myocardial infarction, and stroke in high risk patients. BMJ. 2002;**324**:71-86

[59] ASCEND Study Collaborative Group, Bowman L, Mafham M, Wallendszus K, Stevens W, Buck G, et al. Effects of aspirin for primary prevention in persons with diabetes mellitus. The New England Journal of Medicine. 2018;**379**:1529-1539

[60] McNeil JJ, Wolfe R, Woods RL, Tonkin AM, Donnan GA, Nelson MR, et al. Effect of aspirin on cardiovascular events and bleeding in the healthy elderly. The New England Journal of Medicine. 2018;**379**:1509-1518

[61] McNeil JJ, Woods RL, Nelson MR, Reid CM, Kirpach B, Wolfe R, et al. Effect of aspirin on disability-free survival in the healthy elderly. The New England Journal of Medicine. 2018;**379**:1499-1508

[62] Gaziano JM, Brotons C, Coppolecchia R, Cricelli C, Darius H, Gorelick PB, et al. Use of aspirin to reduce risk of initial vascular events in patients at moderate risk of cardiovascular disease (ARRIVE): A randomised, double-blind, placebo-controlled trial. Lancet. 2018;**392**:1036-1046

[63] Gelbenegger G, Postula M, Pecen L, Halvorsen S, Lesiak M, Schoergenhofer C, et al. Aspirin for primary prevention of cardiovascular disease: A meta-analysis with a particular focus on subgroups. BMC Medicine. 2019;**17**(1):198. DOI: 10.1186/s12916-019-1428-0

[64] Zheng SL, Roddick AJ. Association of aspirin use for primary prevention

with cardiovascular events and bleeding events: A systematic review and meta-analysis. JAMA. 2019;**321**(3):277-287. DOI: 10.1001/jama.2018.20578

[65] Mahmoud AN, Gad MM, Elgendy AY, Elgendy IY, Bavry AA. Efficacy and safety of aspirin for primary prevention of cardiovascular events: A meta-analysis and trial sequential analysis of randomized controlled trials. European Heart Journal. 2019;**40**:607-617

[66] Cheng JW, Colucci V, Kalus JS, Spinler SA. Reply: Managing diabetes and preventing heart disease: Have we found a safe and effective agent? The Annals of Pharmacotherapy. 2019 Oct;**53**(10):1072

[67] Bhatt D, Eikelboom J, Connolly S, Steg P, Anand S, Verma S, et al. Role of combination antiplatelet and anticoagulation therapy in diabetes mellitus and cardiovascular disease: insights from the COMPASS trial. Circulation. 9 June 2020;**141**(23):1841-1854

[68] Piepoli MF, Hoes AW, Agewall S, Albus C, Brotons C, Catapano AL, et al. European Guidelines on cardiovascular disease prevention in clinical practice: The Sixth Joint Task Force of the European Society of Cardiology and Other Societies on Cardiovascular Disease Prevention in Clinical Practice (constituted by representatives of 10 societies and by invited experts) Developed with the special contribution of the European Association for Cardiovascular Prevention & Rehabilitation (EACPR). European Heart Journal. 2016, 2016 Aug 1;**37**(29):2315-2381

[69] Arnett DK, Blumenthal RS, Albert MA, Buroker AB, Goldberger ZD, Hahn EJ, et al. 2019 ACC/AHA Guideline on the Primary Prevention of Cardiovascular Disease: A Report of the American College of Cardiology/American Heart Association Task Force on Clinical Practice Guidelines. Journal of the American College of Cardiology. 10 September 2019;**74**(10):e177-e232

[70] Piepoli MF, Abreu A, Albus C, Ambrosetti M, Brotons C, Catapano AL, et al. Update on cardiovascular prevention in clinical practice: A position paper of the European Association of Preventive Cardiology of the European Society of Cardiology. European Journal of Preventive Cardiology. 2020 Jan;**27**(2):181-205

[71] Fanaroff A, Califf R, Windecker S, Smith S, Lopes R. Levels of Evidence Supporting American College of Cardiology/American Heart Association and European Society of Cardiology Guidelines, 2008-2018. Jama. 19 March 2019;**321**(11): 1069-1080

[72] Murphy S, McCarthy CP, McEvoy JW. Aspirin for the primary prevention of cardiovascular disease: Weighing up the evidence. The American Journal of Medicine. 1 September 2019;**132**(9): 1007-1008

[73] Capodanno D, Angiolillo DJ. Aspirin for primary cardiovascular risk prevention and beyond in diabetes mellitus. Circulation. 2016;**134**(20): 1579-1594

[74] Rothwell PM, Cook NR, Gaziano JM, et al. Effects of aspirin on risks of vascular events and cancer according to bodyweight and dose: Analysis of individual patient data from randomised trials. Lancet. 2018;**392**(10145):387-399

[75] Mainous AG 3rd, Tanner RJ, Shorr RI, Limacher MC. Use of aspirin for primary and secondary cardiovascular disease prevention in the United States, 2011-2012. Journal of the American Heart Association. 2014;**3**:e000989

[76] De Berardis G, Lucisano G, D'Ettorre A, Pellegrini F, Lepore V, Tognoni G, et al. Association of aspirin use with major bleeding in patients with and without diabetes. JAMA. 2012;**307**:2286-2294

[77] Wilkins E, Wilson L, Wickramasinghe K, Bhatnagar P, Leal J, Luengo-Fernandez R, et al. European Cardiovascular Disease Statistics 2017 Edition. Brussels: European Heart Network; 2017

[78] GBD 2015 DALYs and HALE Collaborators. Global, regional, and national disability-adjusted life-years (DALYs) for 315 diseases and injuries and healthy life expectancy (HALE), 1990-2015: A systematic analysis for the Global Burden of Disease Study 2015. Lancet, 2016;**388**:1603-1658

[79] Weir HK, Anderson RN, Coleman King SM, Soman A, Thompson TD, Hong Y, et al. Heart disease and cancer deaths - trends and projections in the United States, 1969-2020. Preventing Chronic Disease. 2016;**13**:E157

[80] Benjamin EJ, Virani SS, Callaway CW, Chamberlain AM, Chang AR, Cheng S, et al. Heart disease and stroke statistics—2018 update: A report from the American Heart Association. Circulation. 2018;**137**:e67-e492

[81] Bibbins-Domingo K, U.S. Preventive Services Task Force. Aspirin use for the primary prevention of cardiovascular disease and colorectal cancer: U.S. Preventive Services Task Force recommendation statement. Annals of Internal Medicine. 2016;**164**:836-845

[82] Whitlock EP, Burda BU, Williams SB, Guirguis-Blake JM, Evans CV. Bleeding risks with aspirin use for primary prevention in adults: A systematic review for the U.S. Preventive Services Task Force. Annals of Internal Medicine. 2016;**164**:826-835

[83] Van't Hof JR, Duval S, Walts A, Kopecky SL, Luepker RV, Hirsch AT. Contemporary primary prevention aspirin use by cardiovascular disease risk: Impact of US Preventive Services task Force recommendations, 2007-2015: A serial, cross-sectional study. Journal of the American Heart Association. 2017;**6**:e006328

11

Drug Repurposing and Orphan Disease Therapeutics

Neha Dhir, Ashish Jain, Dhruv Mahendru, Ajay Prakash and Bikash Medhi

Abstract

Drug repurposing (or drug repositioning) is an innovative way to find out the new indications of a drug that already exists in the market with known therapeutic indications. It offers an effective way to drug developers or the pharmaceutical companies to identify new targets for FDA-approved drugs. Less time consumption, low cost and low risk of failure are some of the advantages being offered with drug repurposing. Sildenafil (*Viagra*), a landmark example of a repurposed drug, was introduced into the market as an antianginal drug. But at present, its use is repurposed as drug for erectile dysfunction. In a similar way, numerous drugs are there that have been successfully repurposed in managing the clinical conditions. The chapter would be highlighting the various drug repurposing strategies, drugs repurposed in the past and the current status of repurposed drugs in the orphan disease therapeutics along with regulatory guidelines for drug repurposing.

Keywords: drug repurposing, drug repositioning, orphan drug, orphan disease, a rare disease, regulatory guidelines

1. Introduction

Despite rapid advancement in science and technology, translating these benefits for care and management of human diseases remains a far slower process than expected. Pharmaceutical industries, research and development (R&D) sectors are facing multifold challenges for taking out any new drug in the market including higher attrition rates, long time span and regulatory restrictions [1]. It takes $2 to $3 billion money and about 13–15 years for developing any new drug in the market with a low success rate of approximately 2% only [2, 3]. Drug development process involves six stages: (i) compound screening and identification of lead compound; (ii) preclinical study; (iii) investigational new drug (IND) application for taking approval to conduct trial in humans, only if preclinical data of the drug is found to be shows effective and safe in animals; (iv) clinical study (phase 1, 2 and 3 clinical trials); (v) new drug application (NDA) if the drug is found to be safe and effective in phase 3 clinical trials; and (vi) post marketing surveillance (PMS) for safety monitoring. However, drug repurposing consists of four stages only: (i) selection of target compound; (ii) clinical trial (phase 2 and 3); (iii) NDA application and (iv) PMS (**Figure 1**). Thereby' drug repurposing is a trending way to reduce the effort, cost and time at every step involved in drug development and thus provides an option to bring the new drugs into the market at relatively low investments (**Figure 1**) [3].

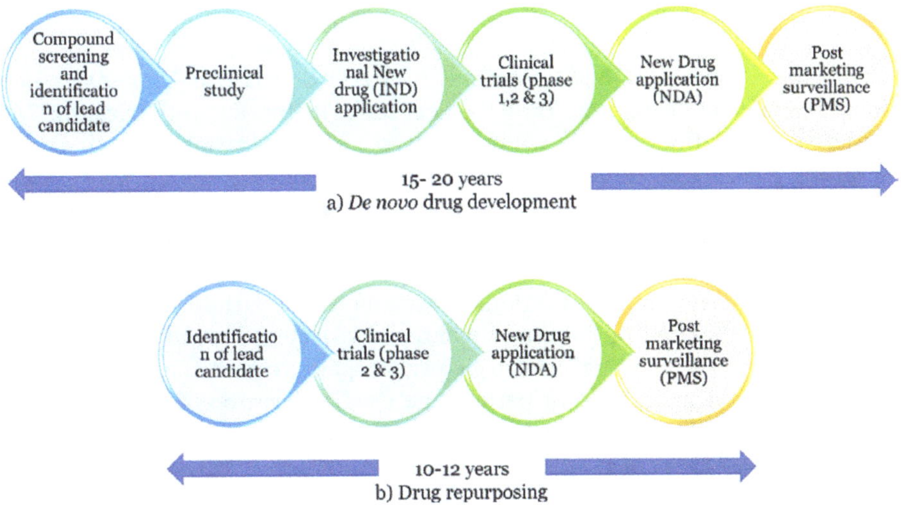

Figure 1.
Phases in drug development.

1.1 Drug repurposing

'Drug repurposing' (or 'drug repositioning') is an effective way to find new targets or new indications of any drug that is already FDA approved and existing in the market. It is an excellent alternative over the *de novo* drug development process which is relatively time consuming and money involved procedure [4]. Since the data including drug efficacy, safety, bioavailability, route and formulation of administration, pharmacokinetic and pharmacodynamic (PK-PD) profile, toxicological data and associated adverse effects, are well known with already approved drugs. Thus, the evaluation process for drug candidates gets facilitated with drug repurposing and drug enters the clinical market for new therapeutic indications. Also, drug repurposing reduces the risk of development failure into the market, thus reducing the cost of the overall drug development process. At present, in the U.S approximately 30% of newly FDA approved drugs are repurposed only [5]. History witnessed numerous drug candidates that have been repurposed either opportunistic or serendipitous. Sildenafil is one of the blockbusters in the history of drug repurposing. Sildenafil, a phosphodiesterase type 5 (PDE5) inhibitor, was introduced in the market in the 1980s by Pfizer for the treatment of coronary artery disease (CAD), hypertension and angina pectoris. During phase-1 trials of sildenafil, it was observed that the patients suffered from marked penile erection. In 1988, the drug was repurposed and approved by FDA for erectile dysfunction in the US market after the drug failed to prove its efficacy in phase-2 trials in angina patients [6]. Another big hit example is thalidomide. In 1957, the drug was developed by German pharmaceutical company named Grünentha for treatment of motion sickness in pregnant women. Soon the drug was withdrawn from the market as its use lead to serious birth defects (malformations of the limbs) and death in approximately 10,000 children in around 46 countries. Subsequently in 2006, the drug was re-approved by FDA for the treatment of multiple myeloma [4]. In the 1960s, amantadine was developed as an antiviral drug to treat influenza infections. After a few years, a patient who was suffering from Parkinson's disease (PD) had taken amantadine for her flu infection. It was seen that the patient was having improvement in her PD symptoms after taking amantadine. From there, it has been concluded that the drug can be used in treating neurological disorders. Years later, amantadine received FDA approval for treatment of PD [7].

1.2 Off-label use of drugs

"Off-label drug use (OLDU)" defines to prescribe the drug beyond the conditions for which the drug is holding the license for its market authorization. More specifically, off-label means using a drug for indications, dosage form, dose strength, route of administration or in that patient age group which are not approved by FDA [8]. FDA approves a drug to market only if it shows to be effective and safe in preclinical as well as clinical studies, refers to as "on-label drug use". However, OLDU is being extensively practiced by physicians in situations: first, when two therapeutic conditions possessing same pathophysiology; second, to treat any life-threatening condition where no treatment is available and thereby provide off-label use may be proven helpful to patient; and third, drug has not been studies in specific group or patient age (pediatrics, pregnancy or geriatric). There are many examples of drugs which have been prescribed commonly as "off-label" drugs (**Table 1**) [9].

1.3 Orphan diseases and drugs

There is no defined definition for orphan diseases (ODs). In the US it is defined as if the disease prevalence affects less than 1 in <200,000, in Japan <50,000 and in Australia <2000. WHO defines the prevalence of less than 6.5–10 in 10,000 [10]. The drug which is used in the treatment of orphan disease is referred to as an orphan drug. For example; haem arginate, is being used to treat porphyria (acute intermittent, variegate and hereditary), ibuprofen to treat patent ductus arteriosus in neonates [11] and N-acetylcysteine for paracetamol poisoning. In orphan diseases (ODs) and their management, the count for orphan diseases exists approximately 6000 but the efforts that are putting off by phar-maceutical and R&D sectors for developing new drugs in their management are negligible cause the huge amount involved in *de novo* drug development [12]. Only 5% of pharmaceutical industries are taking interest in developing new drugs in orphan disease management [12]. At present, approximately 325 drugs are available in the market, which are being used to treat only 5% of orphan diseases. Drug

Drug	Class of drug	Approved use	Off-label use
Desmopressin	Antidiuretic hormone	Central diabetes insipidus	Nocturnal enuresis
Atenolol, propranolol, metoprolol	Beta blockers	Hypertension	Migraine prophylaxis
Imipramine, amoxapine	Tricyclic antidepressant	Depression	Insomnia, Bulimia, neuropathic pain symptoms
Aspirin	NSAIDs	Analgesic	Antithrombosis in atrial fibrillation
Indomethacin	NSAIDs	Analgesic	Closure of patent ductus arteriosus
Erythromycin	Macrolide antibiotic	Haemophilus and Legionella infection, whooping cough, atypical pneumonia	Gastroparesis

Table 1.
Examples of off-label drug use (OLDU).

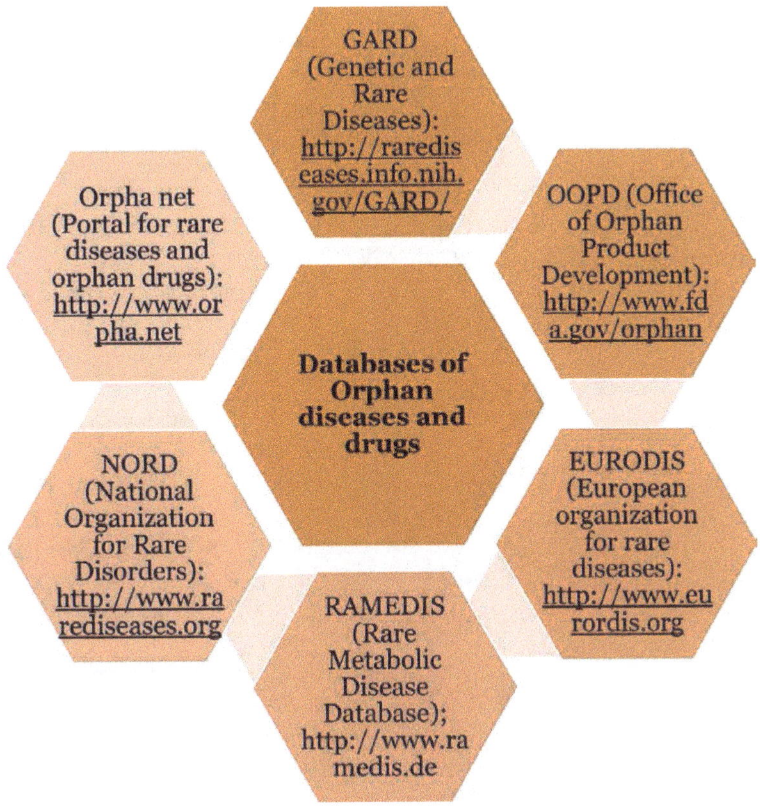

Figure 2.
Resource database for orphan diseases (ODs) and drugs.

repurposing provides one of the best faster and economical ways to find new treatment options in ODs (**Figure 2**). To facilitate drug development and treatment options in orphan disease management FDA Orphan Drug Act (ODA) 1983, has provided many of the benefits or incentives to pharmaceutical and research companies including (i) tax credits (ii) clinical research aids, (iii) fast-track marketing authorization procedures (FDA approval), and (iv) marketing exclusivity [13].

2. Approaches for drug repurposing

In drug repurposing, three major steps are involved which consist of (i) identification of target candidate for new indication (generation of new hypothesis for new indication or new target), (ii) exploration of mechanism or signaling pathway involved in drug or disease and (iii) finally proving the efficacy of drug in phase 2 and 3 clinical trials. Among all steps, identification of lead candidate is one of the most critical steps. This is the step where the most sophisticated and systematic approaches are needed to be implicated for generation of new hypothesis in drug repurposing. Drugs can be repurposed via multiple ways which may be either experimentally, clinical based or computationally (**Figure 3**). Computational approach is '*in silico*' based drug repurposing which is further subclassified as either drug-centric or disease-centric. In drug-centric, we find new indications for existing drugs while in disease-centric approach, we try new drugs for an existing disease.

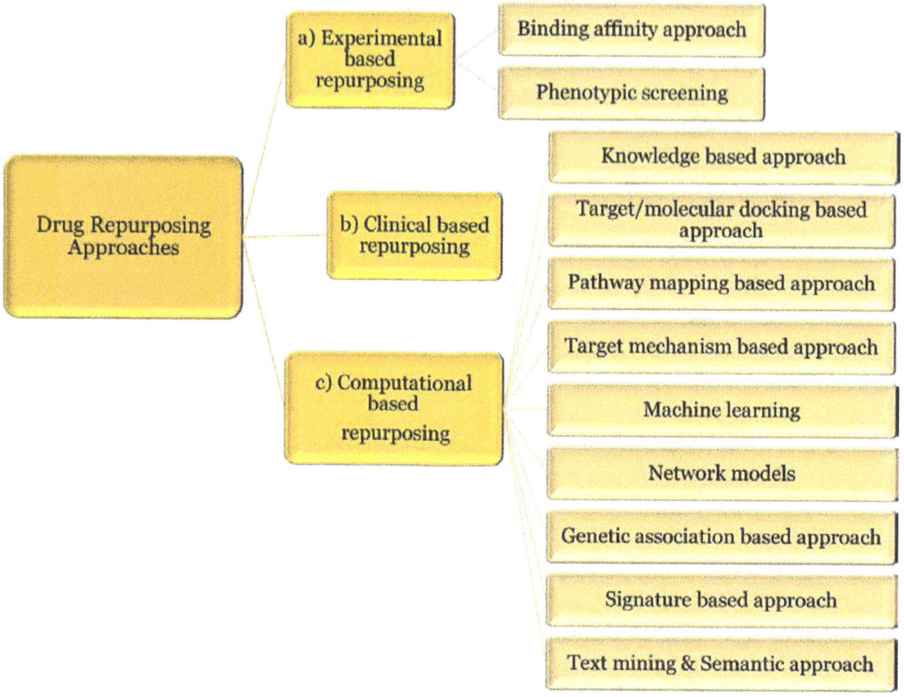

Figure 3.
Approaches for drug repurposing. (a) Experimental based, (b) clinical based and (c) computational based drug repurposing.

2.1 Experimental strategies in drug repurposing

2.1.1 Binding assays to identify target candidate

Techniques like chromatography and mass spectrometry are being used to find all possible binding targets of drug candidates. Brehmer et al. conducted a study using HeLa cell extract to identify possible protein targets of gefitinib. The results of mass spectrometry revealed that the drug can interact with 20 different protein kinases which may be treated as possible targets of gefitinib [14].

2.1.2 Phenotyping screening

In the world of drug discovery and development, the term phenotyping screening is used to describe the ways adopted to identify the biological effects of a drug which is either directly or indirectly linked to a disease. With the development of robotic and sensitive screening tools, the approach is used to screen thousands of chemical drug libraries in a single go. It involves the screening of target drug candidates either using cell-based screens (high throughput screening (HTS)) or even whole organism [15]. Cell based assays involve cell lines derived from human or animals, immortalized cell lines or induced pluripotent cells lines (iPSCs), etc. For example, Iljin et al. [16] performed HTS of approximately 5000 small molecules using prostate cancer epithelial cell lines. In this experiment, disulfiram was found to possess selective antineoplastic property which was validated later using genome wide gene expression studies [16]. Important cell-based assays that are being performed in drug discovery and repurposing include: cell viability assay, signaling pathways assay and disease related mechanistic assay. Other cell assays that are being performed routinely in drug development include cell apoptosis, infection, cell motility, cell cycle arrest and many more [17]. Cousin et al. [18] have used zebrafish model to evaluate the efficacy of compounds against tobacco dependence. In this study the authors have found that the agents like apomorphine may be useful in modifying nicotine or ethanol induced dependence behavior [18]. Over the decades in drug discovery, these approaches are getting shifted more toward molecular targets based on phenotypic methods, which rely mainly on molecular targets of drugs and diseases and related mechanisms for hypothesis generation.

2.2 Clinical perspective

2.2.1 Clinical analysis (human experiments)

Clinical trials providing positive outcomes are quite rare as most of the drugs fail during Phase II/III trials. But many drugs which already have been marketed during post-marketing surveillance provides different outcome. Some may display different adverse events and some may treat specific kinds of disease with no labeled indication. Many drugs have been repurposed with the help of these trials. Some such examples are apomorphine was indicated for Parkinson's disease and it was repurposed for erectile dysfunction, drospirenone—oral contraceptive and repurposed for hypertension, dapoxetine—analgesia and depression and repurposed for hypertension [3]. These are very few examples of clinically repurposed drugs, there are many such drugs which have been repurposed with many new indications [1].

2.3 Computational perspective

2.3.1 Knowledge-based repurposing

This approach is based on already available data such as ligands and receptors. Specific models can be developed in order to locate the targets that have not been discovered/explored yet. These models are developed to discover the novel biomarkers, pathophysiology and receptors for various diseases. This kind of approach could also be beneficial in predicting different adverse reaction related to drugs, their structure activity relationships (SAR), ligands targeting the different pathways, etc., So, this could be mechanism based, pathway-based, receptor-based repositioning of drugs [1].

2.3.2 Target/molecular docking-based drug repurposing

In-silico screening of various compounds by generating drug library could find a lead molecule resulting targeted therapies. Drug compounds of specific interest from drug libraries can be selected by molecular docking or ligand-based screening which incorporates high-throughput screening (HTS) as large number of compounds are screened in this method [19]. The other methods include standard precision (SP), extra precision (XP).

During this screening there is no incorporation of information related to any biological or pharmacological as the screening is blinded. Target-based approach links the targets such as any receptor with the pathophysiology behind the disease and therefore the process of drug-discovery revamps. Withstanding to this target-based approach cannot predict the novel/unknown mechanism with the currently available targets of the disease [1].

2.3.3 Pathway mapping/pathway-based drug repurposing

Information such as protein-protein interaction, cell signaling and metabolic pathways can be useful for predicting the intersection between disease and drugs. The best possible example could be data available from the central database of patients can define the pathways involved in the specific disease are possibly reconstructed for drugs repositioning [19].

2.3.4 Target mechanism-based drug repurposing

Predicting the novel mechanism of action by this approach and resulting in drug repurposing for existing drugs. This is possible by gathering information from signaling pathway information, interaction networks of various proteins and also by data obtained from omics. Additionally, this will contribute to precision medicine. As, increasingly the individuals with their respective diseases have different pathophysiology among them. Precision medicine is upcoming solution for all these unique disease specific pathophysiological individuals. Advantages for drug repurposing by these approaches can discover not only different pathophysiological mechanisms but also providing treatment to them with respective drugs [19].

2.3.5 Machine learning

Machine learning (ML) techniques such as deep learning (DL), gradient boosted machine with trees (GBM), random forest (RF), support vector machine (SVM), logistic regression with elastic net regularization (EN), deep neural networks (DNN) have been usually applied for repositioning of various drugs [20, 21].

2.3.6 Network models

The various interaction patterns such as protein-protein, drug-disease, disease-gene, drug-target, drug-drug, disease-disease and transcriptomes and cell signaling networks are usually procured from different databases, which are interpreted computationally. The network models represent each and everything like drug, disease, gene and related products and their interaction patterns, for example, nodes (drug, disease and genes) and edges (interaction patterns of nodes). Network models are divided in to two types, these includes: network-based cluster approaches and network-based propagation approaches [19].

2.3.6.1 Network-based cluster approaches

These kinds of approaches have been proposed in order to determine the mechanism/relationships between the drug and the disease or the drug and the target/receptor. The biological interaction pattern in our human body has a characteristic network. The entities such as disease, drug and the protein share similar kind of interaction pattern in the network-based cluster approaches. This approach has been incorporated to develop various kinds of modules using the network topology-based cluster algorithms such as cliques/clusters/groups, subnetworks. They portray relationships or pattern of interaction between drug-drug, disease, target/receptors. The overlapping clusters cannot be detected by CLIQUE, OPTICS, DBSCAN and STING [20]. These modules are most commonly used network-based cluster approaches. Examples of repurposed drugs using network approach are atomoxetine indicated for Parkinson's disease and repurposed for attention deficit hyperactivity disorder (ADHD), etanercept indicated for rheumatoid arthritis and repurposed for asthma [3].

2.3.6.2 Network-based propagation approaches

These approaches have been categorized as another important approach under network strategies. They can be classified in two types: local and global approach. The information under this approach circulates from node (source) to all the nodes which are networked to each other and followed by subnetwork nodes [19].

Many studies have stated that these techniques are really being helpful and providing some useful results in obtaining interaction patterns/relationships between the drug—target/receptor, gene, disease. Local propagation procures small/fewer amount of data from the database and displays improper results. In opposing to this global approach gathers all of the data from database/network and make correct predictions. Currently, researchers are working on global approach for drug repurposing/repositioning [1, 19].

2.3.7 Genetic association

Genome-wide association studies (GWAS) has been widely used to determine the genetic alterations in whole genome which contribute to specific diseases and provides the pathophysiology of various diseases. The data obtained from the GWAS helps to identify novel targets which contributes to the specific diseases can provide repositioning of several drugs. Human Genome Project has already been completed and vast amount of data is available for specific diseases. So, there is a huge opportunity for various drugs that could be repositioned and provide beneficial outcome. However, the data available from GWAS does not provide exact pathophysiological mechanism and the available data is not appropriate due to the gene variant. As, there many still thousands of genes hidden which is yet to be discovered and these hidden genes may be contributing largely behind pathophysi-ology of various diseases [1].

2.3.8 Signature-based repurposing

Signature inversion method is defined as the approaches which screens the inverse relationships/interaction pattern of drug and the disease by correlating the gene expression information between the drug-disease. As defined this method utilizes the expression of genes to discover off-target mechanisms as well as novel pathophysiological mechanisms related to diseases. One of the prime advantages of these approaches is that they identify unique/novel mechanisms of action for drugs. Additionally, unlike knowledge-based methods that use the databases to predict the mechanism or action of drugs, more molecular- and/or genetic-level mechanisms are involved in signature-based repurposing methods [1].

2.3.9 Text mining (data mining) and semantic approach

The data available in the literature contains large and varied amount of information/data for all the drugs in the database as well as for the diseases (including orphan/rare diseases) which are commonly occurred in individuals. Through these data one can potentially predict the new indications of existing drugs via text mining approach. Gene ontology/biological ontology allows us to correlate the available information and analyze all the biological data from different databases. One such example of repurposed drug is Everolimus indicated for immunosuppressant and repurposed for pancreatic neuroendocrine tumors [3].

Semantic inference incorporates techniques like topic modeling which utilizes different databases for the discovery of repurposing of existing drugs. Example of repurposed drug was amphetamine which was indicated for CNS stimulant and repurposed for hyperkinesis in children (ADHD) [3].

3. Drug repurposing/repositioning for orphan diseases/disorders

Approximately 7000 rare diseases are currently present in the world and more than 95% among these lack therapeutic agents approved by US-FDA [1]. The concept behind orphan disease might be many yet they have a single key point which is common that is the disease affects a minor part of the population. The definition of orphan diseases differs in different countries. In US, orphan disease is the one affecting fewer than 2 lakh people, in Japan the disease should affect fewer than 50,000 people to be called as orphan disease and in Europe the prevalence should be 5 in 10,000 [1, 22].

It is very challenging to develop new drugs for the treatment of rare diseases because the number of patients suffering from these diseases are very limited and are distributed over a vast geographical area. Another issue is of high variability among these diseases, influenced mostly by genetic factors. Financially, the development and subsequent production of these drugs is not viable for the pharmaceutical companies therefore drug repurposing for orphan diseases is a good option [22]. The patients requiring immediate treatment also do not have the luxury of more time at their disposal therefore a new strategy is needed so that the drugs are made available faster and cheaper to these patients. The pathology and various biochemical pathways of many orphan diseases are not very well known. Computational techniques will be a helpful option in the case where the underlying mechanism of the disease is not well understood. The advancement of the huge scale genomic sequencing project may lead to the understanding of the genetic variations that may be the cause of these diseases and it may lead to possibility of repurposing the drugs which are targeting the concerned protein [1]. There are few examples of repurposed drugs described in **Table 2**.

The approved drugs have already undergone intense testing like the safety studies, bioavailability studies and PK/PD studies and therefore drug repurposing leads to significant cost cutting and faster development [22]. Hence, this is an attractive prospect for the pharmaceutical industry as well. A total of 51 new medications reaching the market in 2009, the drugs which came to the market via the strategy of drug repurposing were 30% [23].

There are particular regulations designed to promote the research into orphan diseases and these rules could give market exclusiveness in circumstances repurposed agents cannot be protected by the patent. The Orphan Drug Act (ODA; 1983) was introduced for the first time which reflected the issues regarding the economics of drug development for orphan disease and how it was unfavorable. FDA has licensed about 360 agents for rare diseases since 1983 as compared to less than 50 agents before 1983 [24]. US legislation provides for faster FDA approval, tax incentives and funding support for research in orphan diseases. Market protection is also one of the incentives in which a generic form is not allowed to come to the market for 7 years. Tax concession, waiving of the regulatory fees are also the incentives which are provided. Similar legislation has been implemented in Singapore, Japan, Europe and Australia after the success of ODA, with each jurisdiction having a little bit of difference in the definition of the indication and the incentives to be provided [1].

Drug	Original indication	New indication
Thalidomide	Morning sickness	Erythema nodosum leprosum and multiple myeloma
Sildenafil	Angina	Erectile dysfunction
Minoxidil	Hypertension	Hair loss
Zidovudine	Cancer	HIV/AIDS
Celecoxib	Pain and inflammation	Familial adenomatous polyps
Atomoxetine	Parkinson disease	ADHD
Aspirin	Analgesia	Colorectal cancer
Ketoconazole	Fungal infections	Cushing syndrome
Topiramate	Epilepsy	Obesity
Dapoxetine	Analgesia and depression	Premature ejaculation
Raloxifene	Osteoporosis	Breast cancer
Rituximab	Cancers	Rheumatoid arthritis
Duloxetine	Depression	Stress urinary incontinence.
Fingolimod	Transplant rejection	Multiple sclerosis
Bupropion	Depression	Smoking cessation
Lidocaine	Local anesthetic	Arrhythmia

Table 2.
A few examples of repurposed drugs with their new indication.

Another area of concern is the broad group of infectious diseases known to affect more than 1 billion population in tropical and subtropical areas [22]. Populations that are severely impacted are the people living below poverty line, not having appropriate sanitary conditions and in direct contact with contagious vectors or domestic animals [25]. The therapies currently present have many drawbacks like pricing and increase probability of drug resistance. Moreover, there are not much financial gains for investing money in developing drugs for these diseases as the patient population is unable to afford them [26]. Subsequently, given that the profit-making companies produce almost all the drugs, these firms will hardly be having any interest in investing in drug research and development which will not produce high financial returns. For this reason, development of therapies for these diseases becomes increasingly necessary. As discussed earlier that drug repurposing is an effective method due to various reasons, it can also be effectively used in this area where resources are limited and there is a huge need for productive therapies. Miltefosine, used for visceral leishmaniasis originally was antineoplastic agent whereas Amphotericin B used to treat fungal infections was repurposed for treating visceral leishmaniasis [22]. Other examples include Tamoxifen (agent for breast cancer) has shown to have anti-leishmanial activity, eflornithine (topical agent for hirsutism) has shown to be effective for sleeping sickness and auranofin (drug for rheumatoid arthritis) has shown to be effective against lymphatic filariasis and Onchocerca volvulus induced river blindness [27].

These days, multiple researches have demonstrated encouraging results in terms of repositioning supported by computational methods like chemical genomics screening for developing agents for such kind of diseases like schistosomiasis [28]. Some other examples where drug repurposing has shown promise for these diseases are vandetanib, trametinib and atorvastatin [29, 30].

Drug repurposing strategies have also been used in the cases of viral diseases like Zika virus where FDA approved drug for hepatitis C which is Sofosbuvir has shown promising results [22]. The target of this drug is RNA polymerase which is present in Hepatitis C and Zika virus and has shown to reduce viral load in experimental studies [31, 32]. The same is the case with prochlorperazine by targeting the binding and the entry of the virus to host cells has shown to have a strong antiviral activity against dengue virus [22].

Drug repurposing is cheaper and faster than the conventional methods and thus gives hope to the patients where the population suffering from the disease is much smaller and making the traditional model of drug discovery nonviable. A collective effort is required among all the stakeholders if already available drugs have to be repurposed. This approach helps in reducing the potential risks and the expense of developing a new agent, therefore having the ability of revolutionizing the drug market of orphan diseases.

4. Regulatory considerations for drug repurposing

In the US, to get permission for drug repurposing, research and pharma companies need to file applications under suitable sections including 505(b)(1), or 505(b)(2) or 505(j), depending upon the regulatory paths. Further, the company needs to fill NDA type 6 and sNDA (supplemental new drug application) for new indication of drug, NDA type 3 for new dosage form and NDA type 4 for drug new combination in drug repurposing [1, 33].

5. Future perspectives of drug repurposing in orphan disease therapeutics

As orphan disease affects a small percentage of the population, research and pharma companies face great challenge and burden in developing drugs for its management because of small market potential. Patients fail to get proper care, diagnosis and treatment. Even if the treatment is available, it is relatively expensive. Thus, drug repurposing can be of great help in orphan disease therapeutics. It saves both' the time and money involved in the drug development process. In October 2010, "Dr Ruxandra Draghia-Akli, the Directorate-General for Research and Innovation (DG RTD) of the European Commission (EC) and Dr Francis Collins, US National Institutes of Health (NIH)" at Reykjavík (Iceland), launched the International Rare Diseases Research Consortium (IRDiRC) to look after the drug and research development in orphan/rare diseases [34]. This consortium unites both government and private research funding societies to advance the drug development for orphan diseases at global level including task forces and drug repurposing in orphan disease therapeutics.

The research in rare diseases has already changed the global approach because earlier researchers were not much interested in repurposing the existing drug but some global breakthrough has really changed the minds of pharma companies and examples are alglucerase that was obtained from human placental tissue and was widely used for Type I Gaucher disease as a "first enzyme replacement therapy" and, it was also approved by FDA in 1991. However, it was withdrawn from the market due to adverse effect and already available drugs in the market which are prepared from recombinant DNA technology which are safe to use [35]. Fomivirsen which is an antisense oligonucleotide and was approved by FDA for

Cytomegalovirus in 1998 but it has been withdrawn from the market due to the development of highly active antiretroviral therapy (HAART) but this was the "first antisense oligonucleotide therapy" [35]. Imatinib was approved by FDA in 2001 for Philadelphia chromosome-positive chronic myelogenous leukemia (CML) as "first targeted cancer therapy" [35]. Alipogene tiparvovec was the "first targeted gene therapy" to be approved in Europe in 2012 for reversing lipoprotein lipase deficiency (LPLD) in patients with pancreatitis [35]. Strimvelis was the "First ex-vivo gene therapy" approved for patients with Severe Combined Immunodeficiency due to Adenosine Deaminase deficiency (ADA-SCID) [35]. USFDA has approved Holoclar as orphan drug for the treatment of limbal stem cell deficiency (LSCD). Currently, this drug is in Phase IV trial and completing in mid of the year 2020 [36].

To overcome R&D-associated financial challenges and clinical trials-related failures of novel drugs, at present scenario, pharmaceutical companies are much more interested in switching to "drug repurposing" or "drug repositioning" drug development by adopting various computational approaches rather than going for de novo drug discovery, which is relatively expensive, risky and time consuming [37]. According to Southall et al. [35], the global market for drug repositioning will possibly be hiked to over $31 billion by 2020, up from about $24 billion in 2015, thus representing large commercial possibility [35].

6. Conclusion

De novo drug development is being time consuming, costly and risk-prone venture 'drug repurposing' has drawn attention of all pharma companies and R and D sectors which offers faster and cheaper ways for bringing new drugs into the market especially for targeting ODs. Based upon the benefits provided by drug repurpos-ing, the development of more sophisticated and systematic approach is required to find more drug candidates that can be fitted into the picture of promising targets for repurposing.

Notes/thanks/other declarations

None.

Author details

Neha Dhir†, Ashish Jain†, Dhruv Mahendru†, Ajay Prakash and Bikash Medhi*
Department of Pharmacology, Postgraduate Institute of Medical Education and Research (PGIMER), Chandigarh, India

*Address all correspondence to: drbikashus@yahoo.com

† All authors have equal contribution.

References

[1] Pushpakom S, Iorio F, Eyers PA, Escott KJ, Hopper S, Wells A, et al. Drug repurposing: Progress, challenges and recommendations. Nature Reviews. Drug Discovery. 2019;**18**(1):41-58

[2] Scannell JW, Blanckley A, Boldon H, Warrington B. Diagnosing the decline in pharmaceutical R&D efficiency. Nature Reviews. Drug Discovery. 2012;**11**(3):191-200

[3] Xue H, Li J, Xie H, Wang Y. Review of drug repositioning approaches and resources. International Journal of Biological Sciences. 2018;**14**(10):1232-1244

[4] Ashburn TT, Thor KB. Drug repositioning: Identifying and developing new uses for existing drugs. Nature Reviews. Drug Discovery. 2004;**3**(8):673-683

[5] Novac N. Challenges and opportunities of drug repositioning. Trends in Pharmacological Sciences. 2013;**34**(5):267-272

[6] Osterloh IH. The discovery and development of Viagra® (sildenafil citrate). In: Dunzendorfer U, editor. Sildenafil. Basel: Birkhäuser Basel; 2004. pp. 1-13

[7] Schwab RS, Poskanzer DC, England AC Jr, Young RR. Amantadine in Parkinson's disease. Review of more than two years' experience. Journal of the American Medical Association. 1972;**222**(7):792-795

[8] Oberoi SS. Regulating off-label drug use in India: The arena for concern. Perspectives in Clinical Research. 2015;**6**(3):129-133

[9] Wittich CM, Burkle CM, Lanier WL. Ten common questions (and their answers) about off-label drug use. Mayo Clinic Proceedings. 2012;**87**(10):982-990

[10] Aronson JK. Rare diseases and orphan drugs. British Journal of Clinical Pharmacology. 2006;**61**(3):243-245

[11] Hift RJ, Meissner PN. An analysis of 112 acute porphyric attacks in Cape Town, South Africa: Evidence that acute intermittent porphyria and variegate porphyria differ in susceptibility and severity. Medicine. 2005;**84**(1):48-60

[12] Sardana D, Zhu C, Zhang M, Gudivada RC, Yang L, Jegga AG. Drug repositioning for orphan diseases. Briefings in Bioinformatics. 2011;**12**(4): 346-356

[13] Lavandeira A. Orphan drugs: Legal aspects, current situation. Haemophilia. 2002;**8**(3):194-198

[14] Brehmer D, Greff Z, Godl K, Blencke S, Kurtenbach A, Weber M, et al. Cellular targets of gefitinib. Cancer Research. 2005;**65**(2):379-382

[15] Aulner N, Danckaert A, Ihm J, Shum D, Shorte SL. Next-generation phenotypic screening in early drug discovery for infectious diseases. Trends in Parasitology. 2019; **35**(7):559-570

[16] Iljin K, Ketola K, Vainio P, Halonen P, Kohonen P, Fey V, et al. High-throughput cell-based screening of 4910 known drugs and drug-like small molecules identifies disulfiram as an inhibitor of prostate cancer cell growth. Clinical Cancer Research. 2009;**15**(19):6070-6078

[17] Zheng W, Thorne N, McKew JC. Phenotypic screens as a renewed approach for drug discovery. Drug Discovery Today. 2013;**18**(21-22): 1067-1073

[18] Cousin MA, Ebbert JO, Wiinamaki AR, Urban MD, Argue DP, Ekker SC, et al. Larval zebrafish model for FDA-approved drug repositioning for tobacco

dependence treatment. PLoS ONE. 2014;**9**(3):e90467

[19] Park K. A review of computational drug repurposing. Translational and Clinical Pharmacology. 2019; **27**(2):59-63

[20] GNS HS, Saraswathy GR, Murahari M, Krishnamurthy M. An update on drug repurposing: Re-written saga of the drug's fate. Biomedicine & Pharmacotherapy. 2019;**110**:700-716

[21] Zhao K, So HC. A machine learning approach to drug repositioning based on drug expression profiles: Applications to schizophrenia and depression/anxiety disorders. arXiv preprint arXiv:1706.03014. 2017

[22] Oliveira EAM, Lang KL. Drug repositioning: Concept, classification, methodology, and importance in rare/ orphans and neglected diseases. Journal of Applied Pharmaceutical Science. 2018;**8**(08):157-165

[23] Graul AI, Sorbera L, Pina P, Tell M, Cruces E, Rosa E, et al. The year's new drugs & biologics—2009. Drug News & Perspectives. 2010;**23**(1):7-36

[24] Xu K, Coté TR. Database identifies FDA-approved drugs with potential to be repurposed for treatment of orphan diseases. Briefings in Bioinformatics. 2011;**12**(4):341-345

[25] World Health Organization. Neglected Tropical Diseases. Available from: https://www.who.int/neglected_diseases/diseases/en/ [Accessed: 17 February 2020]

[26] Berenstein AJ, Magariños MP, Chernomoretz A, Agüero F. A multilayer network approach for guiding drug repositioning in neglected diseases. PLoS Neglected Tropical Diseases. 2016;**10**(1):e0004300

[27] Klug DM, Gelb MH, Pollastri MP. Repurposing strategies for tropical disease drug discovery. Bioorganic & Medicinal Chemistry Letters. 2016;**26**(11):2569-2576

[28] Neves BJ, Braga RC, Bezerra JCB, Cravo PVL, Andrade CH. In silico repositioning-chemogenomics strategy identifies new drugs with potential activity against multiple life stages of *Schistosoma mansoni*. PLoS Neglected Tropical Diseases. 2015;**9**(1):e3435

[29] Rojo-Arreola L, Long T, Asarnow D, Suzuki BM, Singh R, Caffrey CR. Chemical and genetic validation of the statin drug target to treat the helminth disease, schistosomiasis. PLoS One. 2014;**9**(1):e87594

[30] Cowan N, Keiser J. Repurposing of anticancer drugs: In vitro and in vivo activities against *Schistosoma mansoni*. Parasites & Vectors. 2015;**8**:417

[31] Sacramento CQ , de Melo GR, de Freitas CS, Rocha N, Hoelz LVB, Miranda M, et al. The clinically approved antiviral drug sofosbuvir inhibits Zika virus replication. Scientific Reports. 2017;**7**(1):40920

[32] Ferreira AC, Zaverucha-do-Valle C, Reis PA, Barbosa-Lima G, Vieira YR, Mattos M, et al. Sofosbuvir protects Zika virus-infected mice from mortality, preventing short- and long-term sequelae. Scientific Reports. 2017;**7**(1):9409

[33] Dhir N, Sinha S, Medhi B. Drug repurposing. In: Medhi B, Prakash A, editors. Advanced Pharmacology. 2nd ed. India: PharmaMed Press. pp. 630-640

[34] Dawkins HJS, Draghia-Akli R, Lasko P, Lau LPL, Jonker AH, Cutillo CM, et al. Progress in rare diseases research 2010-2016: An IRDiRC perspective. Clinical and Translational Science. 2018;**11**(1):11-20

[35] Southall NT, Natarajan M, Lau LP, Jonker AH, Deprez B, Guilliams T, et al. The use or generation of biomedical data and existing medicines to discover and establish new treatments for patients with rare diseases–recommendations of the IRDiRC Data Mining and Repurposing Task Force. Orphanet Journal of Rare Diseases. 2019;**14**(1):1-8

[36] Fda.https:/wwwaccessdatafdagov/scripts/opdlisting/oopd/detailedIndexcf m?cfgridkey=632218 [Online]. Available from: https://www.accessdata.fda.gov/scripts/opdlisting/oopd/detailedIndex. cfm?cfgridkey=632218 [Accessed: 28 February 2020]

[37] Yella JK, Yaddanapudi S, Wang Y, Jegga AG. Changing trends in computational drug repositioning. Pharmaceuticals. 2018;**11**(2):57

12

Drug Repurposing Techniques in Viral Diseases

Ran Zhang, Rick Oerlemans, Chao Wang, Lili Zhang and Matthew R. Groves

Abstract

Since the advent of the twentieth century, several severe virus outbreaks have occurred—H1N1 (1918), H2N2 (1957), H3N2 (1968), H1N1 (2009) and recently COVID-19 (2019)—all of which have posed serious challenges to public health. Therefore, rapid identification of efficacious antiviral medications is of ongoing paramount importance in combating such outbreaks. Due to the long cycle of drug development, not only in the development of a "safe" medication but also in mandated and extensive (pre)clinical trials before a drug can be safely licensed for use, it is difficult to access effective and safe novel antivirals. This is of particular importance in addressing infectious disease in appropriately short period of time to limit stress to ever more interlinked societal infrastructures; including interruptions to economic activity, supply routes as well as the immediate impact on health care. Screening approved drugs or drug candidates for antiviral activity to address emergent diseases (i.e. repurposing) provides an elegant and effective strategy to circumvent this problem. As such treatments (in the main) have already received approval for their use in humans, many of their limitations and contraindications are well known, although efficacy against new diseases must be shown in appropriate laboratory trials and clinical studies. A clear in this approach in the case of antivirals is the "relative" simplicity and a high degree of conservation of the molecular mechanisms that support viral replication—which improves the chances for a functional antiviral to inhibit replication in a related viral species. However, recent experiences have shown that while repurposing has the potential to identify such cases, great care must be taken to ensure a rigourous scientific underpinning for repurposing proposals. Here, we present a brief explanation of drug repurposing and its approaches, followed by an overview of recent viral outbreaks and associated drug development. We show how drug repurposing and combination approaches have been used in viral infectious diseases, highlighting successful cases. Special emphasis has been placed on the recent COVID-19 outbreak, and its molecular mechanisms and the role repurposing can/has play(ed) in the discovery of a treatment.

Keywords: viral infectious disease, COVID-19, drug development, drug repurposing, drug repurposing strategies, applications

1. Introduction

The development of a new drug is an extensive, intricate, highly risky and expensive process. According to the study of 12,728 transitions over the last decade

(2011–2020), the success rates of clinical drug development were 52.0% (Phase I), 28.9% (Phase II) and 57.8% (Phase III) separately [1]. Most of the candidates failed in the early drug development process for reasons of efficacy and safety concerns [2]. This causes a huge cost in drug development, ranging from tens of millions to billions. In addition, it typically takes at least 10 years from initial laboratory evaluation for a new drug to be approved. All these factors lead to low output disproportionately to the high input and make it challenging for the pharmaceutical industry to respond to emergent infectious diseases within a time frame that is able to impact the course of an outbreak. As a result, the development of vaccine candidates will likely remain to be the optimal mechanism to address outbreaks in the immediate future. Notwithstanding the extraordinary developments in vaccine technology—exemplified by recent events [3, 4]—there still remains a need for therapeutics as a sufficiently successful virus will rapidly become pan/endemic, creating a constant need for treatment of those unfortunate enough to not have access to a vaccine due to socioeconomic, age or immunostatus issues. Indeed, in the case of a pandemic, there is likely to be constant strain on health systems to treat patients, which will significantly enhanced in the absence of an effective therapy as it will instead rely heavily on patient support technologies such as ventilation or oxygen therapy.

A potential solution to this conundrum is the examination of already proposed (ideally approved) medications—repurposing—to assess their potential in the treatment of an emergent diseases. Drug repurposing as a strategy to identify potential new indication areas of approved/old drugs has many advantages. Firstly, low risk. Most repurposed drugs have at least been tested in early clinical trials. Hence, the failure rate of repurposing candidates caused by safety is very low. Secondly, low cost. Most old or approved drugs have clear safety, pharmacokinetics and pharmacodynamics data, which reduces the studies that need to be performed before the drugs extension to a novel indication. Thirdly, a higher success rate. The drugs used for repurposing are enriched from previous studies. This means less promising compounds are filtered out, allowing for a higher success rate [5]. Finally, while the molecular complexity of the protein targets of diseases is extremely broad, areas of essential molecular function can be identified as conserved in many diseases. For example, tyrosine kinase activity is a frequent target for the development of cancers from highly diverse tissues. A common feature of all kinases is the presence of an ATP-binding site, which has resulted in a large number of targeted cancer therapies (tyrosine kinase inhibitors, TKIs) which have a strong resemblance to ATP on the molecular level. This has further resulted in the clinical testing of TKIs for cancers distinct to those for which they were developed, as the evolutionary pressure to retain a function ATP-binding site provides a precondition for potential TKI cross-reactivity [6].

In the past decades, the successful application of drug repurposing shows a promising direction for drug development. For example, Thalidomide was firstly synthesized by Ciba in 1953 and came on to the market to relieve morning sickness in 1957. In 1961, Thalidomide was taken off the market due to the severe teratogenic effect on the developing fetus. In the following years, an Israeli researcher found that thalidomide could be used as a treatment against autoimmune diseases. In 1998 it was approved by FDA for the repurposed use in the treatment of ENL [7–9]. In this chapter, we present an overview of the benefits and drawbacks of drug repurposing in viral disease, including approaches, applications and outlook.

2. Drug repurposing

Drug repurposing is the process of identifying new indications and uses for approved/existing drugs [10]. It mostly involves approved drugs or compounds under study, which have clear pharmacokinetics and pharmacodynamics that provide data on metabolic stability, tissue distribution and clearance rates. In the past decades, a large quantity of new molecular entity drugs was approved or studied, meaning that not only the ~2000 FDA approved compounds can be screened [11, 12], but also a much larger potential library of compounds that have been developed to have appropriate physico-chemical properties for their use as drugs, but that may have failed clinical trials due to lack of action in their original disease class. This, perhaps, is the key benefit of repurposing—as all potential repurposing candidates possess "drug-like" properties. However, these properties should be borne in mind by the researcher as they strongly impact the potential of repurposed compounds in clinical use.

The classic description of "drug-like" properties has grown significantly since the original introduction of the "Rule of 5" by Lipinski (Ro5) [13]. This initial classification arose from the observation that successful drugs shared common properties: low molecular weight (Mw), a relative scarcity of potential electrostatic interactions (H-bond donors and acceptors) and a partition coefficient (logP) that indicated the molecules would be able to passively diffuse across cell membranes. While, the most important descriptors remain unchanged a summary of Lipinski's and others rules is provided in **Table 1** [13–17]. As repurposing candidates will be drawn from compounds that are likely to be enriched for these properties and therefore the potential route of administration for the repurposed disease should be compatible with these. For instance, compounds that are a good fit to Ro5 would be relatively poorly applied to diseases for which administration would be via inhala-tion [18]. Thus, the availability of this pharmacological information and likely route of administration is of key importance in deciding on which compounds should be assessed for repurposing.

In summary, these studies provide a wealth of information about the clinical application and mechanism of action, aiding the rapid development of the drug repurposing. When compared with *de novo* drug discovery, drug repurposing accelerates the development process and significantly reduces development risk [19].

2.1 Drug repurposing approaches

At its broadest level drug repurposing approaches can be divided into two geneal types: computer-based and experimental techniques [20, 21]. Within both these approaches there are three main angles of attack, drug-centric, target-centric and disease-centric methods [22]. As indicated by its name, drug-centric approaches start from the point of view of a drug, with the aim to find efficacy against dis-eases other than the initial indication. In the case of a disease-centric approach the disease is the focus, with the purpose being to identify and repurpose a drug

RO5	RO3	Ghose rules	Veber's Rules	MDDR-like rules
MW ≤ 500	MW < 300 Da	160 ≤ MW ≤ 480	NRTB < 10	RNG ≥ 3
HBD ≤ 5	HBD ≤ 3	−0.4 ≤ logP ≤5.6	PSA < 140 Å	RGB ≥ 18
HBA ≤ 10	HBA ≤ 3	30 ≤ AMR ≤ 130		NRTB ≥6
LogP ≤ 5	cLogP ≤3	20 ≤ NA ≤ 70		
	NRTB ≤3			

Abbreviations: MW, molecular weight; HBD, H-bond donor; HBA, H-bond acceptor; logP, octanol-water partition coefficient; clogP, calculated octanol-water partition coefficient; AMR, molar refractivity; PSA, total polar surface area; RGB, the number of rigid bond; HB, hydrogen bond; NAT, the number of atoms; NRTB, number of rotatable bonds; RNG, number of rings.

Table 1.
Summary of 'druglikeness' rules applied in drug development.

specifically against that disease. Target-centric methods utilize drugs that bind to well-characterized targets that are known to be, or at least suspected to be, involved in other diseases besides the drugs' original indication. What they have in common is that at the core these strategies often employ similarity assessment to identify drugs that can potentially be repurposed.

2.1.1 Computer-based approaches

Traditional drug repurposing often relies on the in vitro/in vivo identification of active drugs or alternative targets. Whilst this can provide promising compounds with reliable, desired activity, it can be expensive, involves physical access to the drug libraries and requires setup and optimization of the assays [23]. With the rapid development of bioinformatics and the accumulation of vast amounts of experimental data, the development of drug repurposing, especially the initial stage, has moved from traditional biological experiments towards an increasing diversity of computational screening approaches, partially due to the lower cost and lower barrier to entry [24].

2.1.1.1 Virtual screening

Virtual screening is an essential computational approach in drug discovery, and particularly in drug repurposing. It involves the use of computer programs to evaluate compound libraries on a specified criterion, usually similarity or calculated binding energy. Virtual screening can be classified into two categories: ligand-based and structure-based virtual screening [25, 26].

Ligand-based screening focuses on analyzing the structure-activity information of known active ligands against a certain indication to identify other potentially effective drugs. This analysis relies on similarity in the form of pharmacophores and geometric shape which can be informed by structural knowledge of the ligand-target complex to identify key pharmacophores or without structural information, relying on the structure-activity relationship information from experimental approaches to identify the pharmacophores [27]. Pharmacophores are the chemical moieties of drugs that play essential roles in the interaction with their targets. Pharmacophore features—including features such as hydrogen bond donors, hydro-gen bonds acceptors, charge groups, aromatic rings and hydrophobic centroids are then identified together with their spatial characteristics and mapped into a string [28]. This string can serve as a fingerprint, which can be used for easy similarity matching between different drugs, potentially identifying drugs that are also active against the disease.

This approach can be successful for small molecules as they are relatively simple molecules from a chemical perspective. Their pharmacophoric features are limited and usually rely on a few strong, deeply buried interactions with the target, making it easy to map and identify drugs with similar characteristics [29]. In contrast, biologics, such as peptides and antibodies, are far less suitable to these techniques as their method of actions typically dependent on mimicking protein-protein interactions, which are characterized by large, flat interaction surfaces [30, 31]. This makes them highly specific for their target, allowing for targeted therapies with typically less side-effects, but that specificity also prevents them from being repurposed for a different target.

In contrast, structure-based virtual screening uses the three-dimensional structure of a target of therapeutic interest [32, 33], which is screened against a virtual library of approved drugs in order to identify those that show interactions with this novel target. Drugs are docked against the target and interaction analysis is performed based on binding energy and binding geometry. Many different docking software packages have been developed with the key differences being in the docking methodologies and the scoring functions used to rank the drugs [34]. Classical scoring functions usually rely on experimental data or prior information to rank the drugs. However, these have been consistently getting outperformed by machine learning based scoring functions, especially when specific target data is available to train on [35, 36].

Developments in computational power have made virtual screening approaches highly accessible to labs all over the world as they do not require nearly the amount of financial resources compared to wet-lab experiments. In addition, due to the speed at which the screenings can be performed nowadays, huge libraries containing 100's of millions of compounds can be screened against a target rapidly massively increasing the chemical space explored [37]. Though these advances are very useful in early drug discovery, where it can be used to screen fragment and compound libraries that cover a diversity in chemical space, they are less impactful when it comes to drug repurposing since the amount of approved drugs is limited and does not comprise wide chemical space. A downside of structure-based screening is the need for the actual structural information, which can be difficult to obtain for novel targets. Fortunately the number of entries available in the PDB has been growing at an exceptional rate, more than doubling in the last decade [38], meaning more and more targets have structural information available. In addition, the recent achievements of AlphaFold [39], including the prediction of the 3-dimensional structures of the entire human proteome, might alleviate this issue [40]. Overall this still has a positive impact on drug repurposing strategies as the more struc-tural information is available the better scoring functions can be become, aiding both ligand-based and structure-based methods in identifying drugs that can be repurposed.

2.1.1.2 Machine learning approaches

Machine learning is an overarching term used to describe diverse algorithms that use data sets to perform intelligent predictions [41]. The algorithms can be trained on large datasets to identify patterns and interactions. The trained algorithm can then be applied to novel data to identify or predict outcomes or interactions.

Computer based drug repurposing techniques utilizing machine learning have been gaining a lot of traction due to a large increase in available omics data in a variety of databases and the development of sophisticated algorithms that can utilize this data [42–44]. It is carried out using computational biology, bioinformatics and database tools, which allows for economical and high efficiency drug discovery [45]. Machine learning techniques used for drug repurposing include: k-nearest neighbor algorithms, decision tree, random forest, artificial neural networks, k-means clustering and principal component analysis [20, 46, 47].

In recent years researchers have not been able to keep up with the amount of information being generated by omics experiments, creating a need for different data analysis methods. Where previously they would manually comb through the data looking for patterns and connections, there has been a shift towards big data analysis utilizing machine learning approaches, which have shown several specific applications in drug repurposing [48].

Signature matching is an approach where complex patterns and profiles—signatures—are generated for diseases and drugs by machine learning algorithms from large omics datasets. By looking for negative correlations between differential signatures resulting from diseases and from drug treatments, drugs can be identified that can serve as treatments for those diseases outside of their original indication [5, 20]. Simultaneously, drug signatures can also be compared with the signatures of structurally dissimilar drugs, with the idea being that if drugs show a similar signature they can share a therapeutic application irrespective of chemical similarity. For both these applications there is an alternative signature that can be compared, the clinical phenotype signature. Even though some diseases or drugs might show little to no similarities in direct transcriptomic, metabolomics or pro-teomic patterns, they could still have similar clinical phenotypic outcomes, which can also allow for the identification of repurposing uses of drugs [49].

Another use of signature matching is in finding similar chemical features of drugs and mapping a network based on shared features. This allows for the identification of drugs that may potentially be repurposed—as similarity in pharmacophores tends to correlate with a similarity in biological activity.

Related to signature-based methods, application of genome-wide association studies (GWAS) have also shown to be valuable within the field of drug repurposing [50]. GWAS data can be analyzed using machine learning approaches to identify interaction and association patterns of genes linked to diseases [51]. Genes identi-fied by GWAS to associate with a disease tend to be enriched with druggable targets. By cross-referencing the disease enriched genes with databases containing drug-target information drugs can be found that inhibit specific genes that are involved in other indications but also seemingly play a role in the GWAS investigated disease, potentially being able to reuse that drug. In addition if a gene is shown to be associ-ated with a disease it could become a novel drug target, which can be screened against using approved drug libraries.

Even though GWAS identified genes can be associated with a disease that does not mean that the target is druggable. Pathway mapping could be a potential tool to leverage the information gained with GWAS and expand upon it [52]. By analyzing the pathways or protein interaction networks up and/or downstream of the GWAS identified genes, other, previously elusive, proteins can be identified that could play a role in disease progression. This can either yield new drug targets or repurpos-ing opportunities of drugs that already inhibit the elucidated target. For example, pathway analysis was performed on data sets containing gene expression data from human hosts infected with many different respiratory viruses. This identified 67 conserved biological pathways that could play an important role in respiratory viral infections. Comparing these pathways to a drug-target database resulted in drugs like pranlukast and amrinone, drugs with a different indication, that could poten-tial be used in treating viral infections [53].

2.1.2 Experiment-based approaches

Empirical evidence is still highest order of evidence and remains the golden standard for drug screening, including drug repurposing. Since experimental assays provide the most immediate evidence of drug activity [51] they are not only used to discover potential repurposing candidates from libraries but they are also essential in validating hits from computational approaches.

Inhibition assays can serve to identify target-specific drug efficacy, including inhibition constants. Binding assays are very powerful as they can also provide binding constant information [54]. Immediate use can be made of the identified binding drug that might not be highly specific or effective but it could serve as a temporary stop gap in emergency situations (like pandemics). Whilst the repurposed drug is being used as a sort of band aid, drug development can be undertaken in parallel, using the drug as the starting point. Rapid SAR approaches can then be utilized to improve the drug binding and efficacy [55]. The fact that the resulting drug would ideally be quite similar to the approved drug could lead to accelerated approval processes.

2.1.2.1 Binding assays

Binding assays aim to detect the interaction(s) between two (bio)molecules, such as protein-protein, peptide-protein, nucleic acid-protein, small molecule-protein, or small molecule-nucleic acid and ideally also evaluate the degree of the interaction [56]. These assays can be used in two ways, in screening approaches to qualitatively identify hits that interact with the target and in a quantitative way to characterize the binding affinity.

There are many examples of different types of qualitative assays that have been used in drug repurposing approaches. Among the most common are immobilization or affinity chromatography, where either the target or the drug are immobilized on a matrix or column followed by exposure to a drug library or potential binding targets [57]. The complexes that have formed can then be eluted and identified using analytic methods. DNA-encoded libraries encompassing wide chemical space have been used in such approaches. After eluting complexes binding compounds are identified by sequencing the DNA-barcode attached to the binding compound. This technique can also be applied to approved drug libraries [58].

The aforementioned assays are aimed at screening large libraries for hits. However, obtaining detailed binding information such as dissociation constants (K_D), is crucial in the identification and development of potent drugs. Several biophysical techniques are available to quantify these interactions. Microscale Thermophoresis (MST) can be used to measure binding affinity by detecting changes in molecular motion in a temperature gradient in the presence and absence of different compound concentrations [59]. Differential scanning fluorimetry (DSF) can be used to measure protein unfolding temperature by monitoring in fluorescence of a probe that binds to hydrophobic moieties in a denaturing temperature gradient. Upon binding of drugs to the protein it can stabilize the complex, leading to a shift in unfolding temperature. By using a range of drug concentrations and measuring the effect on the thermal shift the K_D can be calculated [60]. Surface plasmon resonance (SPR) is a technique in which the target or drug of interest is immobilized on a thin metal film. A light source is aimed at the other side of the film and the surface Plasmon resonance angle is detected. When a drug or target binds to the immobilized partner the local mass at the sensor surface changes, causing a shift in the angle of reflection proportional to the mass. By measuring these changes in the presence and absence of drug or target, association and dissociation constants can be determined [61]. Isothermal titration calorimetry (ITC), one of the golden standards in K_D determination, can directly measure all binding parameters by measuring heat transfer. When binding of drug to target occurs, enthalpy changes (heat absorbed or released) of the system can be measured by a highly sensitive calorimeter. By titrating ligand against the target of interest the Kd, stoichiometry, enthalpy and entropy can be directly measured in the native states of the binding partners since no modifications are required [62].

2.1.2.2 Phenotypic screening

Where binding assays are typically focused on identifying target-drug interactions, phenotypic screening takes a more disease-centric approach. Phenotypic assays aim to identify compounds that show effects on disease-relevant outcomes [63]. These are usually performed on cell lines or organelles engineered to function as disease mod-els. Since the assay is target agnostic less, or no, information about specific targets is obtained. However, the fact that it is agnostic also means that there are more potential targets available within this complex environment, which could lead to the discovery of new targets that would otherwise be left unexplored [63]. There are also additional benefits to this approach in the context of drug repurposing. Since the assays are disease based and compounds are approved drugs or clinical candidates it means that if positive outcomes are obtained the drug already has positive properties and shown efficacy in more complex systems, which is beneficial to real world applications [64].

2.1.3 Side effect based or "serendipitous" drug repurposing

One of the most frequent reasons for drugs failing in (pre)clinical trials is the determination of a side effect that cannot be ignored. Most commonly this is determined to be a dangerous side effect that argues against further clinical investigation of the compound. However, one man's meat is another man's poison. These drugs with unwanted side effects can be given new indications through a drug repurposing strategy. Side effects-based drug repurposing links indications with clinical effect and is one of the common strategies employed for drug repurposing [65, 66]. A key example in this area is Sildenafil, which was originally entered into clinical trials as a drug to treat hypertension and angina [65, 67–70]. Unfortunately, Phase I clinical trials suggested that it had little effect on angina. However, use of Sildenafil causes a significant side effect: marked penile erections. This lead to the discovery that Sildenafil could be used as a treatment for erectile dysfunction (ED) [71]. In 1988, Sildenafil was approved by the FDA for the treatment of ED. Such repurposing approaches could be termed serendipitous repurposing, as the new indication area is revealed during clinical trials. As a result, such repurposing is relatively rare.

3. Drug repurposing in viral diseases

Over the last decades the world has seen multiple severe viral outbreaks resulting in millions of deaths. Among the deadliest were the Influenza pandemics such as H1N1 (1918), H2N2 (1957), H3N2 (1968) and H1N1 (2009). The HIV/AIDS epidemic that was first recognized in the 1980s and went global has also caused up to an estimated amount of 36 million deaths and is still ongoing. Besides the large, deadly pandemics there have been smaller but very impactful localized epidem-ics such as Dengue virus (DENV), Zika virus (ZIKV), Ebola virus (EBOV) and Middle East respiratory-syndrome corona virus (MERS-CoV) which pose serious challenges to public health. Most recently in 2019 there was an outbreak of Severe acute respiratory syndrome coronavirus 2 (SARS-CoV-2) which caused the COVID- 19 pandemic, affecting nearly every country in the world with over 226 million reported cases to date [72]. Despite the advances in controlling viral pathogens that come with the widespread mass vaccination, there are no approved specific (effec-tive) therapies for the treatment of most viral infections.

By exploring new targets and mechanisms, drug repurposing provides new indications for old drugs. The major time advantage of repurposing is that this approach allows repurposed drugs to quickly enter clinical trials, which is of significant importance in reacting to disease outbreaks, especially in the case of worldwide pandemics.

3.1 Drug repurposing for COVID-19

The outbreak of COVID-19, caused by SARS-CoV-2, has spread across the world. There is, as yet, no specific treatment for COVID-19 approved. Drug repurposing provides a fast and economical option for the identification of medications target-ing SARS-CoV-2.

SARS-CoV-2 is a member of of the betacoronaviruses family. It is a single-stranded RNA virus, characterized by large crown-like spikes protruding on the viral surface and an unusually large RNA genome which encodes four main structural proteins: spike (S), envelope (E), membrane (M), and nucleocapsid (N) [62, 73, 74]. Like other coronaviruses, SARS-CoV-2 cell entry is mediated by the spike glycoprotein. The spike glycoprotein is composed of two subunits, S1 and S2, which mediate viral-host attachment and viral-host membrane fusion cascade, respectively [75]. SARS-CoV-2 spike recognizes and binds to the human ACE2 (hACE2) receptor through its receptor-binding domain (RBD) and is primed and activated by proteolytic cleavage by enzymes such as Furin and transmembrane serine protease 2 (TMPRSS2) [76, 77]. Spike, ACE2, Furin and TMPRSS2 have been shown to play a key role in mediating viral-host fusion attachment and fusion, and the Furin cleavage site on the Spike protein has been indicated as one of major reasons SARS-CoV-2 is so infectious [78, 79]. This makes these potentially promising drug targets for COVID-19 treatment [80, 81].

3.1.1 Drug repurposing targeting viral fusion

Inhibition of the Spike-Ace2 interaction is a primary target for drug repurposing as it is crucial to viral entry. *In silico* approaches have been performed and identified Simeprevir, an HCV NSP3A/4 protease inhibitor, as a potential blocker of Spike-Ace2 interaction by binding the RBD [82]. However, other *in vitro* studies showed that Simeprevir is not necessarily active against the RBD but is targeting the viral replication [83].

Another promising target is TMPRSS2, a serine protease. TMPRSS2 is associated to the host endothelial cell surface and cleaves the viral spike glycoprotein after binding to ACE2, activating it. The activation of spike protein then facilitates viral entry [84]. Camostat mesilate (a serine protease inhibitor) has been approved for the treatment of chronic pancreatitis, postoperative reflux esophagitis and kidney or liver disease fibrosis [81, 84, 85]. Since it is an established serine protease inhibitor it is a prime candidate to inhibit the TMPRSS2. An *in vitro* study indeed showed that camostat mesilate can suppress viral replication by halting the fusion of virus-cell membranes through the inhibition of TMPRSS2 [84]. Clinical trials using this drug are currently ongoing [86]. However, recently the results of a small double-blind randomized clinical trial using camostat mesi-late performed in patients hospitalized with COVID-19. The trial determined no adverse effects of treatment with camostat but also no increase in positive clinical outcomes [87].

3.1.2 Drug repurposing targeting endocytosis of SARS-CoV-2

Besides direct membrane fusion, SARS-CoV-2 can also invade cells via endocytosis [88, 89]. This route involves several proteins that play an important role in endosome formation, such as two-pore channel 2 (TPC2), Cathepsin L (CTSL) and Vacuolar-type ATPase (V-ATPase) [90]. These proteins are indicated to be potentially interesting therapeutic targets for COVID-19 treatment.

Tetrandrine is a bisbenzylisoquinoline and calcium channel blocker, known for its anti-inflammatory, immunosuppressive, oncological, and cardiovascular bioactivity [48–49]. The compound has been shown to be effective in the treatment of silicosis [90–92]. According to an *in vitro* study, tetrandrine is a low micromolar inhibitor of viral replication that functions by blocking the two-pore channel 2 (TPC2), which impedes Ca^{2+} release which in turn prevents acidification of the endosome [92].

The now infamous anti-malarial drugs chloroquine (CQ) and hydroxychloroquine (HCQ) were also posited to inhibit endocytosis of SARS-CoV-2 [93, 94]. CQ and HCQ are potentially involved in blocking cleavage of spike by raising the pH of the endosomes, preventing cathepsin L-mediated proteolysis, which is a key element in membrane fusion after binding ACE2. Whilst many potential mechanisms of action have been suggested, none have been rigorously demonstrated. In addition, a recent large meta-data analysis has shown that there is no evidence that treatment with CQ or HCQ reduces COVID-19 mortality in patients [95]. To the contrary, evidence is available that shows HCQ is responsible for a small increase in mortality outcomes. These compounds garnered lots of attention when the presidents of prominent countries started promoting CQ and HCQ as wonder drugs that could combat COVID-19 [96]. However, as mentioned before most evidence points towards the contrary and the WHO recommends against the treatment with these drugs [97]. These cases have shown an important risk in the use of drug repurpos-ing: in the age of hyper connectivity and social media echo chambers dangerous, unfounded ideas can avoid scrutiny and rigorous investigation, leading to large groups of people self-medicating with alternative treatments that have no scientific basis. This poses a problem in general drug development but even more so in drug repurposing cases where these compounds tend to be far more easily obtainable by the general public as they are approved and often available for purchase in pharmacies.

3.1.3 Drug repurposing targeting viral replication

After invading host cells, the coronavirus comes into the next stage of its life cycle: translation, replication, transcription and Assembly. This process mainly involves five different proteins: Mpro, RdRp, nsp14, MTHFD1 and Plpro, which have different functions [74, 98]. Mpro is also known as 3C-likeprotease (3CLpro) and proteolytically processes the majority of the polyprotein into functional polypeptides [99]. Similar to 3CLpro, Plpro is a viral protease that is responsible for cleaving polyproteins to generate a function replicase complex [100]. RNA synthesis, critical for viral replication, is performed by RdRP and its cofactors nsp7 and nsp8. Nsp14 has an exonuclease activity that supports RNA synthesis with an unusual RNA proofreading function. A study performed by Tinghua University showed that knockdown of MTHFD1, a key enzyme in cellular production of purine, dTMP and methyl groups, significantly inhibits viral replication [101]. As a result of their key functions in the viral life cycle these proteins are promising potential targets for antiviral drugs development. Clofazimine is an anti multi-bacillary leprosy drug which was approved for medical use in 1986. A recent study performed by The University of Hong Kong showed that clofazimine inhibits both viral spike glycoprotein mediated cell fusion and replication of SARS-CoV-2 *in vitro* [102].

Genome analysis has demonstrated that SARS-CoV-2 and SARS-CoV genes globally share >80% nucleotide identity and >89% similarity [73, 103, 104]. As a result, the key steps in the CoV family viral life cycle within the host cell are likely to be highly conserved. A key feature of this process is the expression of non-struc-tural proteins (nsps). Subsequent to cell entry, two extended polypeptides (pp1a and pp1ab) from the CoV viral genome are generated by the host cell translation machinery [105, 106]. These two polypeptides then self-cleave into 37 distinct non-structural (nsp) proteins [107] and anaylsis has demonstrated that the CoV family possesses several proteases involved in this essential self-cleavage process: the papain-like protease (PLpro), and the 3C-like proteinases (3CLpro or Mpro) [108]. CoV generally encode two PLpros within nsp3, with the exception of gamma-CoV,

SARS-CoV, Middle East respiratory syndrome coronavirus (MERS-CoV) and SARS-CoV-2 [100]. Thus, 3d unlike structural/accessory protein-encoding genes, which can show significant sequence variation in order to select between different potential host cell receptors, CLpro plays a central and critical role in CoV replication in host cells and the similarity in essential function leads to a high sequence similarity between the proteases of the CoV family, in particular beta-CoV [105, 106]. This increased similarity in the structure of the 3CLpro has the consequence of high structural between 3CLpro of different CoV family members—and the concomi-tant increased likelihood of cross-species function of CoV 3CLpro inhibitors and the potential to repurpose these inhibitors. The high sequence homology within Cov 3CLpros also provided high quality model templates—subsequently supported by the availability of high-resolution diffracting crystals—to perform both computational docking experiments, as well as molecular validation by X-ray crystallography [109]. There also exists the potential for the discovery and the development of a pan-anti-CoV inhibitor [110, 111].

This potential has been partially realized in not only the discovery of entirely novel SARS-CoV2 3CLpro inhibitors [99, 112, 113] (refs), but also in a number of reports describing successful identification of potential repurposing candi-dates [109].

For example, we and others have previously reported the results of a molecular docking experiment that indicated a class of well tolerated compounds (gliptins) as potential SARS-CoV2 inhibitors. For example, Anagliptin, a DPP4 inhibitor, is a well-established treatment for diabetes that is used by millions of patients. It has an excellent safety profile [114]. Computational docking demonstrated an efficient binding, with predicted H-bonds made to the backbone atoms of Gly163, Gly271, and Tyr268 and the side chain of Tyr273. Docking experiments also proposed that α-ketoamide inhibitors of hepatitis C virus (HCV) protease would be potential inhibitors of SARS-CoV-2 3CLpro. Efforts were concentrated on boceprevir and telaprevir as the docking poses were supported by experimental structure analyses (**Figure 1**). Subsequent biochemical assays demonstrated that boceprivir indeed displays strong binding to isolated 3CLpro of SARS-CoV2 and inhibits viral replica-tion in cellular assays.

Similarly to CQ and HCQ, ivermectin, originally an anthelmintic, also gained widespread attention as a potential treatment for COVID-19 and some *in vitro* evidence of SARS-CoV-2 replication inhibition in cell cultures has been provided [115]. The suggested mechanism of action is the inhibition of importin alpha/beta-1 nuclear transport proteins which the virus uses to enter the nucleus and is an important part of the replication cycle as it suppresses host-immune response [116]. Despite the in vitro effect no clinical data has supported the therapeutic use of ivermectin at concentrations approved for use in humans. However, it gained attention in the media and people started buying ivermectin meant for use in large animals to self-medicate against the virus [117]. Even though ivermectin is approved for human use and is generally safe, the doses used in the treatment of animals are several times larger than recommended for humans and can cause side-effects ranging from mild diarrhea to seizures and coma. This once again shows the care that needs to be taken when repurposing drugs in how scientific results are communicated to the general public, as it can lead to potential dangerous situations [118].

3.1.4 Drug repurposing targeting immune response modulators to treat SARS-CoV-2

Clinical symptoms resulting from SARS-CoV-2 infection are heterogeneous. Recent reports have shown that the cytokine storm effect may play a significant

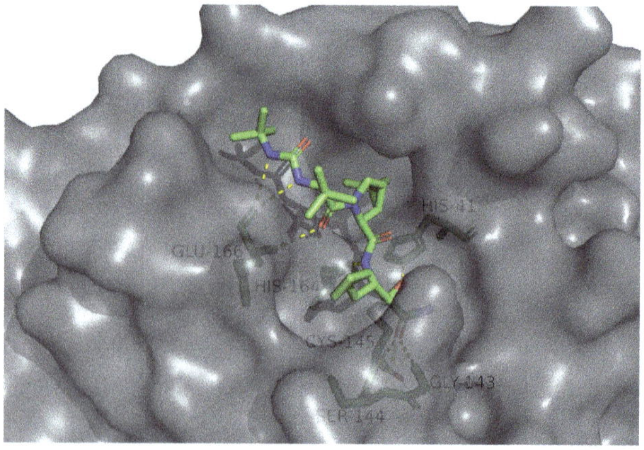

Figure 1.
Boceprevir (green), a HCV NS3/4A protease inhibitor, bound to SARS-CoV-2 3C-like protease (gray surface representation) with several key drug-protein interactions shown. Hydrogen bonds are shown as yellow dotted lines. PDB accession code: 6zru.

role in disease progression, potentially leading to multiple organ failure and death [119]. Immune response-related proteins have been proposed as potential targets for treatment options [120, 121]. Even though effectively suppressing cytokine storm does not directly combat the viral infection itself, it can be a crucial treatment option against COVID-19. It has previously been demonstrated that melatonin has beneficial effects on infection induced models of respiratory disease and associated complications [122]. Recently evidence also surfaced that it can inhibit COVID-19 induced cytokine storm [123]. Tocilizumab, an interleukin antagonist used for rheumatoid arthritis, is an immunosuppressor and was thus posited to be effective at reducing inflammation caused by SARS-CoV-2 [124]. It has recently become one of the first drugs to be recommended by the WHO as an effective treatment against COVID-19 [125]. Even though this is very promising there is an issue with the availability and affordability of this drug [126].

Researchers at Johns Hopkins found that the drug prazosin, an alpha-1 blocker used to treat high blood pressure, can prevent cytokine storms and that it significantly strengthened survival following inflammatory stimuli in preclinical models. This study is now in clinical trials [127].

3.1.5 Drug repurposing targeting pyroptosis

Sepsis is a systemic inflammatory response syndrome reulsting from dysregulation of host immunity. It is one of the deadliest clinical symptoms of severe SARS-CoV-2-infected patients [128]. Sepsis treatment normally mainly relies on the administration of intravenous antibiotics. However, since SARS-CoV-2 viral sepsis is not bacterial in nature the efficacy is low. Treatment is difficult, typically consist-ing of supplying oxygen and assisted breathing using a ventilator. Cocktails of antivirals and immune suppressors are also given but usually only have limited effect [129]. Approximately one-third of the discharged patients will die and one-sixth will suffer severe persistent impairments in the following year [130]. These facts taken together demonstrate the urgency and significance to find new treatments.

Sepsis is associated with pyroptosis (inflammatory programmed cell death) that is triggered by proinflammatory signals [131]. When viruses invade the host cell, inflammasomes are activated which in turn triggers an inflammatory response [132]. Pore-forming protein gasdermin D (GSDMD) is cleaved by activated Caspase-1, releasing its N-terminal domain [133]. The GSDMD N-terminal domain induces the formation of a large plasma membrane pore, resulting in pyroptosis [134]. Under normal circumstances pyropthosis can be good response, being able to trigger cell death of infected cells, releasing the pathogens and stimulating subsequent phagocytosis, protecting against infections [135]. However, excessive activation of pyroptosis will exacerbate sepsis or excessive cell death, causing immunity dysregulation [136, 137].

Disulfiram is approved for the treatment of chronic alcoholism. In a study conducted by Boston Children's Hospital, researchers found that disulfiram posesses inhibiting potential towards GSDMD both in *in vitro* cell assays and in *in vivo* mouse experiments. The experiment results showed that disulfiram inhibit the formation of the GSDMD pore by covalently modifying Cys191 of human GSDMD [138]. These results indicate that disulfiram could potentially be used to combat the pyroptotic effects induced by sars-cov-2 infection, hopefully reducing the negative clinical outcomes.

3.2 Drug repurposing for other viral diseases

Not only large global pandemic diseases are worth investigating for drug repurposing opportunities. Smaller, localized viral epidemics still plague many countries to this date. These diseases tend to fly under the radar since they typically occur in poorer regions of the world, meaning less research money is being spent on novel drug development. Drug repurposing could be the solution for these diseases due to the far faster and cheaper development pipeline.

3.2.1 Dengue virus

Dengue virus (DENV) is a single-stranded RNA virus, enveloped by a bilayer lipid membrane. The premembrane (prM) protein and envelope glycoprotein adhere to the membrane. Dengue virus can infect humans through mosquito bites. Symptoms, that include high fever, severe headache, muscle and joint pain, nausea, vomiting, swollen lymph nodes and rash, usually appear 3–14 days post-infection [139]. Most patients will recover in 2–7 days, while a small number of patients' conditions may worsen accompanied by bleeding, thrombocytopenia and plasma protein effusion. Up to 22,000 people die from Dengue annually and currently there are no therapies to treat this infection [140].

Ulipristal, a FDA approved small molecule, is an elective progesterone receptor modulator (SPRM), that has been demonstrated to be a potent inhibitor of DENV, most likely by blocking viral entry [141]. The antiviral activity was evaluated by *in vitro* DENV infection assay using Vero E6 cells. The results show that ulipristal has an antiviral effect against DENV in Vero E6 cells with an EC50 of 8.3 ± 0.1 μM. The anti-DENV effect of ulipristal was further confirmed using a murine infection model. The ulipristal-treated group presented less weight loss and disease symptoms compared the control group. A significant drop was also detected in the degree of viremia in the blood of the ulipristal-treated group. This study showed that ulipristal has desirable anti-DENV effects *in vitro* and *in vivo* [141].

3.2.2 Zika virus

Zika virus (ZIKV) is another virus that is propagated by mosquitoes and belongs to the genus of flaviviruses. ZIKV infection generally causes only mild symptoms, including fever, rash, conjunctivitis, muscle and joint pain, and headache. However, it has shown severe tetatogenic impacts, being able to cause a range of neurological complications, such as Guillain-Barre syndrome and microcephaly, in the fetuses of infected pregnant women [142].

There are no currently approved specific therapies for ZIKV infection [143]. However, a screening study utilizing 774 approved drugs has shown promising results. In vitro studies showed that ivermectin (anthelmintic), mycophenolic acid (an immunosuppressant), and daptomycin (a lipopeptide antibiotic) can inhibit ZIKV, resulting in reduced infection rates [144].

3.2.3 Ebola virus

Ebola virus is one of numerous hemorrhagic fever viruses, which was first discovered in 1976. It can cause severe viral haemorrhagic fever with case fatality rates vary from 25 to 90% [145]. It is characterized as a non-specific febrile illness (symptoms may include anorexia, arthralgia, headache, malaise, myalgia and rash) in the early infection and progresses to severe gastrointestinal symptoms (nausea, vomiting and high-volume diarrhea) in the first week [146]. To date, a monoclonal antibody (mAb114) and a cocktail of three antibodies (REGN-EB3) have been approved for the treatment of Ebola [147, 148]. Besides these biologics there has also been attempts at drug repurposing for this disease. Several drugs such as Amiodarone (anti-arrhythmia), bepridil (anti-angina pectoris), teicoplanin (antibiotic), amiodarone (ventricular fibrillation/tachycardia) and favipiravir (RNA polymerase inhibitor) have shown therapeutic potential for Ebola, but their efficacy requires further confirmation [149–151].

3.2.4 MERS-CoV

A warning of the potential for a coronavirus pandemic was provided by the Middle East respiratory syndrome coronavirus (MERS-CoV). While the impact of this outbreak was significantly less than that of the current SARS-CoV2 out-break the urgent need for MERS-CoV treatments was recognized, also including a focus on repurposing approaches and a call for the development of pan-corona virus inhibitors [152]. Suggested repurposing agents included GS-5734, which has previously demonstrated antiviral against multiple viral families, including *Coronaviridae*. GS-5734 activity *in vitro* was supported by reduced disease effects in mouse models and, while resistance mechanisms emerged, they were associated with a loss in viral fitness *in vitro* and *in vivo*—supporting the further analysis of GS-5734 as a pan-corona inhibitor [153, 154].

Similarly, lopinavir-ritonavir (a molecule designed as an inhibitor of the HIV-1 protease inhibitor) was proposed as a repurposing target of the 3CLpro of both SARS-CoV and MERS-CoV during their respective outbreaks [155, 156]. Combination therapy approaches in both cases resulted in improved patient outcomes, thereby offsetting the lacking of designed affinity that is a hallmark of repurposed compounds. In the example of SARS-CoV, a study on a combined therapy with ribarivin (a guanosine analog with activity against multiple viral families that inhibits viral RNA synthesis by RdRp) demonstrated both reduced viral load and improved clinical outcomes [157]. Whereas, a clinical trial of lopinavir-rotonavir in combination with IFN-β1b targeted therapies was proposed for MERS-CoV patients in Saudi Arabia [158]. Ribarivin itself was also a focus for repurposing during the SARS-CoV and MERS-CoV outbreaks. However, while efficacy of ribarivin alone could be demonstrated *in vitro* the doses required for a clinical response could not be supported by patients [159, 160].

Screening of an FDA-approved compound subset against viral replication in cul-ture identified lopinavir and an additional 3 compounds with IC50 values in the low micromolar range (chloroquine, chlorpromazine, and loperamide) [156]. This again demonstrates not only the potential for experimentally based repurposing screens to identify potential agents, but also suggests that the relatively limited potency of the agents identified may require the assessment of combination therapies to provoke a clinical response. This additional limitation of identifying appropriate combination therapies may well represent a common theme as a complicating factor in repurposing strategies.

4. Conclusions

In summary, the relatively conserved elements of the viral life cycle offer many opportunities to reexamine compounds developed to address previous outbreaks for efficacy against novel outbreaks. Clear examples are shown in the results against non-structural proteins above, which often maintain significantly higher sequence homology across species due to a conserved mechanism than structural proteins. However, while this sequence conservation indeed leads to a degree of "cross-talk" between nsp inhibitors, the required exquisite and intricate nature of the interaction between a successful drug and its target will almost inevitably reduce the efficacy of a monotherapy. As a result, it is likely that while repurposing can identify promising candidates, care must be taken not to hope for a single effective solution in existing drugs (e.g. Ivermectin, hydroxychloroquinine, etc.). Rather, functional (clinical) solutions are much more likely be found in careful clinical trials of combination therapies of drugs identified through repurposing screens.

The current combination of virtual, *in vitro* and *in vivo* screening is well positioned to perform rapid repurposing experiments on the relatively small number of clinically approved candidate molecules. However, significant research effort should be expended globally to continue to identify potential viral inhibitors and further populate the potential repurposing list.

Response speed is a key factor facing outbreaks. Drug repurposing is a practical solution that provides multiple benefits beyond classical drug discovery. Perhaps the greatest advancement in this area has been the improvements in computational techniques, that has developed in parallel with advances in structural biology—both of which continue to improve. These structural views of the proteins driving disease expand the number of experiments that can be performed *in silico*, providing both an increase in speed of hypothesis generation, as well as an important pre-filter stage to select out candidate molecules for screening. In our opinion a key aspect that should not be overlooked is the *in vitro* validation of a molecular effect on a proposed target. Certain recent experiences have shown that attempts to bypass this stage and short-cut the process by directly jumping into clinical trials can produce conflicting results, leading to confusion and loss of confidence of the public. However, despite successful application of drug repurposing, no single golden standard as yet exists to give relatively predictable results.

Acknowledgements

The authors would like to acknowledge the support of their friends and family over the recent pandemic.

Conflict of interest

The authors declare no conflicts of interest in the contents of this manuscript.

Author details

Ran Zhang, Rick Oerlemans, Chao Wang, Lili Zhang and Matthew R. Groves*
Structural Biology in Drug Design, XB20 Drug Design, Groningen Research Institute of Pharmacy, Groningen, The Netherlands

*Address all correspondence to: m.r.groves@rug.nl

References

[1] Biotechnology Innovation Organization. Clinical Development Success Rates and Contributing Factors 2011-2020 [Internet]. Available from: https://www.bio.org/clinical-development-success-rates-and-contributing-factors-2011-2020

[2] Hwang TJ, Carpenter D, Lauffenburger JC, Wang B, Franklin JM, Kesselheim AS. Failure of investigational drugs in late-stage clinical development and publication of trial results. JAMA Internal Medicine. 2016;**176**(12):1826-1833

[3] Bok K, Sitar S, Graham BS, Mascola JR. Accelerated COVID-19 vaccine development: Milestones, lessons, and prospects. Immunity. 2021;**54**(8):1636-1651. Available from: https://www.sciencedirect.com/science/article/pii/S1074761321003034

[4] Tebas P, Yang S, Boyer JD, Reuschel EL, Patel A, Christensen-Quick A, et al. Safety and immunogenicity of INO-4800 DNA vaccine against SARS-CoV-2: A preliminary report of an open-label, Phase 1 clinical trial. EClinicalMedicine. 2021;**31**:100689. Available from: https://www.sciencedirect.com/science/article/pii/S2589537020304338

[5] Pushpakom S, Iorio F, Eyers PA, Escott KJ, Hopper S, Wells A, et al. Drug repurposing: Progress, challenges and recommendations. Nature Reviews. Drug Discovery. 2019;**18**(1):41-58. Available from: https://www.ncbi.nlm.nih.gov/pubmed/30310233

[6] Paul MK, Mukhopadhyay AK. Tyrosine kinase—Role and significance in cancer. International Journal of Medical Sciences. 2004;**1**(2):101-115. Available from: https://pubmed.ncbi.nlm.nih.gov/15912202

[7] Diggle GE. Thalidomide: 40 years on. International Journal of Clinical Practice. 2001;**55**(9):627-631

[8] Malik S, Cohen PR. Thalidomide—Then and Now: Case Report of a Woman With Thalidomide Embryopathy and Review of Current Thalidomide Uses. Cureus. Aug 2021;**13**(8):e17070

[9] Rajkumar SV. Thalidomide: Tragic past and promising future. Mayo Clinic Proceedings. 2004;**79**(7):899-903. Available from: https://www.sciencedirect.com/science/article/pii/S0025619611621575

[10] Osakwe O. Chapter 2 - Trends in Innovation and the Business of Drug Discovery. In: Social Aspects of Drug Discovery, Development and Commercialization. Cambridge, Massachusetts: Academic Press; 2016. p. 29-55

[11] Kinch MS, Haynesworth A, Kinch SL, Hoyer D. An overview of FDA-approved new molecular entities: 1827-2013. Drug Discovery Today. 2014;**19**(8):1033-1039. Available from: https://www.sciencedirect.com/science/article/pii/S1359644614001032

[12] New Drugs at FDA: CDER's New Molecular Entities and New Therapeutic Biological Products | FDA. [cited 2021 Sep 17]. Available from: https://www.fda.gov/drugs/development-approval-process-drugs/new-drugs-fda-cders-new-molecular-entities-and-new-therapeutic-biological-products

[13] Lipinski CA. Lead-and drug-like compounds: The rule-of-five revolution. Drug Discovery Today: Technologies. 2004;**1**(4):337-341

[14] Jhoti H, Williams G, Rees DC, Murray CW. The "rule of three" for fragment-based drug discovery: Where are we now? Nature Reviews. Drug Discovery. 2013;**12**(8):644. DOI: 10.1038/nrd3926-c1

[15] Bickerton GR, Paolini GV, Besnard J, Muresan S, Hopkins AL. Quantifying

the chemical beauty of drugs. Nature Chemistry. 2012;**4**(2):90-98. DOI: 10.1038/nchem.1243

[16] Oprea TI. Property distribution of drug-related chemical databases. Journal of Computer-Aided Molecular Design. 2000;**14**(3):251-264

[17] Veber DF, Johnson SR, Cheng H-Y, Smith BR, Ward KW, Kopple KD. Molecular properties that influence the oral bioavailability of drug candidates. Journal of Medicinal Chemistry. 2002;**45**(12):2615-2623. DOI: 10.1021/jm020017n

[18] Bin CY, Prausnitz MR. The rule of five for non-oral routes of drug delivery: Ophthalmic, inhalation and transdermal. Pharmaceutical Research. 2011;**28**(5):943-948. Available from: https://pubmed.ncbi.nlm.nih.gov/20967491

[19] Oprea TI, Bauman JE, Bologa CG, Buranda T, Chigaev A, Edwards BS, et al. Drug repurposing from an academic perspective. Drug Discovery Today: Therapeutic Strategies. 2011;**8**(3-4):61-69

[20] Park K. A review of computational drug repurposing. Translational and Clinical Pharmacology. 2019;**27**(2):59-63. Available from: https://www.ncbi.nlm.nih.gov/pubmed/32055582

[21] Cha Y, Erez T, Reynolds IJ, Kumar D, Ross J, Koytiger G, et al. Drug repurposing from the perspective of pharmaceutical companies. British Journal of Pharmacology. 2018;**175**(2):168-180. Available from: https://pubmed.ncbi.nlm.nih.gov/28369768

[22] Parisi D, Adasme MF, Sveshnikova A, Bolz SN, Moreau Y, Schroeder M. Drug repositioning or target repositioning: A structural perspective of drug-target-indication relationship for available repurposed drugs. Computational and Structural Biotechnology Journal. 2020;**18**:1043-1055. Available from: https://www.sciencedirect.com/science/article/pii/S2001037019305021

[23] Oprea TI, Overington JP. Computational and practical aspects of drug repositioning. ASSAY and Drug Development Technologies. 2015;**13**(6):299-306

[24] Xue H, Li J, Xie H, Wang Y. Review of drug repositioning approaches and resources. International Journal of Biological Sciences. 2018;**14**(10):1232-1244. Available from: https://www.ncbi.nlm.nih.gov/pubmed/30123072

[25] Adeshina YO, Deeds EJ, Karanicolas J. Machine learning classification can reduce false positives in structure-based virtual screening. Proceedings of the National Academy of Sciences of the United States of America. 2020;**117**(31):18477-18488

[26] Hamza A, Wei N-N, Zhan C-G. Ligand-based virtual screening approach using a new scoring function. Journal of Chemical Information and Modeling. 2012;**52**(4):963-974

[27] Neves BJ, Braga RC, Melo-Filho CC, Moreira-Filho JT, Muratov EN, Andrade CH. QSAR-based virtual screening: Advances and applications in drug discovery. Frontiers in Pharmacology. 2018;**9**:1275. Available from: https://pubmed.ncbi.nlm.nih.gov/30524275

[28] Qing X, Lee XY, De Raeymaecker J, Tame JRH, Zhang KYJ, De Maeyer M, et al. Pharmacophore modeling: Advances, limitations, and current utility in drug discovery. Journal of Receptor, Ligand and Channel Research. 2014;**7**:81-92

[29] Sanchez G. Las instituciones de ciencia y tecnología en los procesos de

aprendizaje de la producción agroalimentaria en Argentina. El Sist argentino innovación Inst Empres y redes El desafío la creación y apropiación Conoc. ;**2013**(186, October): 659-664

[30] Gao M, Skolnick J. Structural space of protein–protein interfaces is degenerate, close to complete, and highly connected. Proceedings of the National Academy of Sciences. 2010;**107**(52):22517-22522. Available from: http://www.pnas.org/content/107/52/22517.abstract

[31] Lu H, Zhou Q, He J, Jiang Z, Peng C, Tong R, et al. Recent advances in the development of protein–protein interactions modulators: Mechanisms and clinical trials. Signal Transduction and Targeted Therapy. 2020;**5**(1):213. Available from:. DOI: 10.1038/s41392-020-00315-3

[32] Li Q, Shah S. In: Wu CH, Arighi CN, Ross KE, editors. Structure-Based Virtual Screening BT - Protein Bioinformatics: From Protein Modifications and Networks to Proteomics. New York, NY: Springer New York; 2017. pp. 111-124. DOI: 10.1007/978-1-4939-6783-4_5

[33] Maia EHB, Assis LC, de Oliveira TA, da Silva AM, Taranto AG. Structure-based virtual screening: From classical to artificial intelligence. Frontiers in Chemistry. 2020;**8**:343

[34] Pagadala NS, Syed K, Tuszynski J. Software for molecular docking: A review. Biophysical Reviews. 2017;**9**(2):91-102. Available from: https://pubmed.ncbi.nlm.nih. gov/28510083

[35] Li H, Sze K, Lu G, Ballester PJ. Machine-learning scoring functions for structure-based virtual screening. Wiley Interdisciplinary Reviews: Computational Molecular Science. 2021;**11**(1):e1478

[36] Wójcikowski M, Ballester PJ, Siedlecki P. Performance of machine-learning scoring functions in structure-based virtual screening. Scientific Reports. 2017;7(1):46710. Available from:. DOI: 10.1038/srep46710

[37] Lyu J, Wang S, Balius TE, Singh I, Levit A, Moroz YS, et al. Ultra-large library docking for discovering new chemotypes. Nature. 2019;**566**(7743):224-229. DOI: 10.1038/s41586-019-0917-9

[38] PDB. PDB Statistics: Overall Growth of Released Structures Per Year. [cited 2021 Sep 15]. Available from: https://www.rcsb.org/stats/growth/growth-released-structures

[39] Jumper J, Evans R, Pritzel A, Green T, Figurnov M, Ronneberger O, et al. Highly accurate protein structure prediction with AlphaFold. Nature. 2021;**596**(7873):583-589

[40] Tunyasuvunakool K, Adler J, Wu Z, Green T, Zielinski M, Žídek A, et al. Highly accurate protein structure prediction for the human proteome. Nature. 2021;**596**(7873):590-596. DOI: 10.1038/s41586-021-03828-1

[41] Nichols JA, Herbert Chan HW, Baker MAB. Machine learning: Applications of artificial intelligence to imaging and diagnosis. Biophysical Reviews. 2019;**11**(1):111-118. DOI: 10.1007/s12551-018-0449-9

[42] Mohd Hassan KA, Ahmad K, Adil M, Khan ZA, Khan MI, Lohani M. Drug discovery and in silico techniques: A mini-review. Enzym. Eng. 2014;**4**(1):1-3.

[43] Martorell-Marugán J, Tabik S, Benhammou Y, del Val C, Zwir I, Herrera F, et al. Deep learning in omics data analysis and precision medicine. Brisbane: Exon Publication; 2019. pp. 37-53

[44] Krassowski M, Das V, Sahu SK, Misra BB. State of the field in multi-omics research: From computational needs to data mining and sharing. Frontiers in Genetics. 2020;**11**:1598. Available from: https://www.frontiersin.org/article/10.3389/fgene.2020.610798

[45] Ozdemir ES, Halakou F, Nussinov R, Gursoy A, Keskin O. Methods for discovering and targeting druggable protein-protein interfaces and their application to repurposing. In Computational Methods for Drug Repurposing. New York, NY: Humana Press; 2019;**1903**:1-21

[46] Napolitano F, Zhao Y, Moreira VM, Tagliaferri R, Kere J, D'Amato M, Greco D. Drug repositioning: a machine-learning approach through data integration. Journal of cheminformatics. 2013;**5**(1):30

[47] Kim E, Choi AS, Nam H. Drug repositioning of herbal compounds via a machine-learning approach. BMC Bioinformatics. 2019;**20**(Suppl. 10):247. Available from: https://www.ncbi.nlm.nih.gov/pubmed/31138103

[48] Gupta R, Srivastava D, Sahu M, Tiwari S, Ambasta RK, Kumar P. Artificial intelligence to deep learning: Machine intelligence approach for drug discovery. Molecular Diversity. 2021;**25**(3):1315-1360. DOI: 10.1007/s11030-021-10217-3

[49] Paik H, Chen B, Sirota M, Hadley D, Butte AJ. Integrating clinical phenotype and gene expression data to prioritize novel drug uses. CPT: Pharmacometrics & Systems Pharmacology. 2016;**5**(11):599-607. Available from: https://pubmed.ncbi.nlm.nih.gov/27860440

[50] Reay WR, Cairns MJ. Advancing the use of genome-wide association studies for drug repurposing. Nature Reviews. Genetics. 2021;**22**(10):658-671. DOI: 10.1038/s41576-021-00387-z

[51] Nicholls HL, John CR, Watson DS, Munroe PB, Barnes MR, Cabrera CP. Reaching the end-game for GWAS: Machine learning approaches for the prioritization of complex disease loci. Frontiers in Genetics. 2020;**11**:350. Available from: https://www.frontiersin.org/article/10.3389/fgene.2020.00350

[52] Jacobs BM, Taylor T, Awad A, Baker D, Giovanonni G, Noyce AJ, Dobson R. Summary-data-based Mendelian randomization prioritizes potential druggable targets for multiple sclerosis. Brain communications. 2020;**2**(2):fcaa119

[53] Smith SB, Dampier W, Tozeren A, Brown JR, Magid-Slav M. Identification of common biological pathways and drug targets across multiple respiratory viruses based on human host gene expression analysis. PLoS One. 2012;**7**(3):e33174. DOI: 10.1371/journal.pone.0033174

[54] Schenone M, Dančík V, Wagner BK, Clemons PA. Target identification and mechanism of action in chemical biology and drug discovery. Nature Chemical Biology. 2013;**9**(4):232-240. Available from: https://pubmed.ncbi.nlm.nih.gov/23508189

[55] Guha R. On exploring structure-activity relationships. Methods in Molecular Biology. 2013;**993**:81-94. Available from: https://pubmed.ncbi.nlm.nih.gov/23568465

[56] Adams VR, Leggas M. Sunitinib malate for the treatment of metastatic renal cell carcinoma and gastrointestinal stromal tumors. Clinical Therapeutics. 2007;**29**(7):1338-1353

[57] Reinecke M, Heinzlmeir S, Wilhelm M, Médard G, Klaeger S, Kuster B. Kinobeads: A Chemical Proteomic Approach for Kinase Inhibitor Selectivity Profiling and Target Discovery. Target Discovery and

Validation: Methods and Strategies for Drug Discovery. 2019;**78**:97-130.

[58] Chamakuri S, Lu S, Ucisik MN, Bohren KM, Chen YC, Du HC, Faver JC, Jimmidi R, Li F, Li JY, Nyshadham P. DNA-encoded chemistry technology yields expedient access to SARS-CoV-2 Mpro inhibitors. Proceedings of the National Academy of Sciences. 7 Sep 2021;**118**(36):e2111172118

[59] Mani D, Wadhwani A, Krishnamurthy PT. Drug repurposing in antiviral research: A current scenario. Journal of Young Pharmacists. 2019;**11**(2):117-121

[60] Mercorelli B, Palu G, Loregian A. Drug repurposing for viral infectious diseases: How far are we? Trends in Microbiology. 2018;**26**(10):865-876. Available from: https://www.ncbi.nlm.nih.gov/pubmed/29759926

[61] Xu J, Xue Y, Zhou R, Shi PY, Li H, Zhou J. Drug repurposing approach to combating coronavirus: Potential drugs and drug targets. Medicinal Research Reviews. 2021;**41**(3):1375-1426. Available from: https://www.ncbi.nlm.nih.gov/pubmed/33277927

[62] Shang J, Ye G, Shi K, Wan Y, Luo C, Aihara H, et al. Structural basis of receptor recognition by SARS-CoV-2. Nature. 2020;**581**(7807):221-224. DOI: 10.1038/s41586-020-2179-y

[63] Moffat JG, Vincent F, Lee JA, Eder J, Prunotto M. Opportunities and challenges in phenotypic drug discovery: An industry perspective. Nature Reviews. Drug Discovery. 2017;**16**(8):531-543

[64] Zheng W, Thorne N, McKew JC. Phenotypic screens as a renewed approach for drug discovery. Drug Discovery Today. 2013;**18**(21):1067-1073. Available from: https://www.sciencedirect.com/science/article/pii/S135964461300202X

[65] Yang L, Agarwal P. Systematic drug repositioning based on clinical side-effects. PLoS One. 2011;**6**(12):e28025. Available from: https://www.ncbi.nlm.nih.gov/pubmed/22205936

[66] Campillos M, Kuhn M, Gavin AC, Jensen LJ, Bork P. Drug target identification using side-effect similarity. Science (80-). 2008;**321**(5886): 263-266. Available from: https://www.ncbi.nlm.nih.gov/pubmed/18621671

[67] Wermuth CG. Selective optimization of side activities: Another way for drug discovery. Journal of Medicinal Chemistry. 2004;**47**(6):1303-1314. DOI: 10.1021/jm030480f

[68] Jonckers T. Selective optimization of side activities (SOSA) in drug discovery. In: Wermuth CG, Aldous D, Raboisson P, Rognan D, editors. The Practice of Medicinal Chemistry. 4th ed. San Diego: Academic Press; 2015. pp. 473-486. Available from: https://www.sciencedirect.com/science/article/pii/B9780124172050000201

[69] Jern P, Johansson A, Piha J, Westberg L, Santtila P. Antidepressant treatment of premature ejaculation: Discontinuation rates and prevalence of side effects for dapoxetine and paroxetine in a naturalistic setting. International Journal of Impotence Research. 2015;**27**(2):75-80

[70] Goldstein I, Burnett AL, Rosen RC, Park PW, Stecher VJ. The serendipitous story of sildenafil: An unexpected oral therapy for erectile dysfunction. Sexual Medicine Reviews. 2019;**7**(1):115-128

[71] Boolell M, Allen MJ, Ballard SA, Gepi-Attee S, Muirhead GJ, Naylor AM, et al. Sildenafil: An orally active type 5 cyclic GMP-specific phosphodiesterase inhibitor for the treatment of penile erectile dysfunction. International Journal of Impotence Research. 1996;**8**(2):47-52

[72] WHO Coronavirus (COVID-19) Dashboard | WHO Coronavirus (COVID-19) Dashboard With Vaccination Data. [cited 2021 Sep 17]. Available from: https://covid19.who.int/

[73] Wu F, Zhao S, Yu B, Chen Y-M, Wang W, Song Z-G, et al. A new coronavirus associated with human respiratory disease in China. Nature. 2020;**579**(7798):265-269. DOI: 10.1038/s41586-020-2008-3

[74] Fehr AR, Perlman S. Coronaviruses: An overview of their replication and pathogenesis. Methods in Molecular Biology. 2015;**1282**:1-23

[75] Gui M, Song W, Zhou H, Xu J, Chen S, Xiang Y, et al. Cryo-electron microscopy structures of the SARS-CoV spike glycoprotein reveal a prerequisite conformational state for receptor binding. Cell Research. 2017;**27**(1):119-129. DOI: 10.1038/cr.2016.152

[76] Bestle D, Heindl MR, Limburg H, Van Lam T, Pilgram O, Moulton H, et al. TMPRSS2 and furin are both essential for proteolytic activation of SARS-CoV-2 in human airway cells. Life Science Alliance. 2020;**3**(9):e202000786 Available from: https://pubmed.ncbi.nlm.nih.gov/32703818

[77] Yuan M, Wu NC, Zhu X, Lee C-CD, So RTY, Lv H, et al. A highly conserved cryptic epitope in the receptor binding domains of SARS-CoV-2 and SARS-CoV. Science (80-). 2020;**368**(6491):630-633

[78] Xia S, Lan Q, Su S, Wang X, Xu W, Liu Z, et al. The role of furin cleavage site in SARS-CoV-2 spike protein-mediated membrane fusion in the presence or absence of trypsin. Signal Transduction and Targeted Therapy. 2020;**5**(1):92. DOI: 10.1038/s41392-020-0184-0

[79] Peacock TP, Goldhill DH, Zhou J, Baillon L, Frise R, Swann OC, et al. The furin cleavage site in the SARS-CoV-2 spike protein is required for transmission in ferrets. Nature Microbiology. 2021;**6**(7):899-909. DOI: 10.1038/s41564-021-00908-w

[80] Liu S, Xiao G, Chen Y, He Y, Niu J, Escalante CR, et al. Interaction between heptad repeat 1 and 2 regions in spike protein of SARS-associated coronavirus: Implications for virus fusogenic mechanism and identification of fusion inhibitors. Lancet. 2004;**363**(9413): 938-947

[81] Rahbar Saadat Y, Hosseiniyan Khatibi SM, Zununi Vahed S, Ardalan M. Host serine proteases: A potential targeted therapy for COVID-19 and influenza. Frontiers in Molecular Biosciences. 2021;**8**(August):1-13

[82] Trezza A, Iovinelli D, Santucci A, Prischi F, Spiga O. An integrated drug repurposing strategy for the rapid identification of potential SARS-CoV-2 viral inhibitors. Scientific Reports. 2020;**10**(1):13866. DOI: 10.1038/s41598-020-70863-9

[83] Lo HS, Hui KPY, Lai H-M, He X, Khan KS, Kaur S, et al. Simeprevir potently suppresses SARS-CoV-2 replication and synergizes with remdesivir. ACS Central Science. 2021;**7**(5):792-802. DOI: 10.1021/acscentsci.0c01186

[84] Hoffmann M, Hofmann-Winkler H, Smith JC, Krüger N, Arora P, Sørensen LK, et al. Camostat mesylate inhibits SARS-CoV-2 activation by TMPRSS2-related proteases and its metabolite GBPA exerts antiviral activity. eBioMedicine. 2021;**65**:103255

[85] Hoffmann M, Kleine-Weber H, Schroeder S, Krüger N, Herrler T, Erichsen S, et al. SARS-CoV-2 cell entry depends on ACE2 and TMPRSS2 and is blocked by a clinically proven protease inhibitor. Cell. 2020;**181**(2):271-280.e8

[86] Breining P, Frølund AL, Højen JF, Gunst JD, Staerke NB,

Saedder E, et al. Camostat mesylate against SARS-CoV-2 and COVID-19—Rationale, dosing and safety. Basic & Clinical Pharmacology & Toxicology. 2021;**128**(2):204-212

[87] Gunst JD, Staerke NB, Pahus MH, Kristensen LH, Bodilsen J, Lohse N, et al. Efficacy of the TMPRSS2 inhibitor camostat mesilate in patients hospitalized with Covid-19-a double-blind randomized controlled trial. EClinicalMedicine. 2021;**35**:100849. Available from: https://www.sciencedirect.com/science/article/pii/S2589537021001292

[88] Wang H, Yang P, Liu K, Guo F, Zhang Y, Zhang G, et al. SARS coronavirus entry into host cells through a novel clathrin- and caveolae-independent endocytic pathway. Cell Research. 2008;**18**(2):290-301. DOI: 10.1038/cr.2008.15

[89] Bayati A, Kumar R, Francis V, McPherson PS. SARS-CoV-2 infects cells after viral entry via clathrin-mediated endocytosis. The Journal of Biological Chemistry. 2021;**296**:100306. Available from: https://www.ncbi.nlm.nih.gov/pubmed/33476648

[90] Heister PM, Poston RN. Pharmacological hypothesis: TPC2 antagonist tetrandrine as a potential therapeutic agent for COVID-19. Pharmacology Research & Perspectives. 2020;**8**(5):e00653. Available from: https://www.ncbi.nlm.nih.gov/pubmed/32930523

[91] Chen Y, Tsai Y-H, Tseng S-H. The potential of tetrandrine as a protective agent for ischemic stroke. Molecules. 2011;**16**(9):8020-8032

[92] Song M, Wang J, Sun Y, Han Z, Zhou Y, Liu Y, et al. Tetrandrine alleviates silicosis by inhibiting canonical and non-canonical NLRP3 inflammasome activation in lung macrophages. Acta Pharmacol Sin. 2021;**42**:1223-34.

[93] Al-Bari MAA. Targeting endosomal acidification by chloroquine analogs as a promising strategy for the treatment of emerging viral diseases. Pharmacology Research & Perspectives. 2017;**5**(1):e00293-e00293. Available from: https://pubmed.ncbi.nlm.nih.gov/28596841

[94] Satarker S, Ahuja T, Banerjee M, Balaji EV, Dogra S, Agarwal T, et al. Hydroxychloroquine in COVID-19: Potential mechanism of action against SARS-CoV-2. Current Pharmacology Reports. 2020;**6**(5):203-211. DOI: 10.1007/s40495-020-00231-8

[95] Axfors C, Schmitt AM, Janiaud P, van't Hooft J, Abd-Elsalam S, Abdo EF, et al. Mortality outcomes with hydroxychloroquine and chloroquine in COVID-19 from an international collaborative meta-analysis of randomized trials. Nature Communications. 2021;**12**(1):2349. DOI: 10.1038/s41467-021-22446-z

[96] Fraser B. 'Medications should be prescribed by doctors, not the president': leading Brazilian scientist discusses the pandemic. Nature [Internet]. Available from: https://www.nature.com/articles/d41586-020-01506-2. [Accessed 22th May 2020]

[97] Coronavirus disease (COVID-19): Hydroxychloroquine. [cited 2021 Sep 17]. Available from: https://www.who.int/news-room/q-a-detail/coronavirus-disease-(covid-19)-hydroxychloroquine

[98] V'kovski P, Kratzel A, Steiner S, Stalder H, Thiel V. Coronavirus biology and replication: Implications for SARS-CoV-2. Nature Reviews. Microbiology. 2021;**19**(3):155-170

[99] Mengist HM, Dilnessa T, Jin T. Structural basis of potential inhibitors targeting SARS-CoV-2 main protease. Frontiers in Chemistry. 2021;**9**:7. Available from: https://www.frontiersin.org/article/10.3389/fchem.2021.622898

[100] Shin D, Mukherjee R, Grewe D, Bojkova D, Baek K, Bhattacharya A, et al. Papain-like protease regulates SARS-CoV-2 viral spread and innate immunity. Nature. 2020;**587**(7835):657-662. DOI: 10.1038/s41586-020-2601-5

[101] Anderson DE, Cui J, Ye Q, Huang B, Tan Y, Jiang C, Zu W, Gong J, Liu W, Kim SY, Yan BG. Orthogonal genome-wide screens of bat cells identify MTHFD1 as a target of broad antiviral therapy. Proceedings of the National Academy of Sciences. 28 Sep 2021;**118**(39):e2104759118

[102] Yuan S, Yin X, Meng X, Chan JF-W, Ye Z-W, Riva L, et al. Clofazimine broadly inhibits coronaviruses including SARS-CoV-2. Nature. 2021;**593**(7859): 418-423

[103] Zhou P, Yang X-L, Wang X-G, Hu B, Zhang L, Zhang W, et al. A pneumonia outbreak associated with a new coronavirus of probable bat origin. Nature. 2020;**579**(7798):270-273. DOI: 10.1038/s41586-020-2012-7

[104] Zhu N, Zhang D, Wang W, Li X, Yang B, Song J, et al. A novel coronavirus from patients with pneumonia in China, 2019. The New England Journal of Medicine. 2020;**382**(8):727-733. Available from: https://pubmed.ncbi.nlm.nih.gov/31978945

[105] Perlman S, Netland J. Coronaviruses post-SARS: Update on replication and pathogenesis. Nature Reviews. Microbiology. 2009;**7**(6):439-450. Available from: https://pubmed.ncbi.nlm.nih.gov/19430490

[106] Fehr AR, Perlman S. Coronaviruses: An Overview of Their Replication and Pathogenesis Coronaviruses: Methods and Protocols. New York, NY: Springer; 2015. p. 1-23

[107] Kanchan A, John Z, Parvesh W, Mesters JR, Hilgenfeld R. Coronavirus main proteinase (3CLpro) structure: Basis for design of anti-SARS drugs. Science (80-). 2003;**300**(5626):1763-1767. DOI: 10.1126/science.1085658

[108] Mielech AM, Chen Y, Mesecar AD, Baker SC. Nidovirus papain-like proteases: Multifunctional enzymes with protease, deubiquitinating and deISGylating activities. Virus Research. 2014;**194**:184-190. Available from: https://pubmed.ncbi.nlm.nih.gov/24512893

[109] Ma C, Sacco MD, Hurst B, Townsend JA, Hu Y, Szeto T, et al. Boceprevir, GC-376, and calpain inhibitors II, XII inhibit SARS-CoV-2 viral replication by targeting the viral main protease. Cell Research. 2020;**30**(8):678-692. DOI: 10.1038/s41422-020-0356-z

[110] Tahir Ul Qamar M, Alqahtani SM, Alamri MA, Chen L-L. Structural basis of SARS-CoV-2 3CL(pro) and anti-COVID-19 drug discovery from medicinal plants. Journal of Pharmaceutical Analysis. 2020;**10**(4):313-319. Available from: https://pubmed.ncbi.nlm.nih.gov/32296570

[111] Groves M, Domling A, Moreno AJR, Romero AR, Neochoritis C, Velasco-Velázquez M. Gliptin repurposing for COVID-19. ChemRxiv. 2020. Available from: https://chemrxiv.org/ engage/chemrxiv/article-details/ 60c749dd469df4d40af43c4d

[112] Douangamath A, Fearon D, Gehrtz P, Krojer T, Lukacik P, Owen CD, et al. Crystallographic and electrophilic fragment screening of the SARS-CoV-2 main protease. Nature Communications. 2020;**11**(1):5047. DOI: 10.1038/s41467-020-18709-w

[113] Jin Z, Du X, Xu Y, Deng Y, Liu M, Zhao Y, et al. Structure of Mpro from SARS-CoV-2 and discovery of its inhibitors. Nature. 2020;**582**(7811):289-293. DOI: 10.1038/s41586-020-2223-y

[114] Nishio S, Abe M, Ito H. Anagliptin in the treatment of type 2 diabetes: Safety, efficacy, and patient acceptability. Diabetes, Metabolic Syndrome and Obesity. 2015;**8**:163-171. Available from: https://pubmed.ncbi.nlm.nih.gov/25834461

[115] Caly L, Druce JD, Catton MG, Jans DA, Wagstaff KM. The FDA-approved drug ivermectin inhibits the replication of SARS-CoV-2 in vitro. Antiviral Research. 2020;**178**:104787. Available from: https://www. sciencedirect.com/science/article/pii/S0166354220302011

[116] Wehbe Z, Wehbe M, Iratni R, Pintus G, Zaraket H, Yassine HM, et al. Repurposing ivermectin for COVID-19: Molecular aspects and therapeutic possibilities. Frontiers in Immunology. 2021;**12**:1040. Available from: https://www.frontiersin.org/article/10.3389/fimmu.2021.663586

[117] Mega ER. Latin America's embrace of an unproven COVID treatment is hindering drug trials. Nature. 2020;**586**(7830):481-482

[118] Reardon S. Flawed ivermectin preprint highlights challenges of COVID drug studies. Nature. 2021;**2021**: 5967871. Available from: https://www. nature.com/articles/d41586-021- 02081-w

[119] Yang L, Xie X, Tu Z, Fu J, Xu D, Zhou Y. The signal pathways and treatment of cytokine storm in COVID-19. Signal Transduction and Targeted Therapy. 2021;**6**(1):255. DOI: 10.1038/s41392-021-00679-0

[120] Peiris JSM, Chu C-M, Cheng VC-C, Chan KS, Hung IFN, Poon LLM, et al. Clinical progression and viral load in a community outbreak of coronavirus-associated SARS pneumonia: A prospective study. Lancet. 2003;**361**(9371):1767-1772

[121] Nassar M, Bakhrebah MA, Meo SA, Alsuabeyl MS, Zaher WA. Middle East Respiratory Syndrome Coronavirus (MERS-CoV) infection: Epidemiology, pathogenesis and clinical characteristics. European Review for Medical and Pharmacological Sciences. 2018;**22**(15):4956-4961

[122] Wichniak A, Kania A, Siemiński M, Cubała WJ. Melatonin as a potential adjuvant treatment for COVID-19 beyond sleep disorders. International Journal of Molecular Sciences. Jan 2021;**22**(16):8623

[123] Reiter RJ, Sharma R, Ma Q, Dominquez-Rodriguez A, Marik PE, Abreu-Gonzalez P. Melatonin inhibits COVID-19-induced cytokine storm by reversing aerobic glycolysis in immune cells: A mechanistic analysis. Medicine in Drug Discovery. 2020;**6**:100044. Available from: https://pubmed.ncbi.nlm.nih.gov/32395713

[124] Zhang Q, Wang Y, Qi C, Shen L, Li J. Clinical trial analysis of 2019-nCoV therapy registered in China. Journal of Medical Virology. 2020;**92**(6):540-545

[125] WHO recommends life-saving interleukin-6 receptor blockers for COVID-19 and urges producers to join efforts to rapidly increase access. [cited 2021 Sep 17]. Available from: https://www.who.int/news/item/06-07-2021-who-recommends-life-saving-interleukin-6-receptor-blockers-for-covid-19-and-urges-producers-to-join-efforts-to-rapidly-increase-access

[126] Tocilizumab, second drug ever recommended by WHO for COVID-19, will remain unaffordable and inaccessible for most of the world - World | ReliefWeb. [cited 2021 Sep 17]. Available from: https://reliefweb.int/report/world/tocilizumab-second-drug-ever-recommended-who-covid-19-will-remain-unaffordable-and

[127] Konig MF, Powell M, Staedtke V, Bai R-Y, Thomas DL, Fischer N, et al. Targeting the catecholamine-cytokine axis to prevent SARS-CoV-2 cytokine storm syndrome. In: medRxiv. New York, NY: Cold Spring Harbor Laboratory Press; 2020

[128] Olwal CO, Nganyewo NN, Tapela K, Djomkam Zune AL, Owoicho O, Bediako Y, et al. Parallels in sepsis and COVID-19 conditions: Implications for managing severe COVID-19. Frontiers in Immunology. 2021;**12**:602848

[129] Liu D, Wang Q, Zhang H, Cui L, Shen F, Chen Y, et al. Viral sepsis is a complication in patients with Novel Corona Virus Disease (COVID-19). Medicine in Drug Discovery. 2020;**8**:100057. Available from: https://www.sciencedirect.com/science/article/pii/S2590098620300440

[130] Prescott HC, Angus DC. Enhancing recovery from sepsis: A review. Journal of the American Medical Association. 2018;**319**(1):62-75. DOI: 10.1001/jama.2017.17687

[131] Gao YL, Zhai JH, Chai YF. Recent advances in the molecular mechanisms underlying pyroptosis in sepsis. Mediators of inflammation. Oct 2018;**2018**:5823823

[132] He W, Wan H, Hu L, Chen P, Wang X, Huang Z, et al. Gasdermin D is an executor of pyroptosis and required for interleukin-1β secretion. Cell Research. 2015;**25**(12):1285-1298. Available from: https://pubmed.ncbi.nlm.nih.gov/26611636

[133] Franchi L, Eigenbrod T, Muñoz-Planillo R, Nuñez G. The inflammasome: A caspase-1-activation platform that regulates immune responses and disease pathogenesis. Nature Immunology. 2009;**10**(3):241-247. Available from: https://pubmed.ncbi.nlm.nih.gov/19221555

[134] Sborgi L, Ruhl S, Mulvihill E, Pipercevic J, Heilig R, Stahlberg H, et al. GSDMD membrane pore formation constitutes the mechanism of pyroptotic cell death. The EMBO Journal. 2016;**35**(16):1766-1778. Available from: https://www.ncbi.nlm.nih.gov/pubmed/27418190

[135] Wang Q, Imamura R, Motani K, Kushiyama H, Nagata S, Suda T. Pyroptotic cells externalize eat-me and release find-me signals and are efficiently engulfed by macrophages. International Immunology. 2013;**25**(6):363-372. DOI: 10.1093/intimm/dxs161

[136] Aglietti RA, Dueber EC. Recent insights into the molecular mechanisms underlying pyroptosis and gasdermin family functions. Trends in Immunology. 2017;**38**(4):261-271. Available from: https://www.sciencedirect.com/science/article/pii/S1471490617300157

[137] Wang L, Qin X, Liang J, Ge P. Induction of pyroptosis: A promising strategy for cancer treatment. Frontiers in Oncology. 2021;**11**:635774. Available from: https://pubmed.ncbi.nlm.nih.gov/33718226

[138] Hu JJ, Liu X, Xia S, Zhang Z, Zhang Y, Zhao J, et al. FDA-approved disulfiram inhibits pyroptosis by blocking gasdermin D pore formation. Nature Immunology. 2020;**21**(7):736-745. Available from: https://www.ncbi.nlm.nih.gov/pubmed/32367036

[139] Botta L, Rivara M, Zuliani V, Radi M. Drug repurposing approaches to fight Dengue virus infection and related diseases. Frontiers in Bioscience-Landmark. 2018;**23**(6):997-1019

[140] About Dengue: What You Need to Know | Dengue | CDC. [cited 2021 Sep 17]. Available from: https://www.cdc.gov/dengue/about/index.html

[141] Shin H, Park S-J, Kim J, Lee J-S, Min D-H. A graphene oxide-based fluorescent nanosensor to identify antiviral agents via a drug repurposing screen. Biosensors & Bioelectronics. 2021;**183**:113208

[142] Yun SI, Lee YM. Zika virus: An emerging flavivirus. Journal of Microbiology. 2017;**55**(3):204-219

[143] Treatment | Zika virus | CDC. [cited 2021 Sep 17]. Available from: https://www.cdc.gov/zika/symptoms/treatment.html

[144] Barrows NJ, Campos RK, Powell ST, Prasanth KR, Schott-Lerner G, Soto-Acosta R, et al. A screen of FDA-approved drugs for inhibitors of zika virus infection. Cell Host & Microbe. 2016;**20**(2):259-270. Available from: https://www.ncbi.nlm.nih.gov/pubmed/27476412

[145] Ebola virus disease. [cited 2021 Sep 17]. Available from: https://www.who.int/news-room/fact-sheets/detail/ebola-virus-disease

[146] Jacob ST, Crozier I, Fischer WA, Hewlett A, Kraft CS, de La VM-A, et al. Ebola virus disease. Nature Reviews Disease Primers. 2020;**6**(1):13. DOI: 10.1038/s41572-020-0147-3

[147] Gaudinski MR, Coates EE, Novik L, Widge A, Houser KV, Burch E, et al. Safety, tolerability, pharmacokinetics, and immunogenicity of the therapeutic monoclonal antibody mAb114 targeting Ebola virus glycoprotein (VRC 608): An open-label phase 1 study. Lancet. 2019;**393**(10174):889-898

[148] Markham A. REGN-EB3: first approval. Drugs. 2021;**81**(1):175-8

[149] Sweiti H, Ekwunife O, Jaschinski T, Lhachimi SK. Repurposed therapeutic agents targeting the ebola virus: A systematic review. Current Therapeutic Research, Clinical and Experimental. 2017;**84**:10-21. Available from: https://www.ncbi.nlm.nih.gov/pubmed/28761574

[150] Dyall J, Johnson JC, Postnikova E, Cong Y, Zhou H, Gerhardt DM, et al. In vitro and in vivo activity of amiodarone against Ebola virus. The Journal of Infectious Diseases. 2018;**218**(suppl. 5): S592-S596

[151] Oestereich L, Lüdtke A, Wurr S, Rieger T, Muñoz-Fontela C, Günther S. Successful treatment of advanced Ebola virus infection with T-705 (favipiravir) in a small animal model. Antiviral Research. 2014;**105**:17-21

[152] Totura AL, Bavari S. Broad-spectrum coronavirus antiviral drug discovery. Expert Opinion on Drug Discovery. 2019;**14**(4):397-412. DOI: 10.1080/17460441.2019.1581171

[153] Agostini ML, Andres EL, Sims AC, Graham RL, Sheahan TP, Lu X, et al. Coronavirus susceptibility to the antiviral remdesivir (GS-5734) is mediated by the viral polymerase and the proofreading exoribonuclease. MBio. 2018;**9**(2):e00221-e00218. Available from: https://pubmed.ncbi.nlm.nih.gov/29511076

[154] Sheahan TP, Sims AC, Graham RL, Menachery VD, Gralinski LE, Case JB, et al. Broad-spectrum antiviral GS-5734 inhibits both epidemic and zoonotic coronaviruses. Science Translational Medicine. 2017;**9**(396):eaal3653. Available from: https://pubmed.ncbi.nlm.nih.gov/28659436

[155] Wu C-Y, Jan J-T, Ma S-H, Kuo C-J, Juan H-F, Cheng Y-SE, et al. Small molecules targeting severe acute respiratory syndrome human coronavirus. Proceedings of the National Academy of Sciences of the United States of America. 2004;**101**(27):10012-10017. Available from: http://www.pnas.org/content/101/27/10012.abstract

[156] de Wilde AH, Jochmans D, Posthuma CC, Zevenhoven-Dobbe JC, van Nieuwkoop S, Bestebroer TM, et al. Screening of an FDA-approved compound library identifies four small-molecule inhibitors of Middle East respiratory syndrome coronavirus replication in cell culture. Antimicrobial Agents and Chemotherapy. 2014;**58**(8):4875-4884. Available from: https://pubmed.ncbi.nlm.nih.gov/24841269

[157] Chu CM, Cheng VCC, Hung IFN, Wong MML, Chan KH, Chan KS, et al. Role of lopinavir/ritonavir in the treatment of SARS: Initial virological and clinical findings. Thorax. 2004;**59**(3):252-256. Available from: https://pubmed.ncbi.nlm.nih.gov/14985565

[158] Arabi YM, Alothman A, Balkhy HH, Al-Dawood A, AlJohani S, Al Harbi S, et al. Treatment of middle east respiratory syndrome with a combination of lopinavir-ritonavir and interferon-β1b (MIRACLE trial): Study protocol for a randomized controlled trial. Trials. 2018;**19**(1):81. Available from: https://pubmed.ncbi.nlm.nih.gov/29382391

[159] Hart BJ, Dyall J, Postnikova E, Zhou H, Kindrachuk J, Johnson RF, et al. Interferon-β and mycophenolic acid are potent inhibitors of Middle East respiratory syndrome coronavirus in cell-based assays. Journal of General Virology. 2014;**95**(Pt 3):571-577. Available from: https://pubmed.ncbi.nlm.nih.gov/24323636

[160] Barnard DL, Day CW, Bailey K, Heiner M, Montgomery R, Lauridsen L, et al. Enhancement of the infectivity of SARS-CoV in BALB/c mice by IMP dehydrogenase inhibitors, including ribavirin. Antiviral Research. 2006;**71**(1):53-63. Available from: https://pubmed.ncbi.nlm.nih.gov/16621037

Permissions

All chapters in this book were first published by InTech Open; hereby published with permission under the Creative Commons Attribution License or equivalent. Every chapter published in this book has been scrutinized by our experts. Their significance has been extensively debated. The topics covered herein carry significant findings which will fuel the growth of the discipline. They may even be implemented as practical applications or may be referred to as a beginning point for another development.

The contributors of this book come from diverse backgrounds, making this book a truly international effort. This book will bring forth new frontiers with its revolutionizing research information and detailed analysis of the nascent developments around the world.

We would like to thank all the contributing authors for lending their expertise to make the book truly unique. They have played a crucial role in the development of this book. Without their invaluable contributions this book wouldn't have been possible. They have made vital efforts to compile up to date information on the varied aspects of this subject to make this book a valuable addition to the collection of many professionals and students.

This book was conceptualized with the vision of imparting up-to-date information and advanced data in this field. To ensure the same, a matchless editorial board was set up. Every individual on the board went through rigorous rounds of assessment to prove their worth. After which they invested a large part of their time researching and compiling the most relevant data for our readers.

The editorial board has been involved in producing this book since its inception. They have spent rigorous hours researching and exploring the diverse topics which have resulted in the successful publishing of this book. They have passed on their knowledge of decades through this book. To expedite this challenging task, the publisher supported the team at every step. A small team of assistant editors was also appointed to further simplify the editing procedure and attain best results for the readers.

Apart from the editorial board, the designing team has also invested a significant amount of their time in understanding the subject and creating the most relevant covers. They scrutinized every image to scout for the most suitable representation of the subject and create an appropriate cover for the book.

The publishing team has been an ardent support to the editorial, designing and production team. Their endless efforts to recruit the best for this project, has resulted in the accomplishment of this book. They are a veteran in the field of academics and their pool of knowledge is as vast as their experience in printing. Their expertise and guidance has proved useful at every step. Their uncompromising quality standards have made this book an exceptional effort. Their encouragement from time to time has been an inspiration for everyone.

The publisher and the editorial board hope that this book will prove to be a valuable piece of knowledge for researchers, students, practitioners and scholars across the globe.

List of Contributors

Xiao-Yuan Mao
Department of Clinical Pharmacology, Xiangya Hospital, Central South University, Changsha, P.R. China
Hunan Key Laboratory of Pharmacogenetics, Institute of Clinical Pharmacology, Central South University, Changsha, P.R. China
Engineering Research Center of Applied Technology of Pharmacogenomics, Ministry of Education, Changsha, P.R. China
National Clinical Research Center for Geriatric Disorders, Changsha, Hunan, P.R. China

Farid A. Badria
Department of Pharmacognosy, Faculty of Pharmacy, Mansoura University, Mansoura, Egypt

Abdullah A. Elgazar
Department of Pharmacognosy, Faculty of Pharmacy, Kafrelsheikh University, Kafrelsheikh, Egypt

Mithun Rudrapal, Shubham J. Khairnar and Anil G. Jadhav
Institute of Pharmaceutical Sciences, Sandip Foundation, Mahiravani, Nashik, India

Ravirajsinh N. Jadeja
Department of Biochemistry and Molecular Biology, Medical College of Georgia, Augusta University, Augusta, GA, USA

Folami L. Powell
Department of Biochemistry and Molecular Biology, Medical College of Georgia, Augusta University, Augusta, GA, USA
James and Jean Culver Vision Discovery Institute, Augusta University, Augusta, GA, USA

Alkeshkumar Patel
Department of Pharmacology, Ramanbhai Patel College of Pharmacy, CHARUSAT, Anand, Gujarat, India

Matteo Conti
Public Health Department, Ausl Imola, Imola, Italy

Pamela M. Martin
Department of Biochemistry and Molecular Biology, Medical College of Georgia, Augusta University, Augusta, GA, USA
James and Jean Culver Vision Discovery Institute, Augusta University, Augusta, GA, USA
Department of Ophthalmology, Medical College of Georgia, Augusta University, Augusta, GA, USA

James Ronald Lawrence, Gwendoline Joan Baxter and John Robert Paterson
Research and Development Support Unit, Dumfries and Galloway Royal Infirmary, Cargenbridge, Dumfries, Scotland

Sho Tamai, Nozomi Hirai, Shabierjiang Jiapaer and Mitsutoshi Nakada
Department of Neurosurgery, Graduate School of Medical Science, Kanazawa University, Kanazawa, Japan

Takuya Furuta
Department of Pathology, Kurume University, Kurume, Japan

Andrea Vila Domínguez, Manuel Enrique Jiménez Mejías and Younes Smani
Institute of Biomedicine of Seville (IBiS), University Hospital Virgen del Rocío/CSIC/University of Seville, Seville, Spain

Deepak Kumar Dash, Anil Kumar Sahu, Rajnikant Panik and Vaibhav Tripathi
Royal College of Pharmacy, Raipur, Chhattisgarh, India

Vishal Jain
University Institute of Pharmacy, Pt. Ravishankar Shukla University, Raipur, Chhattisgarh, India

Neha Dhir, Ashish Jain, Dhruv Mahendru, Ajay Prakash and Bikash Medhi
Department of Pharmacology, Postgraduate Institute of Medical Education and Research (PGIMER), Chandigarh, India

Ran Zhang, Rick Oerlemans, Chao Wang, Lili Zhang and Matthew R. Groves
Structural Biology in Drug Design, XB20 Drug Design, Groningen Research Institute of Pharmacy, Groningen, The Netherlands

Index

www.ingramcontent.com/pod-product-compliance
Lightning Source LLC
LaVergne TN
LVHW062130200926
848484LV00007B/1791